SURGICAL AND
INTERVENTIONAL ULTRASOUND

SURGICAL AND INTERVENTIONAL ULTRASOUND

Beth Schrope, MD, PhD, FACS, RDMS

Assistant Professor of Surgery
Department of Surgery
Columbia University College of Physicians and Surgeons
New York, New York

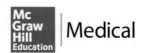

Medical

New York   Chicago   San Francisco   Lisbon   London   Madrid   Mexico City
Milan   New Delhi   San Juan   Seoul   Singapore   Sydney   Toronto

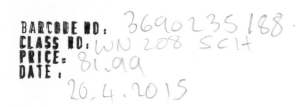
Surgical and Interventional Ultrasound

1 2 3 4 5 6 7 8 9 0   CTP/CTP   18 17 16 15 14 13

Set ISBN 978-0-07-176760-6
Set MHID 0-07-176760-6
Book ISBN 978-0-07-176762-0
Book MHID 0-07-176762-2

This book was set in Berling by Thomson Digital.
The editors were Brian Belval and Brian Kearns.
The production supervisor was Richard Ruzycka.
Project management was provided by Garima Sharma, Thomson Digital.
The cover designer was Thomas De Pierro.
China Translation & Printing Services, Ltd. was printer and binder.

This book is printed on acid-free paper.

Library of Congress Cataloging-in-Publication Data

Schrope, Beth, author.
  Surgical and interventional ultrasound / Beth Schrope.
    p. ; cm.
  Includes bibliographical references.
  ISBN-13: 978-0-07-176762-0 (book : alk. paper)
  ISBN-10: 0-07-176762-2 (book : alk. paper)
  ISBN-13: 978-0-07-176760-6 (set : alk. paper)
  ISBN-10: 0-07-176760-6 (set : alk. paper)
  [etc.]
  I. Title.
  [DNLM: 1. Ultrasonography. 2. Ultrasonography, Interventional. WN 208]
  RC78.7.U4
  616.07'543—dc23
                                    2013018982

McGraw-Hill books are available at special quantity discounts to use as premiums and
sales promotions, or for use in corporate training programs. To contact a representative
please e-mail us at bulksales@mcgraw-hill.com.

CONTENTS

▶ **Corollos S. Abdelshehid, MD**
Education Fellow
Department of Urology
University of California Irvine
Irvine, California
Genitourinary Ultrasound

▶ **Preya Ananthakrishnan, MD**
Assistant Clinical Professor of Surgery
Department of Surgery
Columbia University Medical Center
New York, New York
Breast Ultrasound

▶ **Jerome A. Byam, MD**
Fellow, Abdominal Organ Transplantation
Department of Surgery
University of Chicago
Chicago, Illinois
Hepatobiliary Ultrasound

▶ **John Chabot, MD, FACS**
David V. Habif Professor of Clinical Surgery
Department of Surgery
Columbia University College of Physicians and Surgeons
New York, New York
Ultrasound of the Pancreas

▶ **Anis Dizdarevic, MD**
Clinical Assistant Professor
Anesthesiology and Pain Management
New York Presbyterian Hospital
Columbia University
New York, New York
Ultrasound-Guided Regional Anesthesia

▶ **Eugene Garvin, MD**
Anesthesiology Resident
Anesthesiology and Pain Management
Columbia Presbyterian Medical Center
New York, New York
Ultrasound-Guided Regional Anesthesia

▶ **Rondi B. Gelbard, MD**
Clinical Fellow
Division of Trauma
Emergency General Surgery and Surgical Critical Care
USC + LAC Medical Center
Los Angeles, California
Abdominal Ultrasound
Trauma Ultrasound

▶ **Stephanie L. Goff, MD**
Resident
General Surgery
Columbia University Medical Center
New York, New York
Ultrasound of the Neck: Thyroid and Parathyroid

▶ **Joseph A. Graversen, MD**
Minimally Invasive Urology Fellow
Department of Urology
University of California Irvine
Irvine, California
Genitourinary Ultrasound

▶ **Mark A. Hardy, MD, FACS**
Auchincloss Professor of Surgery
Director Emeritus & Founder, Transplantation Program
Department of Surgery
Columbia University College of Physician and Surgeons
New York, New York
Abdominal Ultrasound

▶ **Mohammad A. Helmy, MD**
Assistant Professor
Department of Radiology
University of California Irvine
Irvine, California
Genitourinary Ultrasound

▶ **David A. Iannitti, MD**
Chief, HPB Surgery
Department of Surgery
Carolinas Medical Center
Charlotte, North Carolina
Hepatobiliary Ultrasound

▶ **Christopher M. Jones, MD**
Assistant Professor of Surgery
Division of Transplantation
Hiram C. Polk, Jr, MD, Department of Surgery
University of Louisville/Jewish Hospital
Louisville, Kentucky
Hepatobiliary Ultrasound

▶ **Adam Kaplan, MD**
Resident
Department of Urology
University of California Irvine
Irvine, California
Genitourinary Ultrasound

▶ **Farhan Khan, MD**
Chief Resident
Department of Urology
University of California Irvine
Irvine, California
Genitourinary Ultrasound

▶ **Jaime Landman, MD**
Chairman
Department of Urology
University of California Irvine
Irvine, California
Genitourinary Ultrasound

▶ **John C. Lantis II, MD, FACS, RPVI**
Chief of Division of Vascular/Endovascular Surgery
Vice Chairman
Department of Surgery
St Luke's-Roosevelt Hospital
Clinical Professor of Surgery
Columbia University
New York, New York
Vascular Ultrasound

▶ **Simon Lavotshkin, MD**
Postdoctoral Residency Fellow
Department of Surgery
New York Presbyterian Hospital; Columbia
New York, New York
Ultrasound of the Pancreas

▶ **James A. Lee, MD**
Assistant Professor of Surgery
Chief, Endocrine Surgery
Department of Surgery
Columbia University Medical Center
New York, New York
Ultrasound of the Neck: Thyroid and Parathyroid

▶ **Achim Lusch, MD**
Minimally Invasive Urology Fellow
Department of Urology
University of California Irvine
Irvine, California
Genitourinary Ultrasound

▶ **Aimee Mackey, MD**
Assistant Professor
Department of Surgery
Duke University Medical Center/Duke Cancer Institute
Durham, North Carolina
Breast Ultrasound

▶ **Arunthathi Oormila Mahendran, MBBS, MRCS**
Fellow in Abdominal Organ Transplantation
Assistant Instructor in Surgery
Department of Surgery
Abdominal Organ Transplant & Hepatobiliary Surgery
New York Presbyterian Hospital
Columbia University College of Physicians and Surgeons
New York, New York
Abdominal Ultrasound

▶ **Cameron Marshall, MD**
Resident Physician, Anesthesiology and Pain Medicine
Department of Anesthesia
New York Presbyterian Hospital
New York, New York
Ultrasound-Guided Regional Anesthesia

▶ **Michael R. Marvin, MD**
Transplant and Hepatobiliary Surgeon
Chief, Associate Professor of Surgery
Division of Transplantation
University of Louisville
Louisville, Kentucky
Hepatobiliary Ultrasound

▶ **Phillip Mucksavage, MD**
Minimally Invasive Urology Fellow
University of California Irvine
Irvine, California
Genitourinary Ultrasound

▶ **Oliver Panzer, MD**
Assistant Professor
Director, Perioperative Ultrasound Education
Department of Anesthesiology
Division of Intensive Care Medicine
Columbia University Medical Center
New York, New York
Critical Care Ultrasonography

▶ **Beth Schrope, MD, PhD, FACS, RDMS**
Assistant Professor of Surgery
Department of Surgery
Columbia University College of Physicians and Surgeons
New York, New York
Ultrasound Physics
Instrumentation, Scanning Techniques, and Artifacts
Advanced Technologies
Ultrasound of the Pancreas
Therapeutic Ultrasound
Documentation, Coding, Billing, and Compliance
Credentialing

▶ **Christina J. Seo, MD, FACS, FASCRS**
Staff Surgeon
Department of Colorectal Surgery
Barash-White, MD, PA
Englewood, New Jersey
Anorectal Ultrasound

▶ **Amrita Sethi, MD**
Assistant Professor of Medicine
Division of Digestive and Liver Diseases
Columbia University Medical Center
New York Presbyterian Hospital
New York, New York
Endoscopic Ultrasound: Foregut Including Esophagus,
*   Stomach, Small Intestine, and Pancreaticobiliary*

▶ **Steven Yap, MD**
Attending
Department of Anesthesiology
New York Cardiovascular Anesthesiologists
St Francis Heart Hospital
Roslyn, New York
Ultrasound-Guided Regional Anesthesia

This book is intended for surgeons and other physicians who use ultrasound to guide their interventions. Although diagnosis may be part of the exam, it is ultrasound that helps to more precisely and effectively deliver a biopsy instrument or therapy that is the focus of this work.

During my practice in academic surgery over the past decade or so, I have often appreciated the learning opportunity afforded by my interactions with physicians in other specialties. I have discovered new "toys" or techniques that I can apply to "my" organs, whether it is a suturing device that I saw my urology colleague using when working together on a joint case, or a particular coding strategy for appropriate reimbursement.

This book spans a number of interventional specialties that use ultrasound, with specific emphasis on image-guided procedures. Following a foundation on the basics of ultrasound physics, imaging techniques, and instrumentation, the subsequent chapters are written by experienced practitioners of ultrasound in their fields, including breast surgery, neck surgery, endoluminal ultrasound, urology, critical care, pain management, and liver and pancreas surgery. Undoubtedly a surgical oncologist would turn his or her eyes to the pancreas and breast chapters first, perhaps, but then may wander to the endoscopic ultrasound chapters if not to expand his or her practice, but at least to understand their patients' workup. Clearly a urologist would not likely endeavor to image the thyroid, yet a perusal of this chapter may present insights into improving technique, offer alternative approaches, or expand descriptions of the genitourinary system.

In particular, the emerging advanced technologies chapter presents much prospect for mining other fields for improvements on your own. Just as radiofrequency ablation for the local treatment of solid tumors was first applied in the liver—and subsequently employed in the kidney, lung, bone, and breast—perhaps ultrasound-assisted drug delivery will also enjoy such a widespread application to the benefit of many.

This book also offers instruction into the banal but necessary realties of medical practice, including credentialing and coding. In these sometimes complicated matters a practitioner in one specialty could very well learn from the experiences of those in other specialties. Indeed even regulatory bodies look to precedents in developing new standards and practices.

The seemingly broad span of specialties in this work is also an attestation to the blurring of the lines of practice in today's medicine, where traditionally "hands-on" specialists such as surgeons now share procedures and surgical treatments with their medical colleagues. Thus the direction in the title to the "interventionalist," not just the surgeon.

Enjoy!

ACKNOWLEDGMENTS

It takes a village to produce a work like the one in your hands. Of course I gratefully acknowledge the time and expertise of each of the contributors; although the topic of "surgical ultrasound" may seem to be a highly specialized niche, each of the areas discussed in this book require specific anatomical and medical expertise in addition to the technical aspects of ultrasound. To adequately present such a diverse array of specialties, therefore, I rely upon my cadre of trained and experienced users.

My interest in this field began in my engineering days; my work in graduate school at Drexel University is the root of my experience and interest in the field of medical ultrasound. There I was fortunate to work with a number of pioneers in the field, including Dr. Vernon Newhouse (my dissertation advisor), Dr. P. Mohana Shankar, Dr. Jack Reid, and Dr. Peter Lewin. It is partly on their shoulders that I stand to offer this work; these scholars are responsible for my foundation in ultrasound.

I was attracted to medicine and ultimately surgery as one enjoys more immediate gratification in caring for patients, rather than churning through necessarily but often mundane research efforts. My inspirations are truly numerous to count, but I will make special mention of some of my contemporary colleagues at Columbia University Department of Surgery. There is Dr. John Chabot, who serendipitously led me back to ultrasound. At his urging I formalized our departmental ultrasound educational curriculum, and this has since resulted in my participation in numerous symposia nationwide, as a physician sonographer and member of the American College of Surgeons National Ultrasound Faculty. It was my fortunate and congenial association with Dr. James Lee and his COACH (Comprehensive Online Archived Care Heuristic) program (coachsurgery.com) that exposed one of my ultrasound lectures to the McGraw-Hill editorial staff, and thus the conception of this book. And my last mention among these, but certainly not the least, is that of Dr. Mark Hardy, an adept sonographer in his own right (among many other talents and accolades), but also to me a mentor, an advocate, and a friend.

At the risk of cliché there is no adequate way to acknowledge my family, my husband Ari, and my children Jacob and Isaac, for their support and sacrifice in this and many other endeavors – my absences may be physical but not spiritual; you are all always on my mind. Lastly a nod to my lifelong advocate and support, my sister Vickie – it all began when she taught me how to read...

ULTRASOUND PHYSICS

BETH SCHROPE

In addition to an exquisite appreciation of anatomy, fundamental to an optimal utilization of ultrasound in medicine is an understanding of the physics of ultrasound. One must recognize the nature of acoustic energy, specifically its creation and interactions with its environs, to fully use it as a diagnostic and potentially therapeutic tool.

WAVE PHYSICS

Sound is simply a type of energy that is transmitted through a medium as a mechanical wave (or vibration). Unlike electromagnetic waves (ie, light), which can travel through a vacuum, mechanical waves require a medium in order to transport their energy. Mechanical waves may have one of two forms, longitudinal or transverse (Figure 1-1). Acoustic energy is a longitudinal wave, where particle displacement is parallel to the direction of wave propagation. In contrast, in a transverse wave the particle displacement is perpendicular to the direction of wave propagation. This can easily be understood if one thinks of a Slinky, the metal spring toy. If the Slinky is stretched out and then given a little push along its axis, a longitudinal wave is created, where a zone of compression is propagated along the coil, accompanied by a zone of rarefaction. On the other hand, if the Slinky is swung side-to-side while holding one end fixed, a transverse wave is created (looking much like a sinusoid as the slinky bounces back and forth).

Although a physical depiction of an acoustic wave is more closely related to the Slinky analogy, characterization of the waves is facilitated by a sinusoidal representation. The zone of compression then corresponds to the positive maximum of a sinusoidal wave, and the zone of rarefaction corresponds to the negative minimum. Waves are described by their wavelength, frequency, propagation velocity, amplitude, and phase, each of which has very important considerations in the use of ultrasound in medicine.

The wavelength is defined as the distance a wave travels per one cycle, which is measured between any two corresponding points on the waveform, that is, from peak-to-peak, trough-to-trough, or zero-to-zero (measured from the same slope) (Figure 1-2). Frequency is inversely proportional to the wavelength and is defined as the number of cycles per second; one cycle/second is termed one Hertz. Frequency and wavelength are related by the speed of sound through a medium, which is a defined property of different media, by the following equation:

$$\lambda = \frac{v}{f}$$

where λ is the wavelength in meters, v is the speed of sound through the medium in meters per second, and f is the frequency of the wave, in Hertz (sec^{-1}). For example, the speed of sound through air is 330 m/s, through water, it is 1480 m/s, and through bone, it is 3000 m/s. For a given defined frequency of an ultrasound transducer, therefore, the wavelength will vary according to the material through which the acoustic wave is traveling. Ultrasound strictly means sound frequencies above the audible range of 20 Hz to 20 kHz; typical frequencies used in medical ultrasound imaging range from about 1 MHz to as high as 20 MHz. Using acoustic waves with small wavelengths allows distinction between smaller features, so applying as high a frequency as possible will result in finer detail. The maximum frequency is limited, however, by other properties of the medium described shortly.

The speed of sound through a medium is also critical to accurately determining the depth of returned echoes and, thus, structures within the insonated field. The depth of an object is equal to the product of the time of travel and the speed of sound in the medium. Soft tissues differ very slightly in their speed of sound characteristics as shown in Table 1-1.

It should be noted that these numbers are approximations as a result of natural variation between humans and of the difficulties inherent in making these measurements. The speed of sound is determined by a number

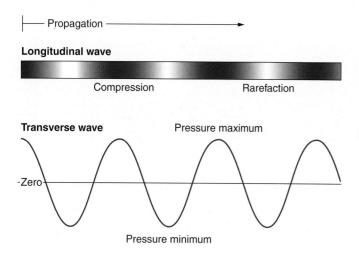

Propagation

Longitudinal wave

Compression   Rarefaction

Transverse wave   Pressure maximum

-Zero

Pressure minimum

Figure 1-1. Physical depiction of the types of mechanical waves.

TABLE 1-1	
Speed of Sound in Different Biological Media	
Medium	**Speed of Sound (m/s)**
Air	330
Fat	1460
Water	1480
Brain	1540
Liver	1580
Kidney	1560
Blood	1580
Muscle	1580
Lens of eye	1640
Bone	3000–4500

of factors including molecular mass, density, and intermolecular forces (elastic modulus). The average speed of sound through soft tissue is often accepted to be 1540 m/s, which is then the assumption used in the calculation of the images obtained in medical ultrasound. Impedance is the product of the density of the material and the speed of sound in that material; impedance mismatches between different materials act as interfaces for reflection or scattering of sound waves and thus can be seen in the reconstruction of the two-dimensional image.

The amplitude of an acoustic wave is a measure of the pressure in the medium as the wave travels. The pressure is positive during the compression stage of the propagation and negative during the rarefaction stage. The logarithm of the square of the amplitude is measured in decibels (dB). The power is the amount of energy generated per unit time and is measured in Watts. Intensity is the power density with an area and is expressed in W/m². It describes the power density within an area (spatial average), or at its peak (spatial peak). However, when considering pulsed ultrasound (which allows for delivery of greater power) one must take into account the duration of the pulse when describing intensity. One could, for example, describe the power delivered only over the duration of the pulse itself (pulse average), or averaged over a period to include the time between pulses (temporal average). From

this discussion it can be seen then that intensity may be described in a number of ways, including I_{SP} (the highest intensity in the beam), I_{SA} (the average value of intensity over a specified area), I_{SATA} (spatial average, temporal average), I_{SAPA} (I_{SATA}/duty cycle), I_{SPTA} (spatial peak, temporal average), or I_{SPPA} (spatial peak, pulse average).

Phase in waves is the fraction of a wave cycle that has elapsed over a given time, and is measured in radians or degrees. Although in ultrasound it is difficult to appreciate the absolute phase of these very tiny waves, the relationship between waves may be critically characterized by their relative phases (Figure 1-3). Two waves that are 180 degrees out of phase, for example, will cancel each other out.

Finally it is important to mention at this juncture that in medical ultrasound, two types of waves are used, continuous and pulsed. Continuous wave devices are the simplest audible probes used for motion detection (fetal heart, arterial pulse, etc) and do not result in two-dimensional images. Pulsed wave ultrasound is most frequently used in

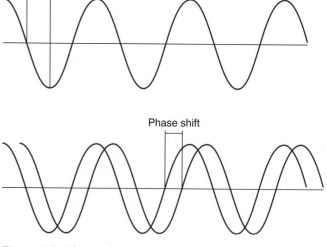

Phase = 90°

Phase shift

Figure 1-3. Phase relationships between sinusoidal waves.

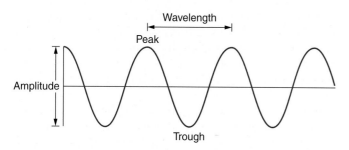

Wavelength

Peak

Amplitude

Trough

Figure 1-2. A sinusoidal wave.

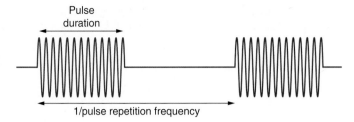

Figure 1-4. A pulsed ultrasound wave.

ultrasound imaging. In this mode, a brief pulse of sound is applied to the medium, and the remaining time is spent "listening" for return echoes. The time duration of the pulse is referred to as the pulse duration, and the time between the initiation of pulses is referred to as the pulse repetition frequency (Figure 1-4). The relevance of this, including the creation of two- and three-dimensional images, will be discussed later in this chapter.

Having described the basic properties of acoustic waves, one must now understand the behavior of these waves as they travel through a medium. Scientifically and philosophically proven, energy is never lost but is simply transformed. Ultrasound, as it travels through a medium, is either transmitted, refracted, absorbed, reflected, or scattered (Figure 1-5). When ultrasound encounters media of different velocity, the proportion of the beam that is not reflected continues to be transmitted but may undergo a change in direction, or refraction. This phenomenon can offer artifacts to the image, or may be used deliberately to enhance certain areas of the region of interest. The "loss" of ultrasound energy, meaning the fraction of energy that is not received as an echo back at the transducer, by the latter three processes is termed attenuation. In soft tissue, acoustic energy is lost at a rate of approximately 0.5 dB/cm/MHz. Absorption occurs when the acoustic energy is transformed to thermal energy. The rarefaction and compression cause vibration in the medium; this translates into friction and heat, which is dissipated through (or absorbed by) the medium. The amount of absorption depends on the transmitted frequency as well as the absorption coefficient of the tissue, an inherent property of all materials. For homogeneous media such as water, absorption is the sole means of attenuation.

Specular reflection occurs at a boundary that is smooth or where the dimensions of the interface are larger than the wavelength, like the diaphragm. A major determinant of reflection is the angle of the incidence. An ultrasound wave hitting a smooth interface at a 90 degree angle will result in a perpendicular reflection. A wave hitting the interface at an angle less than 90 degrees will result in the wave being deflected away from the transducer at an angle equal to the angle of incidence but in the opposite direction (angle of reflection). When this happens, some of the returning echo is lost. Nonspecular or diffuse reflection occurs where the dimensions of the interface are smaller than the wavelength, such as red blood cells or ultrasound contrast media. As will be seen later, when received echoes are "translated" into ultrasound images, these different types of reflection result in different types of images.

Scattering occurs when the interface is irregular, or the reflectors are smaller than the wavelength (thus it is a type of diffuse reflection). Depending on the size, shape, and orientation of the scatterers, scattering can redirect energy in all directions, or it can redirect energy primarily in the same direction as the incident energy (forward scattering) or in the reverse direction (backscattering).

Each of these phenomena is influenced by the frequency of the transmitted wave; that is, the higher the frequency, the greater the energy loss or attenuation. The attenuation coefficient is a unique property of media and, for soft tissue, may be approximated as 0.5 dB/cm/MHz. In the application of medical ultrasound, this influences your choice of transducer; although a higher frequency of sound would result in clearer images, this is limited by the attenuation of the sound wave. In other words, you would use a lower-frequency transducer to reach deeper structures (at the sacrifice of image clarity), and a higher-frequency transducer for more superficial structures (to optimize clarity).

The clarity of an ultrasound image is known as resolution, which is defined as the ability to separate the smallest reflectors from one another. There are two types of resolution: axial resolution and lateral resolution. Axial resolution is the minimum reflector separation along the sound path needed to produce distinct echoes. Also known as range resolution, axial resolution is determined by frequency, wavelength, and pulse duration. In theory, for a minimum pulse duration of 1.5 cycles, of frequency 5 MHz, a propagation velocity of 1500 m/s results in a wavelength of 300 microns and, therefore, an axial resolution of 1.5 × 300 = 450 microns or almost half a millimeter. This theoretical result is limited by other technical factors, and the true resolution is about half the theoretical resolution (so, in our example, the resolution would be closer to one millimeter). Lateral resolution is the ability to distinguish separate echoes perpendicular to the sound path. This depends on transducer diameter and focusing, which often can be electronically manipulated by the user on contemporary ultrasound equipment.

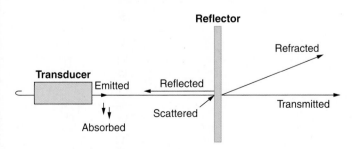

Figure 1-5. Wave behavior in a medium.

An important and well-known acoustic phenomenon is the Doppler effect, described by Christian Doppler, an Austrian physicist, in 1842. When sound is reflected from a moving object (ie, a red blood cell), the frequency of the reflected echo changes in proportion to the velocity of the object. (The classic real-world example is the change in pitch heard as a train passes the listener.) This change in frequency is commonly referred to as the Doppler shift. This observation is governed by the following equation:

$$\Delta f = 2f_0 v \ (\cos\theta)/c$$

where Δf is the frequency shift, f_0 is the incident frequency, c is the speed of sound in the medium, v is the speed of the object, and θ is the angle between the direction of motion of the object and the axis of the ultrasound beam. If the object is moving along the axis of the beam, θ is zero; this is the most accurate technique of determining flow velocity. A negative Doppler shift implies the object is moving away from the receiver; a positive Doppler shift means that the object is moving toward the receiver. Thus, one can use ultrasound to determine blood flow velocity (and other movements) noninvasively.

THE PIEZOELECTRIC EFFECT AND TRANSDUCERS

The application of ultrasound to an object is made possible by the transformation of electrical energy to mechanical energy (vibration) by a piezoelectric material. When electrical energy is applied to a piezoelectric material, pressure is generated; this causes expansion and contraction of the material and thus creates sound waves. This material is the active element of ultrasound transducers, and when the transducer is in passive or listening mode, it can convert the vibration energy back to electrical energy for signal processing and ultimately display of the image. Among other factors, the thickness of the material determines the frequency of the acoustic wave. The original materials employed in ultrasound equipment were barium titanate and lead zirconatetitanate (PZT), although contemporary materials may also include various polymers that allow thinner materials and thus higher frequencies and/or more flexible applications. Most medical ultrasound transducers contain hundreds of piezoelectric elements, each of which can function independently for more rapid acquisition of images and steering and focusing capabilities.

An ultrasound beam has a distinct anatomy, which must also be appreciated in order to understand the interpretation of the images. Two separate regions along the beam can be distinguished, the near field or Fresnel zone and the far field or Fraunhofer zone (Figure 1-6). The near field or Fresnel zone is adjacent to the transducer face and has a converging beam profile due to complex interference patterns close to the face. Lateral resolution is best at the end of the near field. The far field or Fraunhofer zone is characterized by beam divergence and loss of ultrasound intensity. The point of transition between these two zones

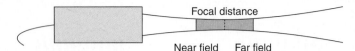

Figure 1-6. Ultrasound beam anatomy.

represents the maximum ultrasound intensity (also known as the spatial peak intensity), and the distance from the transducer face to this point is known as the focal distance. The focal zone is defined as the region over which the width of the beam is less than two times the width of the focal distance. In practical applications, as the frequency of the transmitted energy increases, the length of the near field increases and the angle of or amount of divergence in the far field decreases. Both have the effect of improving lateral resolution. The focal zone can also be manipulated by focusing the beam with a lens or with electronic directional manipulation ("phasing") of multiple piezoelectric elements at the transducer face. The latter represents an array-type transducer, which can be presented in several forms including linear, curvilinear, and sector arrays.

IMAGING MODES

In an ultrasound imaging device, the energy from the received acoustic echoes is converted to electrical energy by the piezoelectric element(s), which is then further manipulated to display the diagnostic information. The basic imaging modes are A-mode, B-mode, Doppler, M-mode and duplex imaging. A-mode, or Amplitude mode, is simply a display of the raw radiofrequency signal over time (much like the figures in the beginning of this chapter used to illustrate wave principles), where the amplitude of the signal is representative of the amplitude of the acoustic waveform. In Figure 1-7, the uppermost picture represents

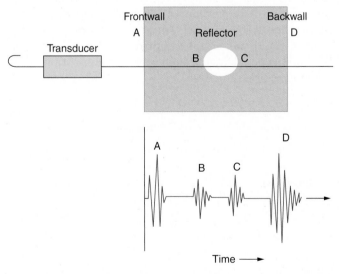

Figure 1-7. A mode imaging.

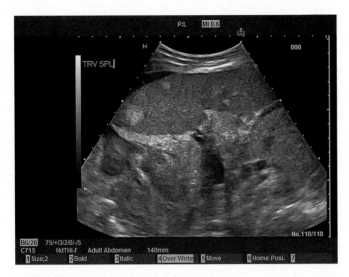

Figure 1-8. B mode image of the liver.

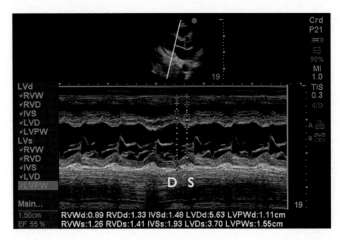

Figure 1-9. M mode image of the fetal heart.

a schematic of an ultrasound transducer emitting a beam into a region of interest. Within the homogeneous medium is an object. The lower picture shows the corresponding A-mode image, where 'A' is the echo from the front wall of the region, 'B' is the echo from the nearest boundary of the object, 'C' is the echo from the far boundary of the object, and 'D' is the backwall of the region. Referring back to the discussion earlier of distance traveled as a function of time and the speed of sound in a medium, one can now see that the timing of the return of the echoes corresponds to the measurements of objects within the tissues.

A B-mode, or Brightness mode, image is the gray-scale image most commonly associated with medical ultrasound imaging. The B-mode image is the two-dimensional reconstruction of the information obtained in the A-mode over a given space at a given time point, where the amplitude of the spikes on the A-mode image are now pixels whose brightness is governed by the amplitude of the received signal (Figure 1-8).

M-mode, or Motion mode, depicts movement of structures as a function of depth and time. This is most often used in mapping the motion of myocardium or cardiac valves, as in Figure 1-9. It has also been described in assessing diaphragmatic motion.

A spectral Doppler image displays velocity (calculated from the frequency shift detected from moving objects) over time. In continuous wave Doppler, an uninterrupted transmission of ultrasound is applied and the return signal (sensed from a different piezoelectric element or array) is displayed as velocities detected at each time point on a time line. Continuous wave (CW) Doppler ultrasound is unable to determine the specific location of velocities (no depth resolution) within the beam and cannot be used to produce color flow images. Pulsed wave (PW) Doppler samples velocities in a specific sample volume and displays them on a time line. PW Doppler is limited to the detection of Doppler frequencies that are half the

pulse repetition frequency. (Thus, CW Doppler is more useful for detecting high flow velocities.) Figure 1-10 shows the rhythmic variation in blood flow through the renal artery.

Finally, duplex ultrasound is a Doppler image and a B-mode image on the same display. The Doppler part can either be a true pulsed Doppler waveform (spectral Doppler) as shown above, or it can be a color flow map ("color Doppler"), where relative speed and direction are shown as colors (often red and blue) with different intensities overlaid on a B-mode image, as shown in Figure 1-11. Clearly the color flow map is not a precise objective measurement, but is very useful in medical imaging when trying to distinguish moving structures from stationary structures or to get a sense of relative flow velocities. Many ultrasound machines can also display the B-mode image, the color flow map, and the Doppler waveform, known as triplex ultrasound. Because one transducer is obtaining all three modes, the frame rate must be decreased and lag in image refreshment is noticeable.

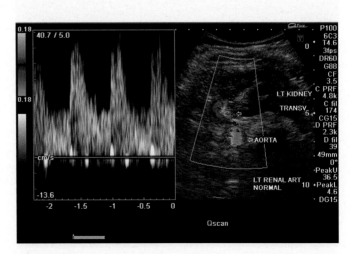

Figure 1-10. Doppler waveform of blood flow through a renal artery.

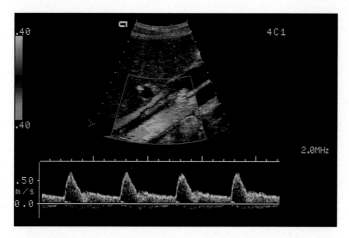

Figure 1-11. Duplex image.

Power Doppler is a display of the magnitude of the color flow, and does not provide information on flow direction (Figure 1-12). Essentially the calculation is the square of the amplitude of the return signal, to "magnify" smaller signals out of noise. However, positive or negative amplitudes (directional information) are lost with this calculation. Power Doppler is useful in detecting low flows and velocities.

SAFETY AND BIOEFFECTS

One of the unique attributes of diagnostic ultrasound is its excellent safety profile. Indeed, its liberal use in fetal examinations without any reported adverse effect attests to this feature. However, responsible use of ultrasound, as with any diagnostic maneuver, beholds the practitioner to consider risk and benefit issues, and to use the lowest energy necessary to produce an adequate study (adhere to the principle of ALARA, As Low As Reasonably Achievable).

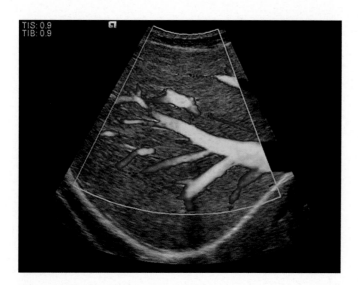

Figure 1-12. Power Doppler image.

Interestingly, when the power is increased above diagnostic levels, the resulting significant bioeffects are exploited for therapeutic uses (as will be discussed elsewhere in this book in detail).

Any effect on biological tissue from ultrasound originates from two processes, thermal and mechanical. The former occurs when the ultrasound energy is absorbed as it travels through tissue and is converted to thermal energy. The amount of tissue heating depends on frequency, intensity, beam area, duration of insonation, and blood perfusion. Higher frequencies and intensities result in greater absorption and thus greater tissue heating. Broader beams result in greater thermal effect. Longer exposure times with ultrasound also increase the thermal effect. Perfusion of blood by either large or small vessels impacts the heating as well, as the blood removes heat from the area of interest. Bone present in the beam area also increases the potential for tissue heating, as absorption is increased at the bone/soft tissue interface.

The World Federation of Ultrasound in Medicine and Biology released an opinion of bioeffects on the fetus in 1992. A conference of experts reviewed the data available at that time and concluded that "a diagnostic exposure that produces a maximum temperature rise of 1.5C above normal (37C) may be used without reservation in clinical examinations." Most commercially available systems approved for diagnostic use fall well below a 1C threshold, with the rare exception of certain peripheral vascular pulsed Doppler systems.

Nonthermal or mechanical effects of ultrasound on tissues are perhaps less intuitive to grasp. These include cavitation and acoustic streaming. Cavitation refers to the formation and behavior of microbubbles in tissue. If certain conditions are met, microbubbles may be formed from dissolved gas in the medium. Or, air cavities may be naturally occurring, such as in the lung alveoli, or bubbles may be iatrogenically introduced, as in ultrasound contrast agents. As the ultrasound wave compresses and rarefacts through the medium, it causes microbubbles in the tissue to contract and expand. The potential for cavitation to occur and its relative magnitude are related to numerous factors, including frequency, amplitude, and pulse duration and pulse repetition frequency.

Acoustic streaming is related to the concept of cavitation, except that it describes the behavior of the medium around the bubbles as a consequence of their vibration. These shear stresses have been shown to be capable of displacing ions and small molecules, potentially rendering cell membranes transiently more permeable, for example. Mechanical effects of ultrasound are exploited for many therapeutic applications including lithotripsy and targeted drug delivery.

When considering the magnitude and relevance of bioeffects at diagnostic levels, it is important to distinguish between imaging and Doppler modes. When an image is acquired, pulses are directed sequentially across the area of interest; thus, the exposure of any single volume of tissue is relatively small and not sustained. In contrast, with Doppler examinations, multiple ultrasound pulses are emitted along a single line of sight; thus, the beam is stationary, the exposure is sustained, and the potential for thermal or nonthermal effects is greater. In addition, in Doppler as opposed to imaging modes, longer pulses as well as shorter pulse repetition frequencies are utilized to avoid aliasing. These factors result in a higher duty cycle, greater overall exposure of the tissue to the ultrasound energy, and, thus, greater potential for the bioeffects described above. Similarly, continuous wave Doppler applications, though generally lower in amplitude, also subject the tissue to greater exposure to ultrasound energy over time.

The Food and Drug Administration has attempted to regulate ultrasound devices with respect to their potential for bioeffects in the past. This had come under criticism, as many users and professional organizations felt that the standards enacted were based on arbitrary interpretations of data. More recently, a voluntary standard was created, supported by the FDA and endorsed by professional organizations, whereby output information relevant to the potential for bioeffects is displayed on the user interface. The thermal index (TI) is the ratio of total acoustic power to the acoustic power required to raise the temperature of tissue 1C. A TI of 1, then, implies to potential of heating the tissue 1C. This calculation was created with the worst-case assumptions, to allow for redundancy in safety. Systems that are not capable of a TI greater than 1 are not required to display the TI. The mechanical index (MI) is defined as the spatial peak of the peak rarefaction pressure, or

$$MI = PNP/\sqrt{F_c}$$

where PNP is the peak negative pressure of the ultrasound wave in MPa, and F_c is the center frequency in MHz. At present the FDA stipulates that the MI cannot exceed 1.9 on diagnostic ultrasound scanners, and those machines incapable of producing an MI greater than 1 are not required to display it in real time.

SUGGESTED READINGS

Edelman, Sidney K. *Understanding Ultrasound Physics*. 3rd ed. E.S.P. Ultrasound; 2004.

Hedrick, Wayne. *Technology for Diagnostic Sonography*. 1st ed. St. Louis, Missouri: Elsevier Saunders; 2012.

Kremkau, Frederick W. *Sonography Principles and Instruments*. 8th ed. St. Louis: Elsevier Saunders; 2010.

TerHaar G. Ultrasound bioeffects and safety. *Proceedings of the Institution of Mechanical Engineers. Part H* 2010;224(2): 363–373.

INSTRUMENTATION, SCANNING TECHNIQUES, AND ARTIFACTS

BETH SCHROPE

Discussions on basic ultrasound instrumentation have historically focused on proper handling of the transducer and adjustment of controls for image optimization. These will of course be addressed in this book, but more importantly in a text concentrating on interventional ultrasound one must also appreciate the dynamic nature of ultrasound as an instrument for achieving the procedure at hand. Special attention will be given to intraoperative and endoscopic techniques, which are solely the realm of the proceduralist. What follows is simply the fundamentals for performing an ultrasound examination and/or guided procedure; familiarity and experience cannot be overemphasized.

INSTRUMENTATION

Any ultrasound system has three basic components: a transducer, or probe; the processing unit, including the controls; and the display. The transducer (Figure 2-1) consists of the piezoelectric material (active element) within a nonconductive housing, which may consist of one solitary element or several hundred elements (known as an array). A piezoelectric material has the property of converting mechanical energy (ultrasound vibrations) into electrical energy, and vice versa. In an ultrasound transducer, the electrical excitation impulse is transmitted to the piezoelectric element, and the returning echoes are then converted into electrical signals by the element and transmitted to the processing unit via a shielded cable for further image processing. The thickness of the piezoelectric element determines the center frequency of the transducer (multiple elements allow for a range of frequencies in a single transducer). Backing material absorbs excess vibration of the received signal (dampening) and its impedance should closely match that of the active element to optimize resolution. To minimize energy loss at the face of the transducer, a matching layer is incorporated of a material with an acoustic impedance somewhere in between that of the piezoelectric material and the tissue under investigation (in medical applications). The thickness of this matching layer should be half that of the element so that waves reflected within the matching layer remain in phase when they exit the layer.

Ultrasound transducers can be divided into two basic types: mechanical and electronic. Mechanical probes contain one or multiple piezoelectric elements that physically oscillate to scan a region of interest, resulting in the classic sector scan image. These are the least expensive type of transducer to manufacture, but scanning and processing options are limited. In the case of radial scanning, such as that employed for endocavity (endorectal, endoanal, and esophageal) applications, rigid mechanical transducers are utilized for a 360 degree view of the luminal structure. They are available in a variety of sizes, frequencies, and lengths (Figure 2-2).

Electronic transducers, or arrays, employ groups of piezoelectric elements working in concert, and can further be divided into linear, curvilinear, phased, and annular, based on the arrangement of the elements in the probe. Biplane and three-dimensional transducers are also of this type. Array transducers have the advantage that both the transmitted ultrasound emission and the received signal can be manipulated much more than in the mechanical probes. Most ultrasound machines for medical use have multiple transducers available for different applications, that is, a higher-frequency linear transducer for neck ultrasound, or a curvilinear array of relatively lower frequency for abdominal applications. Flexible through-the-scope endoscopic ultrasound probes for use in imaging foregut structures (pancreas, bile duct, stomach, and proximal small bowel) are either linear array or radial subtypes.

There are additional considerations for ultrasound-guided procedures. Many of these procedures are

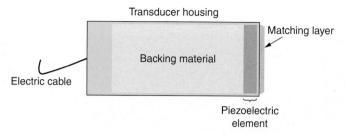

Figure 2-1. Schematic of an ultrasound transducer.

performed sterilely (ie, needle biopsy). In this case, the probe needs to be either sterilized or draped sterilely. Ultrasound transducers cannot be autoclaved, as this may alter their piezoelectric properties. Ultrasound transducers are most often sterilized by immersion in a solution; some transducers can be gas-sterilized. The user is referred to the manufacturer of the probe for specific instructions. Of course care must be taken to thoroughly clean the probe of gross contaminants prior to sterilization. Biopsy guides and other attachments should also be subject to sterilization. An alternative to sterilization by the aforementioned methods is using a sterile drape over the probe. When utilizing this method it is important to be sure to couple the face of the transducers to the inside of the drape with a coupling agent such as gel, water, or oil.

Ultrasound machines from different manufacturers may look very different, but there are certain necessarily common elements amongst them. It is essential of course for users to familiarize themselves with the layout of the control panel, available transducers, various output options, etc. Starting with the control panel, the first step of any ultrasound examination is entering patient identification, at minimum name and another identifier such as date of birth or medical record number. This is best practice in terms of archiving and billing compliance. In fact, some ultrasound machines do not allow scanning without the input of some minimum patient identification.

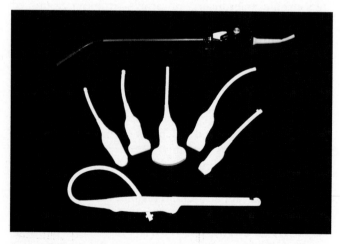

Figure 2-2. Photograph of various ultrasound transducers, including laparoscopic, endorectal, transcutaneous and intraoperative types.

Many ultrasound machines offer *presets* or defaults for certain types of examinations, with titles such as liver, abdomen, breast, etc. These presets are pre-adjusted settings of gain, depth, focus, etc, and are usually quite adequate to at least get the user started on an examination; individual settings can be adjusted as needed as anatomic or patient factors dictate. Many machines also offer the option for custom presets.

The *frequency* of the transducer selected is actually the center frequency, as a typical ultrasound pulse contains a range of frequencies. Most transducers are capable of transmitting over a range of center frequencies as well, enabling a user more flexibility during a single examination. Typically three center frequencies are available, for example, 5.0–7.5–10.0 MHz, and the frequency select button cycles or toggles through the frequencies. The frequency selected will be displayed on the image. (Remember that the improved resolution with higher frequencies comes at the expense of greater attenuation and, thus, poorer imaging of deep structures.)

The *power* control adjusts the strength of the signal delivered to the transducer. This will lead to a brighter image, but may also increase noise and other unwanted artifacts. In addition, although ultrasound is a very safe energy modality to use for imaging, the user must be aware of the principle of ALARA: As Low As Reasonably Achievable, referring to the amount of incident energy needed to produce the optimal image.

Adjusting the *gain* will also deliver a brighter image, but unlike the power setting, the gain control amplifies the returning (instead of the transmitted) signal. Increasing the gain too high can also result in artifactual echoes from surrounding tissues (for example, when in color flow map mode, color may be applied to obviously stationary tissue because the sensitivity is too high).

Gain can be adjusted variably according to depth with the time gain compensation (TGC) controls, which often appear as a group of slide switches on the control panel. To accommodate for the attenuation of the ultrasound energy as it travels through the tissue, back and forth from the transducer, echoes at different time points from the incident pulse are amplified separately.

The *dynamic range* (DR) refers to the range of echo amplitudes processed and displayed by the system, from strongest to weakest, analogous to the concept of contrast in video applications. The strongest echoes received are those from the initial impulse and transducer–skin interface, and will generally be similar for different examinations. As the DR is decreased, the echoes at the weaker end of the spectrum will be lost. For most imaging applications the DR should be kept at its maximum level to maximize the contrast of the image. In situations where low-level noise or artifacts degrade the image quality, however, the DR can be reduced to partially eliminate these appearances.

The *depth* of the insonified region displayed is adjustable as well. For example, imaging the jugular vein will optimally be displayed at a more shallow depth than transabdominal imaging of the gallbladder. Varying the depth will affect the spatial resolution of the image, as a higher pulse repetition frequency (thus greater spatial resolution) is possible for more shallow imaging. The depth control generally allows adjustment from the transducer face to some point in the tissue; many machines also provide controls for displaying only a section of the region ("zoom"), not necessarily starting from the transducer face.

Adjusting the *focus* will optimize the resolution at a selected depth. This means that the beam is being electronically focused or narrowed at the desired location (reference the Physics chapter in this book for a more detailed explanation). The region of focus is generally displayed by indicators at the side of the image. Many ultrasound machines allow multiple areas of focus to be chosen simultaneously.

For measurements or archiving it is most often necessary to *freeze* the image. Measurements are often an integral part of an ultrasound examination. To measure a target, the image is frozen and then *calipers* are selected on the control panel. The target can be measured in as many as four linear dimensions, and volumetrically. The dynamic ultrasound examination is often saved in mini cine loops; therefore, the freeze button does not have to be depressed at the exact moment the image is best. A dial or trackball will then allow review of a few frames back to find the best image for archiving or measurement.

Ultrasound still images can be printed or stored digitally as DICOM (Digital Image in Communication in Medicine) images. In addition, cine-loops can be archived as DICOM.

Another option for ultrasound imaging widely available is tissue harmonics, or *harmonic* imaging. As stated previously, the transducer is excited by an electronic pulse of a certain center frequency, f_0. As the ultrasound energy travels through tissue, it is distorted by inherent properties of the medium, producing weak but detectable echoes at multiples of the incident frequency. As the multipliers increase ($2f_0 \rightarrow 3f_0 \rightarrow 4f_0$, etc), the signal becomes weaker and more difficult to detect. Certain unique properties of different media may provide "signatures" for further characterization of tissues, such as using intravascular contrast agents with strong harmonic echoes to delineate otherwise undetectable subtle tissue perfusion.

SCANNING TECHNIQUES

Although not usually required to perform an examination, for documentation and billing purposes at minimum the patient name and a second identifier (MRN, date of birth) should be inputted.

Transducer selection depends on the region of interest. In general, higher-frequency transducers (7.5 MHz and up) are useful for imaging small structures at shallow depth, such as for thyroid, breast, scrotum, or vascular examinations. In addition, intraoperative probes can be of higher frequency because the probe is placed directly on the organ of interest; likewise, endoluminal probes (endorectal, choledochal) are of even higher frequency. On the other hand, deeper applications such as abdominal imaging require a lower-frequency transducer (2.5-, 3.5-, or 5.0-MHz). Specialized examinations such as transrectal, transvaginal, or endoscopic ultrasound have specialized transducers for these purposes. Transducer footprint or face dimensions also affect the choice of transducer; larger curvilinear transducers are useful for transabdominal imaging, wide linear arrays can be used on the breast or neck, and small articulated probes can be used in the OR for retroperitoneal structures. Biplane probes are available to simultaneously image in two two-dimensional planes, which can enhance procedural accuracy when ultrasound is used for guidance. Three-dimensional and four-dimensional planes (volume plus time) are also available.

It is easiest to get started when a preset appropriate for the application is selected. The names of presets vary according to the manufacturer, but should be fairly apparent. In addition, many ultrasound machines allow saving of custom presets.

For contact imaging, a coupling agent must be used to avoid loss of energy at the interface between the transducer face and the tissue. In transcutaneous imaging, a gel is most often used. For intraoperative imaging, a saline bath in the body cavity is also adequate. For endoluminal applications, natural body fluids (bile, enteric contents) are sufficient. When transducers are draped for use in a sterile field, the interface between the transducer and the inside of the drape must be coupled with gel or oil in addition to the interface between the drape and the tissue. In any case, care must be taken to avoid bubbles in the gel or fluid, which would cause unwanted artifacts in the image.

All transducers have an indicator one side (visible and/or palpable) that corresponds to a certain side of the image. It is extremely important to establish this orientation prior to scanning. One trick is verifying a perturbation on the image when one side of the probe face is touched. By convention on a longitudinal scan, the transducer should be oriented so that the left side of the screen should be cephalad (toward the head) and the right side should be caudad (toward the feet). Sagittal images are oriented with right-sided structures to the left of the image. Since most procedural ultrasound is dynamic and sometimes requires unconventional transducer position, it is probably less important to obey imaging convention than it is to simply be aware of imaging orientation at all times.

Patient position depends on the anatomic area being studied. Since ultrasound is a dynamic measurement, patient cooperation in shifting position, breath-holding, or Valsava, for example, can all be exploited for optimal image acquisition.

ARTIFACTS

Artifacts are phenomena occurring as a result of ultrasound's interaction with the medium. Although artifacts are by definition false images, proper recognition and characterization of artifacts is paramount to optimal image interpretation. It is also important to recognize the fact

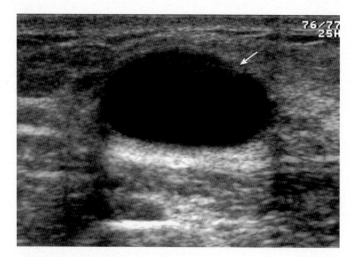

Figure 2-3. Reverberation artifact.

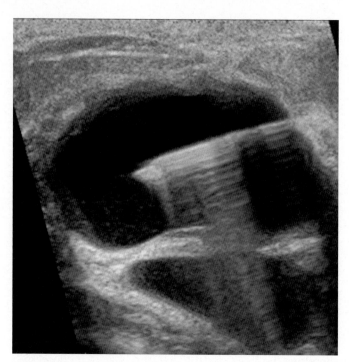

Figure 2-4. Comet tail artifact.

that ultrasound is a dynamic procedure, so artifacts can often be distinguished from genuine by scanning in different planes or by adjusting the system controls.

▶ Reverberation

Reverberation artifact is produced from multiple reflections from an object as the sound energy bounces back and forth between the object and the transducer face or within a structure with high acoustic mismatch. Figure 2-3 depicts a breast cyst, whose walls are strong acoustic reflectors due to the high impedance mismatch between the cyst fluid and surrounding breast tissue. During an examination, the sonographer would image in different planes to assess whether this reflection is an artifact or true anatomic structure.

▶ Comet Tail Artifact

The comet tail artifact is a type of reverberation artifact. It is often seen with metallic objects, which cause a comet tail effect as the metallic substance produces small, tightly bound reverberations or ringing. Figure 2-4 illustrates a biopsy needle in this image-guided aspiration of a breast cyst. Note that the beveled edge of the needle also produces a characteristic echo, known as a flame artifact.

▶ Ring-Down Artifact

This artifact, also a type of reverberation artifact, is produced by small bubbles of air or partial liquids (lipids). Figure 2-5 is a ring-down artifact in a gallbladder with adenomyomatosis. The artifact is due to reverberation of sound within or between the cholesterol crystals, which send several echoes back to the transducer, creating a line of closely spaced echoes in one or two vectors.

▶ Mirror Image Artifact

This artifact occurs when a strong specular reflector (such as the diaphragm) is imaged. If some acoustic energy is transmitted through the reflector, upon its return it can again be reflected at the other (distal) side of the reflector, creating

a mirror image on the other side. Eventually all of those echoes return and are displayed as a false image on the other side of the reflector. In Figure 2-6 the mirror image of the liver could mistakenly be taken for a pleural effusion.

SHADOWING

Shadowing is loss of signal distal (relative to the transducer face) to an object with a large impedance mismatch. A well-known portrayal of shadowing occurs with gallstones

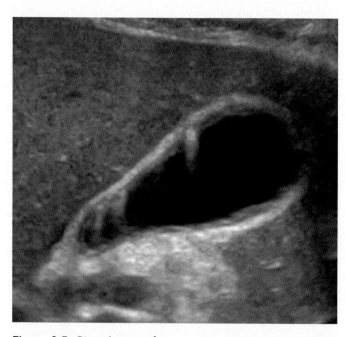

Figure 2-5. Ring-down artifact.

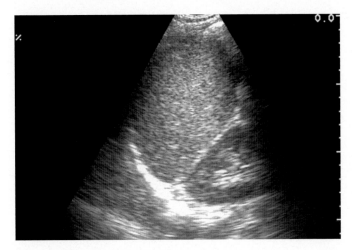

Figure 2-6. Mirror image artifact.

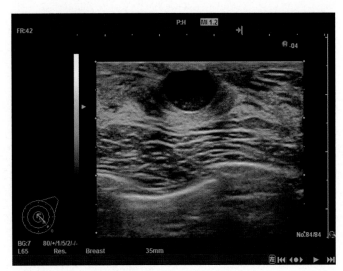

Figure 2-8. Enhancement artifact.

in the gallbladder, as shown in Figure 2-7. Another commonly seen example of shadowing occurs at the transducer face, when it is not coupled properly to the tissue, such as with air bubbles trapped in the coupling gel.

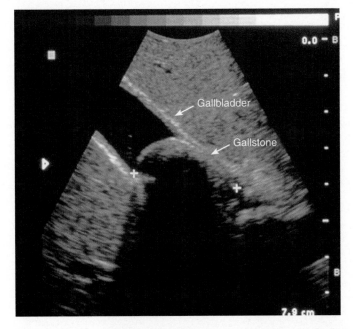

Figure 2-7. Shadowing artifact.

ENHANCEMENT

Enhancement is the appearance of brighter echoes distal to an anechoic object relative to other structures at the same depth. This is due to unattenuated travel of the beam through the anechoic structure. This can be very helpful in situations where suboptimal settings (low power, low gain) might not display subtle but real echoes within a solid tumor; if the posterior enhancement is not appreciated, one must adjust the gain settings to see the true structure. On the other hand, when the power and/or gain is too high, reverberations across an anechoic structure could be mistaken for solid tissue; posterior enhancement will still be seen, however, thus aiding in the differentiation of a fluid-filled structure from a solid structure (Figure 2-8).

ALIASING

In pulsed Doppler applications there may be situations where the velocity of the sampled object is too high to be determined by the Doppler frequency shift. In other words, the Doppler frequency must be within half the pulse repetition frequency (it must be detected before the next pulse is transmitted). Figure 2-9 shows

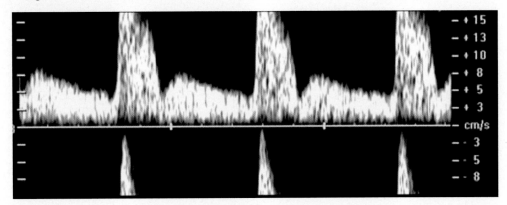

Figure 2-9. Aliasing on a Doppler waveform, a consequence of the Doppler frequency being greater than having the pulse repetition frequency.

the appearance of aliasing on a Doppler waveform, where the signal appears to be wrapped around the display so that the peak of the waveform is displayed below the baseline. This can be corrected by increasing the PRF, increasing the Doppler angle, shifting the baseline, lowering the transmitted frequency, or using a continuous wave transmission. In other words, low velocities (venous flow, microperfusion) should be investigated with low PRFs, with the longer time between pulses to allow time for the low Doppler shift echo to come back to the transducer.

However, if a high-velocity flow occurs in the sample volume, aliasing may occur if the Doppler frequency is greater than half the PRF.

SUGGESTED READINGS

Hedrick, Wayne. *Technology for Diagnostic Sonography*. 1st ed. St. Louis, Missouri: Elsevier Saunders; 2012.

Kremkau, Frederick W. *Sonography Principles and Instruments*. 8th ed. St. Louis: Elsevier Saunders; 2010.

3

ADVANCED TECHNOLOGIES

BETH SCHROPE

There are numerous exciting new technologies beyond the basic physics of ultrasound previously discussed that hold promise for expanding diagnostic, interventional, and therapeutic ultrasound applications. This chapter will review the current state of some of the more popular of these technologies.

THREE-DIMENSIONAL ULTRASOUND

Three-dimensional ultrasound is most familiar to the lay public as the source of beautiful baby pictures *in utero*. An internet image search will yield billions of images of before (fetal) and after (infant) pictures, with remarkable results. The technology is proving itself also quite useful in nonobstetric applications, such as breast, abdominal, thyroid, etc., limited only by the imagination of the user.

Hands-on conventional two-dimensional ultrasound can be construed in and of itself as a three-dimensional technology if one considers the user's manipulations of the beam and mental reconstruction of the image. Over 10 years ago computational speed and power, however, allowed for automatic reconstruction, display, and archiving of these images. In addition, 3D reconstruction allows for imaging awkward or otherwise inaccessible areas of the body. In certain applications, accurate volumetric quantification is essential for disease diagnosis and follow-up.

In the early days of 3D ultrasound, mechanical transducers were employed to sweep the volume of interest. The reconstruction was performed after the examination, at a PACS workstation. Alternatively a conventional 2D transducer was manually ("freehand") swept with the movement either tracked or untracked to build the 3D image. The transducers currently used for 3D ultrasound are electronic probes that steer the beam in pyramid-like volumes to obtain multiplanar image data for the calculation of the 3D image. Now real-time displays are possible. The image may be displayed as a whole volume (volume-rendering), with the user given the ability to rotate the volume, or as individual planes, or as a crossed-plane view (multiplanar reformatting), which may be more intuitive for a user more comfortable with 2D imaging. One advantage is the ability to reconstruct the image "behind" obstructing or shadowing structures, which, in a conventional two-dimensional image, would remain elusive. The addition of time information results in a "4D" image, for use in echocardiography or vascular applications, for instance.

There is a convention for the multiplanar reconstruction. Three-dimensional ultrasound is described as three planes: the A plane, B plane, and C plane (Figure 3-1). The A plane is the plane parallel to the acquisition plane, the B plane is perpendicular to the A plane but still parallel to the ultrasound beam, and the C plane is often referred to as the coronal plane, or the two-dimensional slices at various depths from and parallel to the transducer face (and perpendicular to the ultrasound beam). Many scanners will display these three planes with these monikers in addition to a volumetric rendering (Figure 3-2).

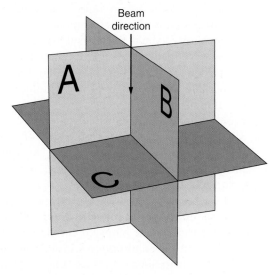

Figure 3-1. Multiplanar image display schematic for 3D ultrasound.

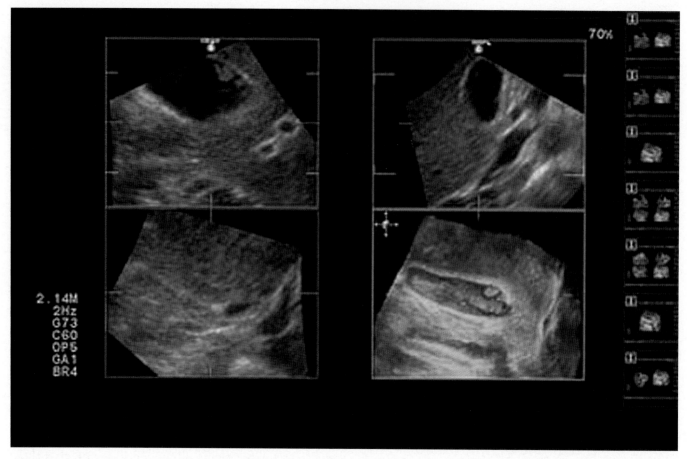

Figure 3-2. Three-dimensional multiplanar and volumetric rendering of a gallbladder polyp. (Used with permission from Hitachi-Aloka.)

As mentioned above, an obvious use of 3D ultrasound lies in stereotactic biopsy. The benefits are increased precision and fewer needle passes and/or overall biopsy events. In addition, unlike conventional radiographic stereotactic biopsies, ultrasound does not use ionizing radiation.

One of the first nonobstetric areas of application for 3D imaging was in the prostate, where both biopsy and treatment planning are benefitted by this technique (Figure 3-3). Often a patient with elevated PSH is subject to random biopsies searching for malignancy. This methodology has a clear disadvantage in terms of a high false negative rate. 3D imaging can perhaps denote areas of sonographic abnormality. More importantly, treatment with seed implants can be precisely directed and repeatedly monitored with real-time 3D ultrasound imaging. Cryotherapy can also be guided with confidence using 3D ultrasound, with attention to sparing surrounding tissue and thus potentially minimizing complications.

The benefits in breast practice are obvious. If a lesion is discovered on mammography, it may be considered for 3D ultrasound-guided stereotactic biopsy if certain conditions are met, that is, it is visible on ultrasound. In addition, in the event of awkward orientations necessitated by anatomy or patient comfort, 3D ultrasound can allow for monitoring of needle placement at all times, even if an oblique angle is

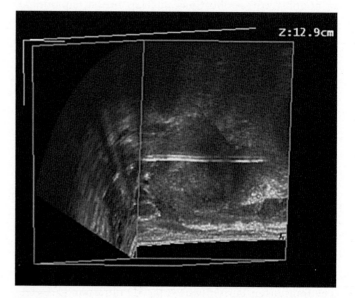

Figure 3-3. Three-dimensional image of prostate, showing needle position. (From Mingyue Ding, Zhouping Wei, Lori Gardi, Donal B. Downey, Aaron Fenster, "Needle and seed segmentation in intra-operative 3D ultrasound-guided prostate brachytherapy," Ultrasonics, Volume 44, Supplement, 22 December 2006, Pages e331–e336.)

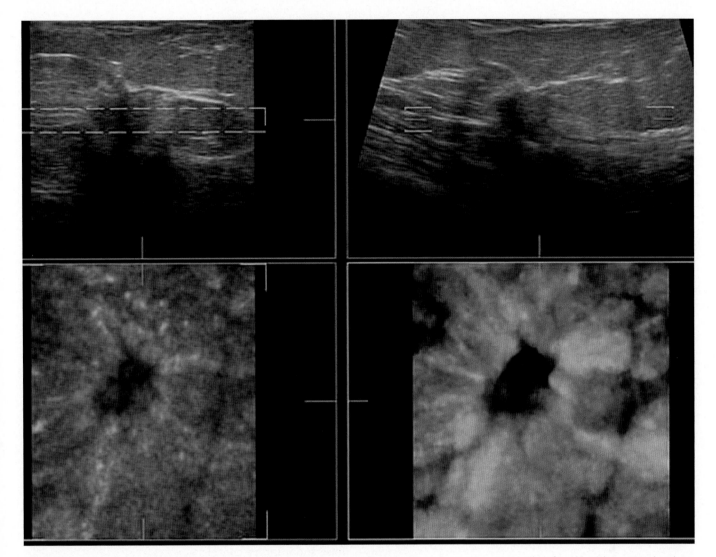

Figure 3-4. Three-dimensional image of breast lesion depicting infiltrating ductal carcinoma with ill-defined borders. (Used with permission from Hitachi-Aloka.)

employed. Figure 3-4 demonstrates a 3D ultrasound view of a breast lesion.

A generally close and superficial space, the neck stands to benefit from more widespread use of 3D ultrasound. Visualization of pathology with respect to its position to vital structures is crucial to safe and accurate needle biopsy as well as operative planning. The regions alongside and behind the esophagus and trachea, previously inaccessible to ultrasound, can be discovered and examined with a 3D modality.

In the liver, both transcutaneously and intraoperatively, 3D ultrasound can deliver an inexpensive yet high-yield method for obtaining a tissue diagnosis of lesions. Similar to the discussion of breast biopsies, awkward needle placement is transformed by the volumetric nature of 3D ultrasound. Determination of tumor position with respect to vascular and biliary structures is also facilitated by 3D ultrasound, useful for planning and guiding definitive surgical intervention (Figure 3-5).

Another interesting concept not fully developed or accepted at the time of this writing is the notion of an ultrasound-rendered cholangiopancreatogram (URCP). Displaying the same information as an ERCP (endoscopic retrograde cholangiopancreatogram), which necessitates patient anesthesia and often significant doses of ionizing radiation, or an MRCP (magnetic resonance cholangiopancreatogram), which requires an expensive, unwieldy and at times intolerable imaging modality, a URCP could potentially supplant these exams in certain cases. Figure 3-6 demonstrates an ultrasound rendering of the biliary tree.

FUSION IMAGING

Combining ultrasound imaging modalities with another cross-sectional imaging technique such as CT or MRI is known as fusion imaging. The main advantage of this technique is its use in image-guided interventions. Consider a lesion that is poorly defined with ultrasound, but distinct on CT. An ultrasound-guided intervention, such as a needle biopsy or lesion ablation, would be beneficial, since it does

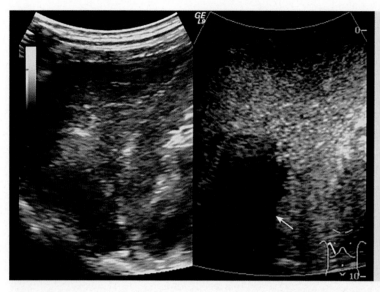
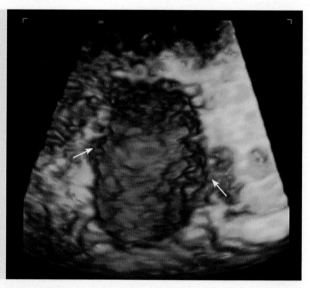

Figure 3-5. Three-dimensional image of liver lesion. (Used with permission from Xu H, et al. Treatment response evaluation with three-dimensional contrast-enhanced ultrasound for liver cancer after local therapies. *Eur J Radiol.* 2010 Oct;76(1):81–88.)

not involve ionizing radiation, and can be performed in real-time and in a wide variety of locations, including the operating room, for example.

The CT or MRI DICOM image data is downloaded to an appropriate ultrasound system. The system employs some type of patient positioning device to enable correlation of the real-time ultrasound images to the DICOM images. Both are displayed during the procedure for greatest accuracy (Figure 3-7).

TISSUE HARMONIC IMAGING

Although the nonlinear response to an acoustic wave is strongest for microbubbles, biologic tissues also exhibit nonlinearity and thus harmonic frequency generation

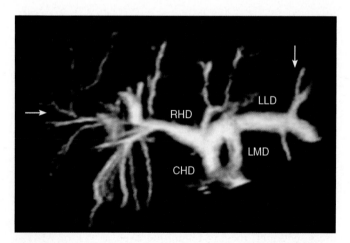

Figure 3-6. Three-dimensional volume rendering of biliary tree, or URCP, ultrasound-rendered cholangiopancreatography. (Used with permission from Zheng R, et al. Evaluating biliary anatomy and variations in living liver donors by a new technique: three-dimensional contrast-enhanced ultrasonic cholangiography. *Ultrasound Med Biol.* 2010 Aug:1282–1287.)

under the right conditions. In conventional ultrasonography, echoes of the same frequency spectrum as the incident beam are used to reconstruct the B-mode image. In harmonic imaging, a multiple of the incident frequency is used to reconstruct the image. For example, second harmonic imaging uses $2f_0$, subharmonic imaging uses $f_0/2$, and ultraharmonic imaging uses $1.5f_0$. This potentially offers some advantages including better lateral resolution with the higher frequencies, and less attenuation since the incident wave is of lower frequency. Additionally, artifacts from weak echoes such as scatter and side lobes reduce noise and improve contrast.

Numerous clinical applications to this technique have emerged, and most commercially available scanners offer harmonic imaging processing. THI or tissue harmonic imaging has been touted as responsible for improved border delineation in solid tumor imaging (Figure 3-8). Decreasing interference from surrounding structures, such as that found with the body wall in kidney imaging, may enable detection of more subtle pathology. Imaging in patients with body mass indices greater than 30, a technical challenge for transcutaneous imaging, may also be improved with THI.

CONTRAST-ENHANCED ULTRASOUND

The notion of contrast agents for ultrasound probably first began with the bubble studies used in echocardiography, where agitated saline was injected intravenously to assess for abnormal blood flow from the right to the left side of the heart (through a patent foramen ovale, for example). Today there are numerous commercially available agents, consisting of various manufactured gas-containing bubbles, as well as "smart" contrast agents whose shells have been manipulated for targeted imaging or therapies. The physics

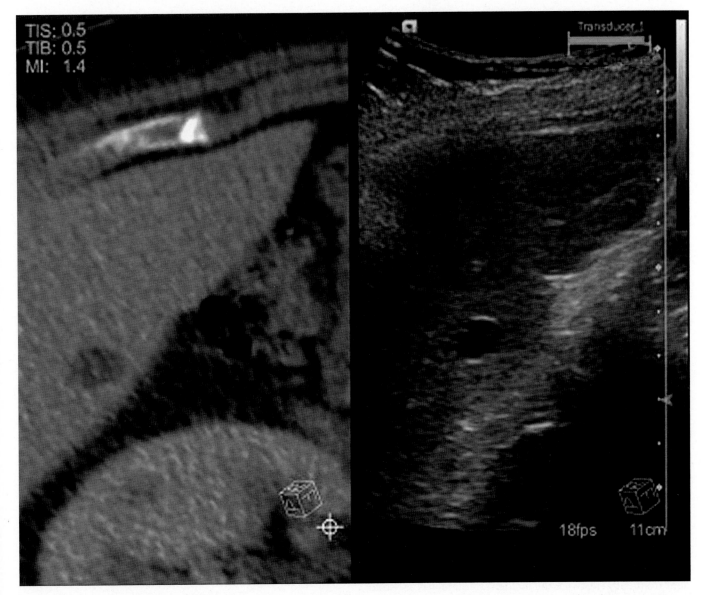

Figure 3-7. Fusion image with CT of liver, showing a hepatic cyst. (Used with permission from Stoll J. Ultrasound fusion imaging. *Perspect Med.* 2012 Sep;1(1–12):80–81.)

of contrast-enhanced imaging is based on the laws of cavitation, which describe the behavior of bubbles under the influence of acoustic energy.

Intuitively, the gas inside the bubble is a strong reflector, so any vessel containing a contrast agent will be strongly echogenic against a background of nonvascularized tissue. Furthermore, bubbles filled with gas will vibrate (shrink and expand) when subject to acoustic excitation. Because the capacity for expansion is greater than the capacity for shrinkage (because the bubble is stiffer when the radius is smaller), this oscillation is termed nonlinear.

Commercially available contrast agents are all composed of a synthetic shell around a gaseous core. The gas core is of course responsible for the enhanced echogenicity afforded by contrast agents, and may consist of air, or of high-molecular-weight gases such as perfluorocarbon or

nitrogen. A high-molecular-weight gas has less tendency to diffuse out of the shell in the circulation, thus permitting a more lasting contrast effect in the circulation. The selection of a shell material is influenced by a number of factors, including elasticity (a more flexible shell is more durable in the circulation and in an acoustic field, thus longer-lived), and whether or not the microbubble will be tagged with a ligand for specialized imaging or therapy. Some shell materials include albumin, lipids, polymers, or galactose.

Detection of microbubble contrast agents as well as distinction from surrounding tissues is augmented by the use of harmonic imaging. Although biological tissue will exhibit harmonics at high amplitudes, in general it behaves linearly in a diagnostic ultrasound application. In contrast, bubbles behave more nonlinearly and thus will preferentially enhance in harmonic imaging when compared to the tissue

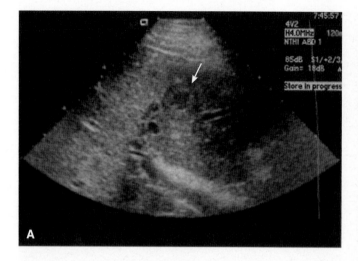

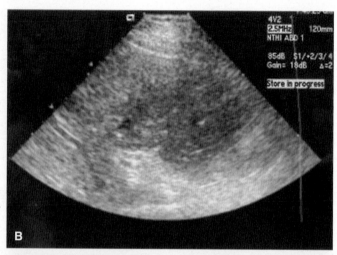

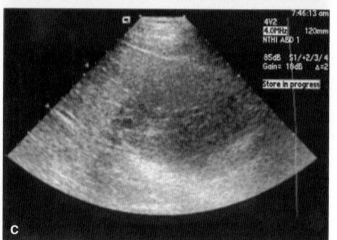

Figure 3-8. 39-year-old man with liver mass. (**A–C**) Sonograms of the same anatomic area in the liver using tissue harmonic imaging (A), 2.5 MHz (B), and 4.0 MHz (C) show that the mass (arrow) is detectable in A, but not in B or C. Images B and C were graded as nondiagnostic. (Used with permission from Shapiro RS, et al. Diagnostic value of tissue harmonic imaging compared with conventional sonography. *Comput Biol Med.* 2005 Oct;35(8):725–733.)

background. Frequency analysis of nonlinear oscillations yields harmonic frequencies that are multiples of the incident frequency (ie, twice the incident frequency is a second harmonic, half the incident frequency is a subharmonic). This property can be exploited for enhancing many imaging applications. An example is shown in Figure 3-9, which displays a dual image of conventional ultrasound on the left side of the figure, where a hyperechoic lesion is noted in the left hepatic lobe. The contrast-enhanced image is on the right, which demonstrates the lesion to be hypoechoic in the late phase, confirming the likelihood that this is a metastasis from this patient's colon carcinoma.

As alluded to above one of the more exciting concepts under development in many centers is the notion of targeted microbubbles. Basically a ligand is affixed to the microbubble shell, which in turn can bind to receptors expressed by specific cells, such as inflammatory cells, tumor cells, antibodies, or other proteins such as vascular endothelial growth factor (VEGF). Detection of bound microbubbles would then delineate the area where the cells of interest as determined by the ligands are, enhancing diagnosis and potentially directing therapies such as gene delivery or drug delivery. This concept ties in very closely to molecular imaging, discussed in detail below.

MOLECULAR IMAGING

Ultrasound imaging in the classic sense offers imaging at the anatomic level, where investigations and interventions are carried out on two- or three-dimensional pictures with a certain resolution. Although numerous efforts at image enhancement, many mentioned above, can improve resolution, ultrasound has finite capability on the order of millimeters. Ultrasound imaging at the molecular or cellular level, however, does not mean that we are magically expanding resolution down to the micron level. Rather, molecular imaging is a method of detecting or highlighting certain molecules, even if the individual molecules are not uniquely defined. The concept is not unique to ultrasound, being employed with nuclear radiology techniques, MRI, and others. Molecular imaging is a complement, not a replacement, to anatomic imaging.

Molecular imaging in ultrasound requires the technology of contrast enhancement. As described elsewhere in this chapter, microbubbles can be tagged with specific ligands that bind with receptors on the cell of interest. In Figure 3-10, for example, a contrast agent is labeled with a ligand for VCAM-1, which is highly expressed on inflamed

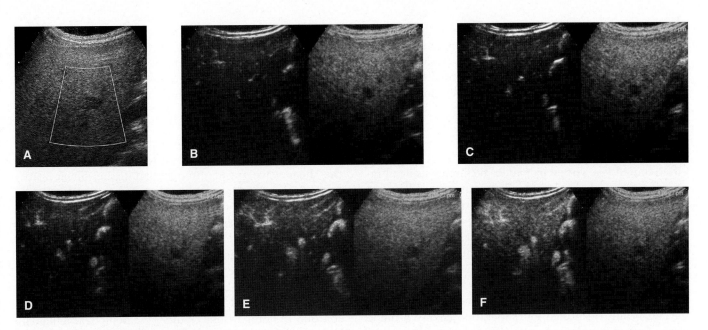

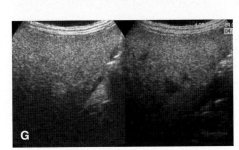

Figure 3-9. Conventional and contrast enhanced images of a lesion in the left lobe of the liver. (**A**) Conventional US scan of the right lobe shows marked steatosis of the liver and an uncharacteristic hypoechoic small focal liver lesion (1.2 cm in diameter). (**B–G**) Contrast-enhanced US with a bolus of 2.4 mL SonoVue demonstrates typical enhancement characteristics at split screen (left side: contrast-enhanced US scans; right side: conventional US information). (B) Very early arterial phase with detection of a centrally located artery only. (C and D) Early arterial phase with spoke-wheel sign. (E and F) Late arterial and portal venous phases with intense globular enhancement. (G) Late phase shows the FNH as slightly hyperechoic. (Used with permission from Rettenbacher T. Focal liver lesions: role of contrast-enhanced ultrasound. *Eur J Radiol.* 2007 Nov;64(2):173–182.)

endothelial cells, indicating atherosclerosis. The upper image shows the duplex image of the major arteries in a mouse model. The middle molecular image reveals significant uptake of the VCAM-1 agent, when compared to a control nontargeted agent in the lower image.

Although still investigational, molecular imaging using ultrasound conceivably has many advantages over other techniques. Ultrasound offers 1–2 mm spatial resolution, good temporal resolution, real-time imaging, no ionizing radiation, cost-effective, and portability. The requirement

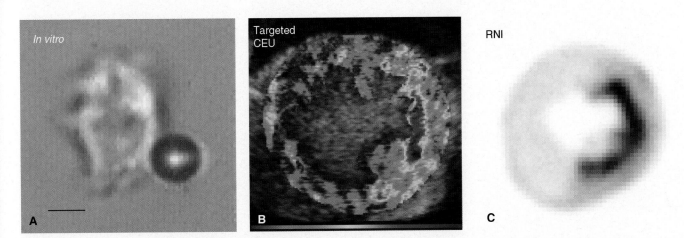

Figure 3-10. Molecular imaging. Imaging of post-ischemic myocardial inflammation with microbubbles targeted to leukocytes by virtue of their lipid shell constituents (phosphatidylserine). (**A**) Microbubble attachment to an activated neutrophil in vitro. (**B**) The contrast-enhanced ultrasound (CEU) image obtained 10 min after intravenous injection of leukocyte-targeted microbubbles in a canine model of ischemia and reperfusion of the left-circumflex coronary artery (scale bar at bottom). The region of CEU enhancement is similar to that obtained with (**C**) leukocyte-targeted radionuclide imaging (RNI). (Used with permission from Kaufman B, Lindner J. Molecular imaging with targeted contrast ultrasound. *Curr Opin Biotechnol.* 2007 Feb;18(1):11–16.)

for intravenous contrast enhancement has the advantage, and disadvantage, of localizing investigations to the intravascular space. In addition to the example provided above, molecular imaging has been proposed for detecting angiogenesis, cancer, stem cell proliferation and differentiation, among others.

SHEAR WAVE ELASTOGRAPHY

Often touted as a "virtual palpation" technique using ultrasound, shear wave elastography determines the stiffness of tissue in an attempt to further characterize tissues. Practitioners all know that a soft tissue lesion can feel "hard" or "soft," and although not a conclusive measure, this can provide a clue as to whether it is benign or malignant. Incident pressure is generated by a focused acoustic beam, which imparts a radiation force to the region of interest in the scan. The tissue's displacement is detected with ultrasound tracking beams, quantified, and superimposed on a B-mode image (either in color or grayscale), as a complement to the discovery and characterization of various lesions. This technique has been under study for about the past decade, and in the last few years several commercial scanners have included this feature. This technique has been applied to characterizing liver fibrosis, breast masses, thyroid masses, and prostate gland.

As stated above, elasticity is a measure of stiffness. It is the tissue displacement caused by the incident pressure pulse that is detected by the ultrasound beam, and this measurement combined with time-of-flight information results in a computation of shear wave velocity. The stiffness of tissue is quantified by the Young's modulus, E (kPa), which can be approximated by

$$E = 3\rho v^2,$$

where ρ is the density of the material and v is the shear wave velocity. In general, the stiffer the tissue, the greater the shear wave speed through that tissue. Shear waves travel perpendicular to the incident pressure pulse, unlike acoustic waves that travel along the axis of the ultrasound beam. In addition, shear waves attenuate much more rapidly than ultrasound waves (on the order of 10,000 times). An "elastogram" can be superimposed on or displayed alongside a B-mode image in real-time, and/or numeric measurements can be displayed, as seen in Figure 3-11, which shows a benign breast mass with a relatively "soft" contour. In comparison, Figure 3-12 depicts a malignant breast mass, and here it can be seen to be stiffer relative to the surrounding tissues, suspicious for malignancy and warranting biopsy.

Diagnosing and monitoring liver fibrosis in patients with chronic liver disease is crucial for prognosticating and tracking treatment effectiveness and progress. The gold standard has been histologic, with tissue being obtained by needle biopsy. This clearly presents obstacles including patient discomfort and potential for major complications.

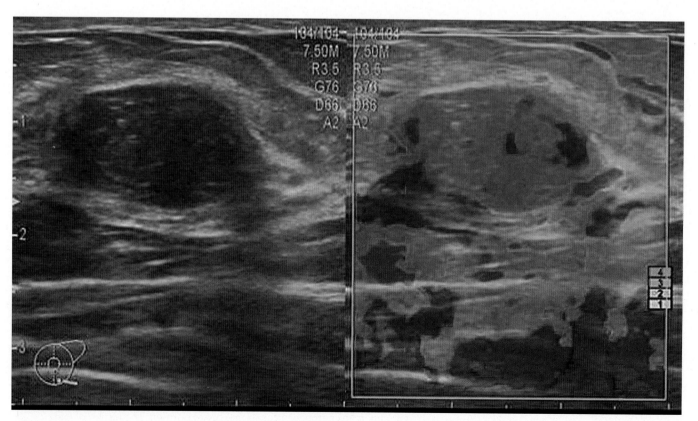

Figure 3-11. An elastography image of a benign breast mass with a relatively "soft" contour. (Used with permission from Hitachi-Aloka.)

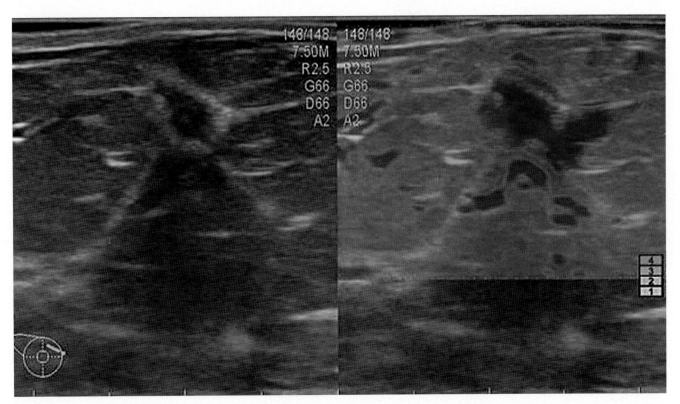

Figure 3-12. An elastography image of a malignant breast mass. Note that the mass is relatively stiffer than surrounding tissues. (Used with permission from Hitachi-Aloka.)

Ultrasound elastography or "fibroscanning" is widely used in Europe for the noninvasive determination of hepatic fibrosis. Although no linear correlation between shear wave velocity and degree of fibrosis has been confirmed, studies have shown the value of elastography in separating patients with little to no fibrosis from those with advanced fibrosis or cirrhosis. The range of values of elastic modulus in the liver extends from 1 to 20 kPa, which is much smaller than that seen in other tissues (breast, for example). In addition, certain confounding factors can hinder an accurate scan, including livers with macronodular cirrhosis, extrahepatic cholestasis, and ascites. Because ultrasound elastography is easily performed with no risk to the patient, it has emerged as a useful clinical tool in the monitoring of hepatic fibrosis, minimizing the need for baseline or repeat needle biopsy.

Perhaps the most clinical experience with elastography is in the breast. A recent study of over 1,800 lesions has demonstrated the value of elastography as an adjunct in the management of breast masses. This study, sponsored by Supersonic Imagine, a manufacturer of an ultrasound elastography platform, sought to insure the reproducibility of shear wave elastography images, and to verify the increased value of its use. Reproducibility is inherent, given the fact that the shear wave is generated by regulated pulses of ultrasound (as opposed to mechanical deformation). In addition, the study confirmed an improvement in lesion characterization for BIRADS 3 and 4 lesions, where specificity of ultrasound diagnosis increased by 28% with no loss in sensitivity, and the PPV for biopsy of the BI-RADS

4a class increased by 155%. These results confirmed numerous other smaller studies that had been reported in advance of this one, suggesting the value of elastography in the management of breast disease.

Early data shows the promise of elastography in the imaging of the thyroid and parathyroid and in the management of diseases of these structures. Along with physical examination, ultrasound has become an essential component of the diagnosis and management of diseases of the thyroid and parathyroid. Ultrasound provides valuable information in the decision for intervention, and certain sonographic features are used to help differentiate malignant versus benign tumors. Hypoechogenicity, microcalcifications, irregular margins, and intranodular vascularity, though not diagnostic in and of themselves, raise suspicion for malignancy. Analogous to its utility in breast disease, elastography thus has shown some preliminary promise in providing yet another criterion for characterizing and following thyroid nodules, although at this writing more studies are needed.

One of the challenges of prostate care is the relative heterogeneity of the organ and its propensity to harbor small, indolent, multifocal malignancy. Clinicians and investigators are looking to elastography as a guide to the often nebulous imaging examination of the prostate. Figure 3-13 shows that although the prostate appeared relatively homogeneous on conventional B-mode imaging, the addition of elastography targets biopsies to the regions of firmer tissue, color-coded in blue.

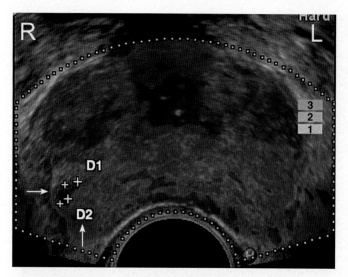

Figure 3-13. Elastogram of the midgland of the prostate. Two areas (arrows) of stiff tissue suspected to be cancerous tissue are visualized in dark blue color in the peripheral zone on the right side of the prostate. (Used with permission from Salomon G, et al. Evaluation of prostate cancer detection with ultrasound real-time elastography: a comparison with step section pathological analysis after radical prostatectomy. *Eur Urol.* 2008 Dec;54(6):1354–1362.)

HISTOSCANNING

Devised initially to address the unique challenges of prostate care already mentioned, histoscanning combines ultrasound imaging with algorithms for tissue characterization in an attempt to identify and localize suspicious lesions. Various sonographically detectable features such as boundary, shape, perfusion, and stiffness are exploited and combined to differentiate tissue across the span of the scan area, which is then color-coded on the final image to guide diagnosis and intervention. Developed by a privately held company, the technology has undergone verification with pathologic specimens in numerous European centers over the past decade, as well as comparison with dynamic contrast-enhanced MRI. A sensitivity of 90% and specificity of 72% when compared with tissue have been reported. Ultimately if widely accepted histoscanning may have the potential to improve biopsy yield and reduce the positive surgical margin rate.

PHOTOACOUSTIC IMAGING

When a medium is subject to externally applied energy that generates heat from absorption, the resulting thermal energy leads to thermoelastic expansion and thus ultrasonic emission. These acoustic emissions can then be sensed by an ultrasonic transducer and used to create two-dimensional or three-dimensional images. When the applied energy is an optical laser, it is called photoacoustic imaging; when RF energy is used, it is called thermoacoustic imaging. Optical energy does not penetrate deeply into tissues, so this modality has the greatest utility in superficial structures, such as skin and peripheral vessels. For example, skin lesions such as suspected melanomas can be characterized and risk-stratified with the assistance of photoacoustic imaging.

SUGGESTED READINGS

Kollman C. New sonographic techniques for harmonic imaging – underlying physical principles. *Eur J Radiol.* 2007;64: 164–172.

McCulloch M, Gresser C, Moos S, Odabashian J, Jasper S, Bednarz J, Burgess P, Carney D, Moore V, Sisk E, Waggoner A, Witt S, Adams S. Ultrasound contrast physics: a series on contrast echocardiography, article 3. *J Am Soc Echocardiogr.* 13:959–967.

Prager RW, Ijaz UZ, Gee AH, Treece GM. Three-dimensional ultrasound imaging. *Proc Inst Mech Eng H.* 2010;224(2): 193–223.

Sebag F, Vaillant-Lombard J, Berbis J, Griset V, Henry F, Petit P, Oliver C. Shear wave elastography: a new ultrasound imaging mode for the differential diagnosis of benign and malignant thyroid nodules. *J Clin Endocrinol Metab.* 2010 December; 95(12):5281–5288.

Simmons L, Autier P, Zat'ura F, Braeckman J, Peltier A, Stenzl A, Treurnicht K, Walker T, Nir D, Moore C, Emberton M. Detection, localization and characterization of prostate cancer by Prostate HistoScanning. E-published ahead of printing in *Br J Urol Int* (BJUI). 2011 May.

4

ULTRASOUND OF THE NECK: THYROID AND PARATHYROID

STEPHANIE L. GOFF & JAMES A. LEE

The evaluation of the patient with thyroid and/or parathyroid pathology is increasingly multimodal and includes history and physical examination, laboratory evaluation, and adjunctive radiologic studies. In particular, ultrasound has become an extension of the physical examination for patients with endocrine diseases of the neck and is often the first step in a radiologic evaluation of neck pathology. In fact, ultrasound is so ubiquitous that it is now commonly performed in the outpatient office setting and can provide immediate information that expedites diagnosis and treatment. Even when a patient presents for consultation with reports from prior ultrasound studies, a real-time sonography can confirm findings in addition to providing an opportunity for immediate image-guided biopsy. Ultrasound of the neck has become such a critical tool for the surgeon that the American College of Surgeons has determined that every surgical practice should include a "working knowledge of ultrasound of the head and neck." Surgeons are typically asked to see a subset of patients with neck pathology. As such, this chapter will address primarily ultrasound for thyroid nodules/multinodular goiter, parathyroid disease, and pathologic lymphadenopathy.

CLINICAL INDICATIONS FOR ULTRASOUND

Indications for neck ultrasonography by the surgeon include:

- Thyroid
  - To delineate the presence, absence, size, and echo-characteristics of thyroid nodules/pathology
  - To differentiate between solid and cystic lesions
  - To delineate ultrasound characteristics that raise the risk of thyroid cancer in thyroid nodules (irregular borders, microcalcifications, hypoechogenicity, hypervascularity)
  - To detect concomitant pathology (lymph node disease, parathyroid disease, etc)
  - To identify the presence or absence of a substernal component, superior extension, or tracheal deviation from a goiter
  - To follow the progression, regression, or stability of thyroid disease
  - To identify characteristic findings of thyroid disease (ie, Hashimoto thyroiditis)
  - To assist in post-thyroidectomy surveillance for thyroid cancer recurrence (ie, thyroid remnant, lymph node recurrence)
  - To plan the location of the incision for surgery
- Parathyroid
  - To identify and localize parathyroid adenoma(s) or hyperplasia
  - To detect concomitant pathology (lymph node disease, thyroid disease, etc)
  - To plan the location of the incision for surgery
- Lymph nodes
  - To delineate the presence or absence of pathologic/benign lymph nodes as well as their precise locations
  - To detect concomitant pathology (thyroid disease, parathyroid disease, etc)
  - To plan the location of the incision for surgery
- Interventions
  - To assist in fine needle biopsy of thyroid nodules, parathyroid glands, and/or lymph nodes
  - To assist in core needle biopsy of thyroid nodules/lymph nodes
  - To guide percutaneous treatments such as radiofrequency ablation, ethanol ablation, etc.

NORMAL ANATOMY

The vast number of structures in the neck can make mastery of neck ultrasound seem a daunting task, but the heterogeneity of those structures makes interpretation easier to learn. The superficial location of the soft tissue components of the anterior neck, as well as today's high-frequency probes, allows physicians to study and delineate the anatomy of the neck clearly and with confidence.

The neck is divided into the lateral and central neck compartments. The central neck comprises the structures anterior to the paraspinous muscles and between the two carotid sheaths, whereas the lateral neck compartments comprise the structures anterior to the paraspinous and scalene muscles and lateral to the medial border of the carotid sheath (Figure 4-1).

▶ Central Neck Compartment

The major components of the central neck include the thyroid, trachea, esophagus, parathyroid glands, and central neck lymph nodes. The thyroid gland lies posterior to the strap muscles (sternohyoid, omohyoid, and sternothyroid), and each lobe is bordered medially by the trachea. The isthmus lies immediately anterior to the trachea approximately a fingerbreadth or two below the cricoid cartilage. Immediately lateral to the thyroid lobes are the carotid sheaths. The longus colli muscle and parathyroid glands lie posterior to the thyroid. The esophagus lies posterior to the left thyroid lobe.

While the parathyroid glands typically lie immediately posterior to the thyroid gland, up to 13% to 20% may be in ectopic locations. The superior parathyroid is normally located on the posteromedial aspect of the thyroid

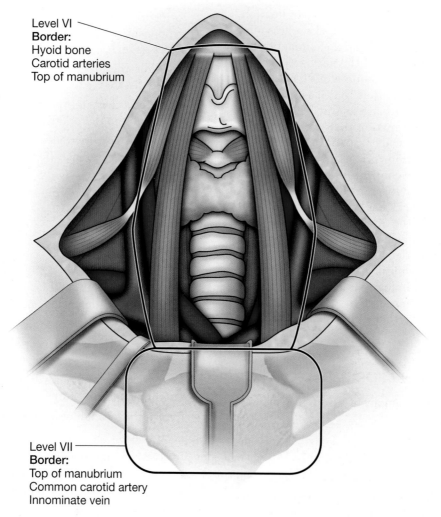

Level VI
Border:
Hyoid bone
Carotid arteries
Top of manubrium

Level VII
Border:
Top of manubrium
Common carotid artery
Innominate vein

Figure 4-1. Schematic of intraoperative anatomy depicting the central neck lymph node compartments. The lateral neck compartments extend from the medial border of the carotid sheath. (Reprinted from Pai S. Central compartment lymph node dissection. *Operative Technique in Otolaryngology – Head and Neck Surgery.* 2009;20:39–43, with permission from Elsevier.)

gland near the tracheoesophageal groove, cephalad to the intersection of the recurrent laryngeal nerve and inferior thyroid artery. The most common ectopic location for an upper parathyroid gland is low in the tracheoesophageal groove, but less common locations include the mediastinum, intrathyroidal position, and high in the neck in the undescended position. Due to the embryonic development and descent, the inferior gland has more variability, but it usually lies on the posterolateral aspect of the inferior pole of the thyroid lobe. The most common ectopic location is in the thyrothymic ligament, but the inferior gland may also be found in the carotid sheath, mediastinum, intrathyroidal position, and high in the neck in the undescended position.

The level VI and VII or central neck lymph nodes include the prelaryngeal (lying anterior to the trachea and between the superior border of the isthmus and hyoid bone, often called the Delphian lymph nodes), pretracheal nodes (lying anterior to the trachea between the innominate artery and the lower border of the isthmus of the thyroid), and juxtathyroid nodes (between the trachea and the medial border of the carotid sheath).

▶ Lateral Neck Compartment

The lymph nodes of the lateral neck are divided into five levels. The mandible, hyoid bone, and posterior belly of the digastric muscle define Level I. Levels II, III, and IV are defined by the lateral margin of the sternohyoid muscle and the posterior border of the sternocleidomastoid muscle, and surround the carotid sheath structures. These three so-called jugular levels are subdivided cranially to caudally by the horizontal plane of the hyoid bone and the inferior edge of the cricoid cartilage. The upper jugular or jugulodigastric nodes are Level II, with midjugular nodes in Level III and lower jugular nodes in Level IV. The posterior triangle of the neck, bordered by the sternocleidomastoid and the trapezius, is level V.

NORMAL APPEARANCE OF ULTRASOUND

A normal thyroid lobe has a homogenous "ground glass" appearance that is slightly hyperechoic and can be identified on transverse scanning by its position between the relatively hypoechoic trachea and carotid artery. Since it is air-filled, the trachea does not transmit acoustic energy; thus, there is a characteristic black void posterior to the anterior border of the trachea and this posterior shadowing artifact may cause difficulty in visualizing posterior and medial structures. In real-time sonography, the carotid artery may be identified by its pulsatile nature, whereas the internal jugular vein can be identified by its compressibility as well as its dilation with a vigorous Valsalva maneuver. The parathyroid glands are not typically identified on ultrasound scanning unless they are enlarged. The esophagus may be seen abutting the posterior border of the left lobe of the thyroid depending on the degree of shadowing from

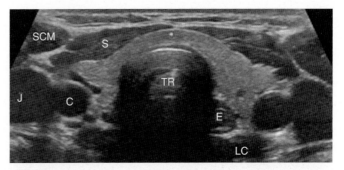

Figure 4-2. Normal ultrasonographic appearance of thyroid. Surrounding structures: (J) internal jugular vein, (C) carotid artery, (SCM) sternocleidomastoid muscle, (S) strap muscles, (TR) trachea, (E) esophagus, (LC) longus colli muscle. (Reprinted from Sholosh B, Borhani A. Thyroid ultrasound. Part I: technique and diffuse disease. *Radio Clin Am*. 2011;49(3): 391–416 with permission from Elsevier.)

the trachea. The esophagus typically has a bulls-eye appearance and with real-time sonography one may see a bright flash as the mucosa apposes with swallowing (Figure 4-2). Normal lymph nodes of the neck are usually too small to be with ultrasound, but benign enlargement may be detected. Enlarged, benign lymph nodes typically have a fatty hilum (seen as a small area of white enhancement in one side), uniform echotexture, and a morphology in which they are wider than they are tall.

In transverse scanning, the width and depth of the thyroid lobes can be measured, while length can be measured in the longitudinal view. A normal thyroid lobe is approximately 2 cm in width and depth, and 4.5 to 5.5 cm in length. A measurement of width in the transverse view should be taken from an imaginary vertical line at the edge of the trachea to the most lateral point of the thyroid at its largest dimension. Within the same image, depth is measured perpendicularly at the maximal anterior-posterior distance in the middle third of the lobe. In the longitudinal view, the length is measured between the maximal cranial to caudal dimension (Figure 4-3A,B). The volume (in mL) is derived from the geometry of a prolate ellipsoid and is calculated by $\pi/6$ ($W \times D \times L$) in cm. The total volume is the sum of the two lobes, barring the presence of an enlarged isthmus. Asymmetry of the lobes is a normal variant, and if asymmetry is present, the left lobe is usually smaller. Hemiagenesis, a benign variant of normal, has an incidence of 1:2500 and 95% of cases describe a "missing" left lobe.

SCANNING TECHNIQUE FOR OBTAINING THESE IMAGES

For uniformity of measurement and appearance, a routine sequence of real-time scanning should be adopted. The patient should be in a supine or recumbent position, with the neck slightly extended. Extension can be assisted with a small roll or pillow behind the shoulders.

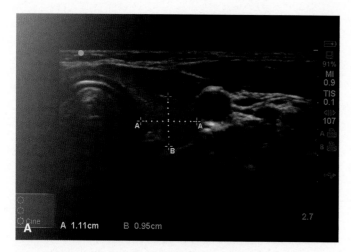
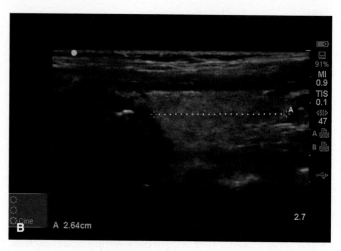

Figure 4-3. Normal ultrasonographic appearance of thyroid with measuring technique applied. (**A**) Transverse; (**B**) longitudinal.

A thorough ultrasound examination of the neck includes systematic examination of the central and lateral neck compartments in both transverse and longitudinal planes.

Selection of transducer shape, size, and frequency is based on the patient's body habitus and the indication for sonography. A linear transducer provides an image without the spatial distortion seen in the curved transducers, but images and measurements are limited by the size of the probe. For the majority of neck ultrasonography, a linear transducer probe with a 3.5 to 5 cm footprint is adequate. A smaller curvilinear probe can be helpful for evaluating structures in the lower neck, at the level of the manubrium and clavicles. Higher-frequency probes provide clear images of superficial structures, but penetration is shallower. A useful probe is a variable-frequency probe ranging from 7.5 to 14 MHz, primarily utilizing the higher frequency settings. For obese patients or to examine deeper neck structures, it may be necessary to use the lower settings.

A typical routine for a thorough examination of the neck progresses as follows.

The neck is palpated to identify the thyroid and cricoid cartilage of the trachea. The probe is then held transversely in the center of the neck between the thyroid and cricoid cartilage. Throughout the preliminary examination, an effort should be made to keep the probe perpendicular to the skin and perpendicular or parallel to the trachea to insure consistent measurements. The probe is drawn inferiorly until the isthmus of the thyroid is identified. The isthmus is assessed for nodules and size. The probe is then placed over the superior extent of the right central neck and drawn inferiorly to scan the right thyroid lobe. The thyroid lobe lies directly between the carotid artery and the trachea. The lobe is assessed in its entirety for size, echotexture, and thyroid nodules. Concomitant lymphadenopathy and/or parathyroid disease may be identified at the same time. The size of the thyroid lobe is measured as previously described. At this point, the probe is placed longitudinally and the carotid artery is identified. The probe is drawn medially and the thyroid lobe is assessed in its entirety for size, echotexture, and thyroid nodules. Concomitant lymphadenopathy and/or parathyroid disease may be identified at the same time. The length of the thyroid lobe is measured as previously described. The same process is repeated in the left central neck compartment with the additional identification of the esophagus as described. At this point, the probe is placed over the superior extent of the right lateral neck compartment (ie, level II). The carotid artery and internal jugular vein are identified. The probe is drawn inferiorly toward the clavicles scanning for lymphadenopathy and other pathology. The probe is then turned longitudinally over the carotid sheath and drawn laterally to identify any lymphadenopathy or pathology. This process is repeated in the left lateral neck compartment.

▶ Sample Report

I performed an ultrasound of the neck in the office using a 12-MHz grayscale ultrasound. The right lobe of the thyroid measured 5 × 2.5 × 4 cm and the left lobe of the thyroid measured 5.2 × 3 × 3 cm. The isthmus measured 0.3 cm. There was a nodule in the right upper-pole of the thyroid that measured 1.5 × 1 × 1 cm (hypoechoic, regular, no increased vascularity, and no calcifications). There was no evidence of enlarged parathyroid glands. There was no evidence of pathologic adenopathy in the central or lateral neck bilaterally.

COMMON FINDINGS/ABNORMALITIES

▶ Thyroid Nodules

It is estimated that 15% to 30% of the US population will have a sonographically visible thyroid nodule. The sonographic appearance of a thyroid nodule, in conjunction with size criteria and clinical history, can help identify nodules that should be biopsied. Suspicious characteristics, as defined by the American Thyroid Association, include presence of microcalcifications, hypoechogenicity, increased vascularity, irregular margins, and appearing taller than wide on transverse view. Associated sensitivities and specificities for malignancy are listed in Table 4-1.

Echogenicity refers to the appearance of the nodule against the background of normal thyroid tissue. Normal thyroid parenchyma is typically slightly hyperechoic and bright when compared to the overlying strap muscles. Nodules are then classified as hypo- (Figures 4-4A and 4-5A), iso-, or hyperechoic (Figure 4-4B) in comparison to normal thyroid tissue. Hypoechoic nodules are more frequently associated with malignancy. In contrast, purely cystic nodules (Figure 4-4C) are anechoic, with

TABLE 4-1

Sonographic Characteristics of Thyroid Nodules: Sensitivity and Specificity for Malignancy

	Median Sensitivity (Range)	Median Specificity (Range)
Microcalcifications	50% (26–73)	85% (69–96)
Irregular margins	55% (17–77)	76% (63–85)
Hypoechoic	80% (49–90)	53% (36–66)
Increased vascularity	67% (57–74)	81% (49–89)

Source: Data from Baskin.

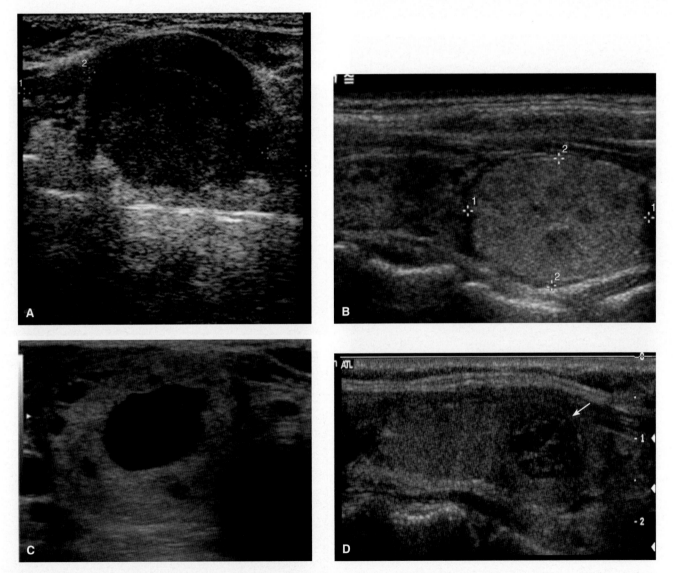

Figure 4-4. Initial descriptions of thyroid nodules remark on comparisons to surrounding adjacent thyroid tissue. (**A**) hypoechoic nodule; (**B**) hyperechoic nodule with size markings; (**C**) cystic nodule; and (**D**) mixed solid-cystic nodule indicated by arrow. (Reprinted from: (A) Kangelaris G, et al. Role of ultrasound in thyroid disorders. *Otolaryngol Clin North Am.* 2012 April;7(2):197–210. (B) Jung A, Grant E. Ultrasound interventions in the neck with emphasis on postthyroidectomy papillary carcinoma. *Ultrasound Clin.* 2009 Jan;4(1):1–16. (C) Rago T, Vitti P. Role of thyroid ultrasound in the diagnostic evaluation of thyroid nodules. *Best Pract Res Clin Endocrinol Metab.* 2008 Dec;22(6):913–928. (D) Jin J, McHenry C. Thyroid iIncidentaloma. *Best Pract Res Clin Endocrinol Metab.* 2012 Feb;26(1):83–96 with permission from Elsevier.)

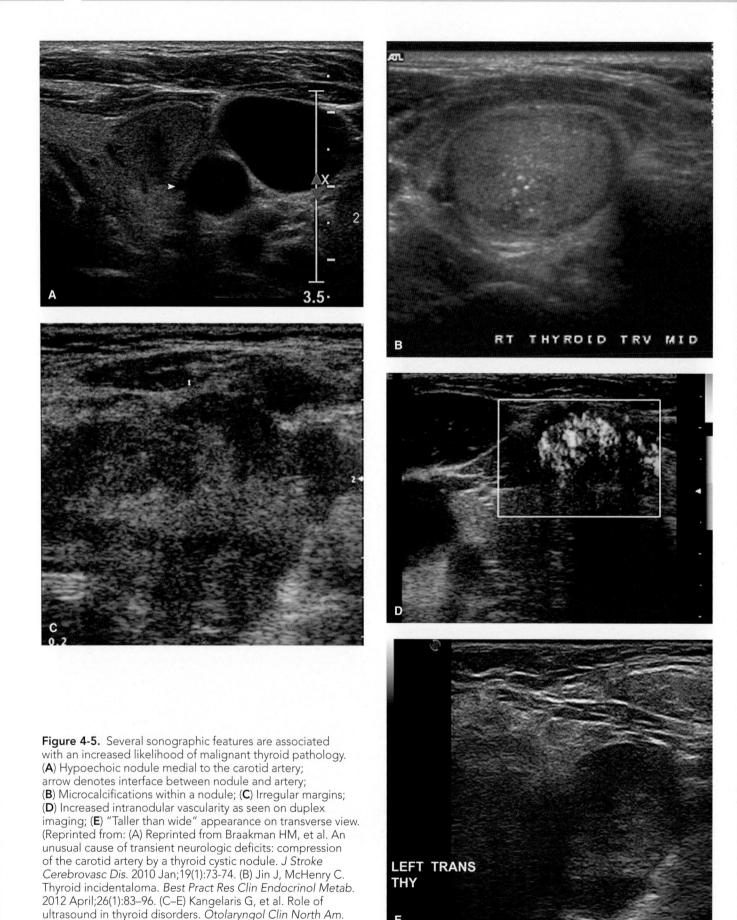

Figure 4-5. Several sonographic features are associated with an increased likelihood of malignant thyroid pathology. (**A**) Hypoechoic nodule medial to the carotid artery; arrow denotes interface between nodule and artery; (**B**) Microcalcifications within a nodule; (**C**) Irregular margins; (**D**) Increased intranodular vascularity as seen on duplex imaging; (**E**) "Taller than wide" appearance on transverse view. (Reprinted from: (A) Reprinted from Braakman HM, et al. An unusual cause of transient neurologic deficits: compression of the carotid artery by a thyroid cystic nodule. *J Stroke Cerebrovasc Dis.* 2010 Jan;19(1):73-74. (B) Jin J, McHenry C. Thyroid incidentaloma. *Best Pract Res Clin Endocrinol Metab.* 2012 April;26(1):83–96. (C–E) Kangelaris G, et al. Role of ultrasound in thyroid disorders. *Otolaryngol Clin North Am.* 2012 April;7(2):197–210 with permission from Elsevier.)

posterior acoustic enhancement, and are more often benign. Mixed solid-cystic nodules (Figure 4-4D) should be defined by the echogenicity of the solid component.

In addition to the echotexture of a nodule, there are a number of findings that may raise the suspicion for malignancy. Calcifications can be present within or surrounding thyroid nodules. Coarse calcifications are usually greater than 2 mm in size and demonstrate posterior acoustic shadowing, whereas microcalcifications are smaller (<1 mm) echogenic foci (Figure 4-5B). Peripheral or "egg-shell" calcifications can be associated with benign or malignant disease, although an area of interruption in a rim calcification is worrisome for invasive malignancy. Assessment of the margins of a thyroid nodule is prone to interobserver variability, hindering the sensitivity of this finding. Most benign nodules have a regular geometric shape (often ellipsoid) and a clearly defined border, whereas the border of malignant nodules may be blurred or have a microlobulated appearance (Figure 4-5C). The vascularity of a nodule can be assessed with the use of real-time color flow Doppler and can be classified as absent (type I), perinodular (type II), or peri- and intranodular (type III). There is an association between intranodular vascularity (Figure 4-5D) and malignant cytology. When assessing a thyroid nodule in the transverse view, a comparison can be made of its dimensions (Figure 4-5E). Although a two-dimensional image cannot fully describe the geometry of a nodule, an increased association with malignancy has been found when a depth to width ratio is greater than 1, ie, "taller than wide." Capelli et al. found this characteristic to be highly sensitive (84%) and specific (82%) for detection of malignancy. A benefit of real-time sonography, rather than office-based review of static imaging, is the ability to fully assess suspicious lesions in three dimensions using transverse and longitudinal views by simply turning the probe in real time.

▶ Parathyroid Adenoma

An ultrasound evaluation for parathyroid pathology should only be performed after a biochemical diagnosis has been made. This strategy helps to reduce the likelihood of false positive findings. Normal parathyroids are usually not visualized with ultrasonography, but the classic parathyroid adenoma is tear-drop shaped along the longitudinal axis and is hypoechoic (Figure 4-6). In contrast to an enlarged lymph node, there should not be a fatty hilum, although the vascular pedicle may be visualized with Doppler. Depending on the expertise of the sonographer, the reported sensitivity of ultrasound for localizing parathyroid adenomas is between 60% to 90%. Certain maneuvers such as repositioning the neck and applying gentle pressure to the central neck may help to identify ectopically located parathyroids. Due to the difficulty in assessing the parathyroid glands with ultrasonography, the neck is often imaged with a variety of modalities, both anatomic and functional, in an attempt to better localize an abnormality. Parathyroid carcinoma is exceedingly rare, but a very large parathyroid

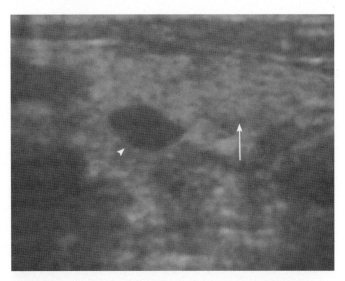

Figure 4-6. A hypoechoic parathyroid adenoma (arrowhead) indenting the capsule of the adjacent thyroid (arrow). (Reprinted from Palestro CJ. Radionuclide imaging of the parathyroid glands. *Semin Nucl Med.* 2005;35:266–276 with permission from Elsevier.)

with evidence of invasion into surrounding structures or irregular borders should raise the suspicion of parathyroid cancer given the proper clinical scenario. In rare cases in which it is not clear from the ultrasound whether a lesion is a parathyroid adenoma or another type of lesion (ie, thyroid nodule or lymph node), fine-needle aspiration biopsy with the measurement of parathyroid hormone levels of the washout of one biopsy may be performed.

▶ Lymphadenopathy

Similar to the evaluation of thyroid nodules, there are specific sonographic criteria that are associated with the presence of malignancy in cervical lymph nodes (Table 4-2). These findings include a cystic appearance, hyperechoic punctuations, peripheral vascularity, loss of a fatty hilum, and a width to depth ratio greater than 1 (ie, "taller than wide" morphology) (Figure 4-7). The presence of suspicious adenopathy should prompt fine-needle biopsy to determine if cancer is present.

TABLE 4-2

Sonographic Characteristics of Lymph Nodes: Sensitivity and Specificity for Malignancy

	Sensitivity (95% CI)	Specificity (95% CI)
Short axis >5 mm	61% (41–78)	96% (82–100)
Cystic appearance	11% (2–28)	100% (88–100)
Hyperechogenic punctuations	46% (28–60)	100% (88–100)
Peripheral vascularity	86% (67–96)	82% (63–94)
Absence of hilum	100% (88–100)	29% (13–49)

Source: Data from Leboulleux et al.

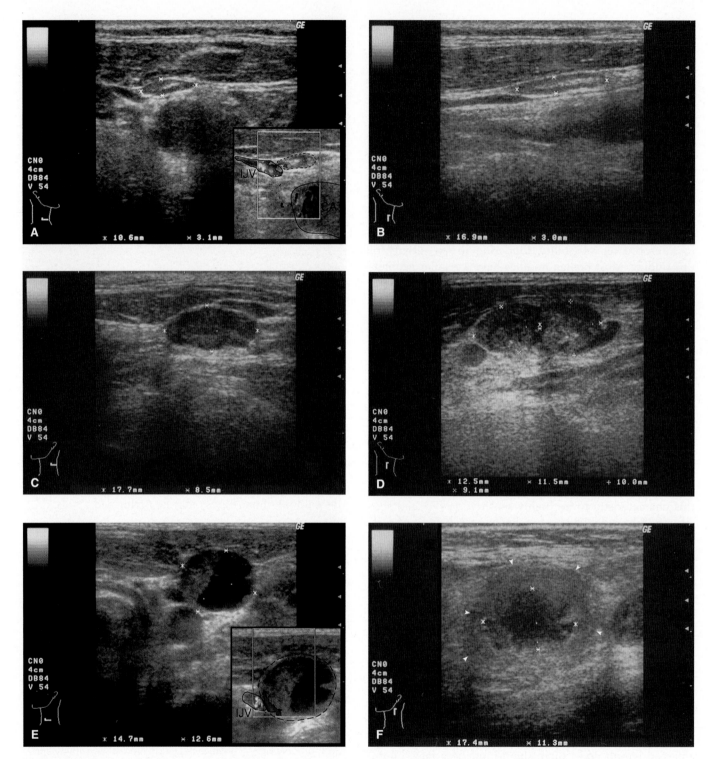

Figure 4-7. Sonographic findings in cervical lymph nodes. (**A**) transverse and (**B**) longitudinal normal lymph node with smooth border, oval shape, echogenic hilum (inset) duplex mode with hilar vascular pattern. Surrounding structures: (IJV) internal jugular vein, (CA) carotid artery; (**C**) loss of echogenic hilum; (**D**) matted nodes with loss hyperechogenic punctuations; (**E**) cystic degeneration and peripheral vascularity demonstrated in duplex mode; and (**F**) cystic degeneration. (Reprinted from Röper B. Tissue characterization of locoregionally advanced head-and-neck squamous cell carcinoma (HNSCC) using quantified ultrasonography. *Radiother Oncol.* 2007;85:48–57 with permission from Elsevier.)

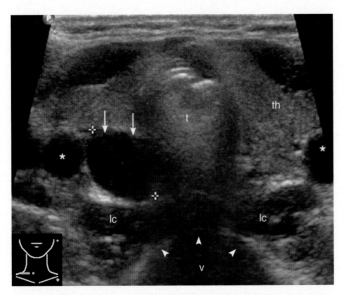

Figure 4-8. A paratracheal lymph node (arrows and calipers) can masquerade as a parathyroid adenoma. Surrounding structures: (th) thyroid, (t), trachea, (v & arrowheads) vertebral body, (lc) longus colli, (*) carotid artery. (Reprinted from Rhys R. Cervical lymph nodes. In: *Clinical Ultrasound*. 3rd ed. Vol. 2. 2011:920–937 with permission from Elsevier.)

COMMON PITFALLS

- Hold the probe either parallel or perpendicular to the trachea to insure consistent measurements.
- Parathyroid adenomas and enlarged lymph nodes may have a very similar appearance and location. FNAB with parathyroid hormone washout and assay may help to differentiate the two (Figure 4-8).
- Autoimmune thyroiditis (a.k.a. Hashimoto thyroiditis) causes a heterogeneous echotexture to the thyroid and can cause pseudonodules.

CLINICAL PEARLS/TIPS

- Always perform the examination in the same sequence.
- When looking for parathyroid adenomas, look for the bright white line that designates the interface between the posterior capsule of the thyroid and surrounding structures. This line will help differentiate between thyroid nodule and parathyroid adenoma.
- Ultrasound can detect concomitant pathology that is present in about 20% to 40% of cases and help guide the extent of surgery.
- If using different gauge needles for FNAB, work from smaller gauge to larger to minimize trauma to the nodule.

THERAPEUTIC MANEUVERS – ULTRASOUND-GUIDED PROCEDURES

Ultrasound can be used to increase the safety and diagnostic accuracy of percutaneous procedures, the most important of which is fine-needle aspiration biopsy (FNAB).

Ultrasound-guided FNAB allows the operator to avoid vascular injuries by clearly identifying the carotid artery and internal jugular vein and to precisely place the needle in the desired structure. Ultrasound-guided FNAB can be performed in one of two ways: either in-plane (parallel) or out-of-plane (perpendicular) to the object being biopsied. The majority of experienced operators prefer performing the biopsy in-plane because it allows them to follow the course of the entire needle into the object. However, with either approach, the procedure should only be attempted when the clinician and ancillary staff are trained in the preparation and handling of the specimens to the specifications of the receiving cytopathology facility. Since thyroid nodules are so common, many organizations have detailed criterion for which lesions should be biopsied. The American Thyroid Association guidelines for biopsy are the most commonly referenced and are detailed in Table 4-3.

Prior to performing an ultrasound-guided FNAB, the patient should be asked specifically about a history of bleeding or any medications that might increase the risk prior to obtaining informed consent for the biopsy. Similar to the diagnostic ultrasound, the patient should be positioned supine with the neck slightly extended by a small roll beneath the patient's shoulders. The ideal setup is to have the operator, lesion, and ultrasound machine screen in-line in order to provide the clinician with the most ergonomic approach. Local anesthetic may or may not be instilled at the discretion of the physician. Cytologic preparation materials generally include multiple glass slides, cytofixative solution, a 10-cc slip tip syringe (preferably with an eccentric tip), and a variety of standard small-gauge needles (23–27 gauge). Prior to inserting the needle, the operator may get a sense as to the trajectory the needle must take by pushing on the skin where the needle is to be inserted.

The in-plane approach entails scanning the neck with the probe in transverse position. When the lesion of interest is targeted, the clinician engages the needle at the midline of the narrow axis of the probe, thus enabling real-time observation of the track of the needle as it traverses the tissue to engage the target lesion (Figure 4-9). The in-plane method is highly recommended as it allows greater visualization of the lesion and the needle.

In the out-of-plane technique the probe is applied in the longitudinal position, scanning medially and laterally until identifying the target lesion. The clinician then engages the lesion by insertion of the needle at the midpoint of the long axis of the probe. The needle is only seen in the ultrasound display when the tip engages the tissue of interest. The majority of the needle is not under direct visualization, and therefore this technique should be used with caution.

Gentle aspiration should draw a column of cells into the needle while engaged in the tissue, which should then be dispersed onto the glass slide. The syringe should be removed from the needle, drawn back, reconnected to the needle, and dispersed again on to the slide.

TABLE 4-3		
ATA Guidelines for FNA of Thyroid Nodules		
Sonographic and Clinical Features	**Threshold Size for Biopsy**	**Strength of Recommendation***
High risk history		
Suspicious sonographic features	>5 mm	A
Without suspicious sonographic features	>5 mm	I
Abnormal cervical lymph nodes	All	A
Microcalcifications	≥1 cm	A
Solid nodule		
Hypoechoic	>1 cm	B
Iso- or hyperechoic	≥1–1.5 cm	C
Mixed cystic-solid nodule		
Any suspicious ultrasound features	≥1.5–2.0 cm	B
Without suspicious ultrasound feature	≥2.0 cm	C
Spongiform	≥2.0 cm	C
Purely cystic nodule	Not indicated	

*A: Strongly recommends. Evidence includes consistent results from well-designed, well-conducted studies demonstrating direct improvement in outcomes; B: Recommends. Evidence is sufficient to determine effects on health outcomes, but the strength of the evidence is limited by the number, quality, or consistency of the individual studies; C: Recommends. The recommendation is based on expert opinion; I: Recommends neither for nor against. The panel concludes that the evidence is insufficient to recommend for or against.

Source: Adapted from US Preventative Services Task Force.

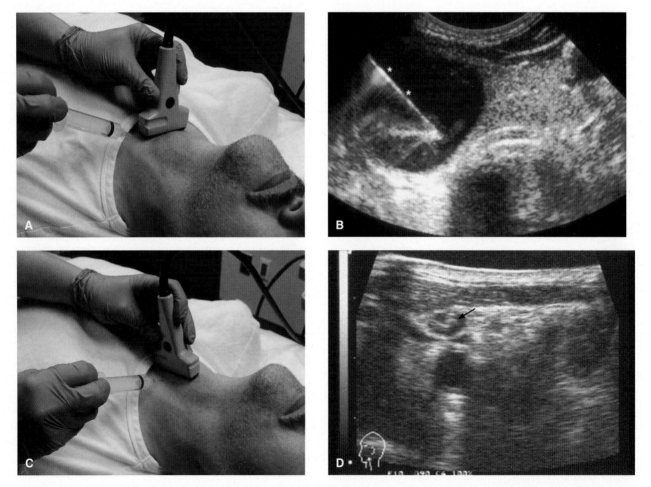

Figure 4-9. Ultrasound-guided fine-needle aspiration. (**A** & **B**) the in-plane approach facilitates visualization of the path of the needle as it traverses the neck; (**C** & **D**) the needle is only identified as it engages the tissue of interest. (Reprinted from: (B) Loevner L, et al. Cross-sectional Imaging of the thyroid gland. *Neuroimag Clin Am.* 2008 Aug;18(3):445–461. (D) Takes R, et al. The value of ultrasound with ultrasound-guided fine-needle aspiration biopsy compared to computed tomography in the detection of regional metastases in the clinically negative neck. *Int J Radiat Oncol Biol Phys.* 1998;40(5):1027–1032 with permission from Elsevier.)

Additionally, an additional sample can be collected for cytospin reduction by dispersion into a collection tube containing fixative solution.

CASE STUDIES

▶ Case 1

A 60-year-old woman presents with an incidental finding in the right neck discovered during a free carotid screening ultrasound. She denies dysphagia, dysphonia, and dyspnea. The patient has no family history of thyroid cancer or radiation exposure. On examination, there is no palpable mass. Diagnostic ultrasound reveals a solitary nodule in the right mid-thyroid lobe and is hypoechoic with a spongiform appearance and no evidence of punctate calcifications or hypervascularity (Figure 4-10). After informed consent, the patient underwent FNAB of the dominant lesion with a cytologic diagnosis of colloid nodule.

Discussion: This case represents one of the most common scenarios for thyroid disease, the solitary thyroid nodule. Given the prevalence of thyroid nodules and the patient's lack of risk factors for thyroid cancer (family history/radiation exposure), she is low risk for thyroid cancer. The physical examination is similarly not worrisome. Incidentally, lesions smaller than 1 to 1.5 cm in size are very difficult to pick up on physical examination unless the patient has a very slender neck. The diagnostic USG also suggested a benign, solitary lesion. The spongiform pattern created by an aggregation of microcystic structures is highly specific for benign disease. Despite all of this, the ATA guidelines suggest that all thyroid nodules over 1 cm in size should have a FNAB. With a FNAB read as a benign lesion, there is a 97% likelihood that this is a benign lesion

that should be followed with serial ultrasound to assess for growth or change in characteristics.

▶ Case 2

A 50-year-old woman presents with a biopsy-proven papillary thyroid cancer in a solitary 3 cm left thyroid nodule. She denies dysphagia, dysphonia, and dyspnea. The patient has no family history of thyroid cancer or radiation exposure. On examination, the mass is located in the left thyroid lobe and is approximately 3 cm in size and is quite hard but mobile. Ultrasound reveals a solitary nodule in the left mid-thyroid lobe and is hypoechoic with punctate calcifications and hypervascularity around the margins. Prior to total thyroidectomy, you perform an office ultrasound looking at the central and lateral neck nodes. In the left central neck, there are two 1 cm lymph nodes without fatty hilum. In the left lateral neck, there is a 0.6 cm mass lateral to the jugular vein in level IV with foci of microcalcifications (Figure 4-11). You perform FNAB of the left lateral neck node and confirm that it is metastatic papillary thyroid cancer.

Discussion: This case illustrates one of the most important aspects of office-based ultrasound by the surgeon. The diagnostic procedure confirmed the presence of a highly suspicious lesion for cancer, but more importantly, the lymph node mapping portion identified level VI (central neck) and left lateral neck adenopathy that is highly

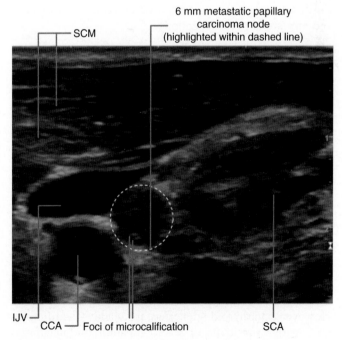

Figure 4-11. Transverse ultrasound at level IV on the left, showing a typical small (6 mm) nodal metastasis from a papillary carcinoma. It is solid, echogenic, and contains foci of microcalcification, despite its size. Surrounding structures: (SCA) scalenus anterior, (SCM) sternocleidomastoid muscle, (CCA) common carotid artery, (IJV) internal jugular vein. (Reprinted from Cozen N. Thyroid and parathyroid. In: *Clinical Ultrasound.* 3rd ed. Vol. 2. 2011: 867–889 with permission from Elsevier.)

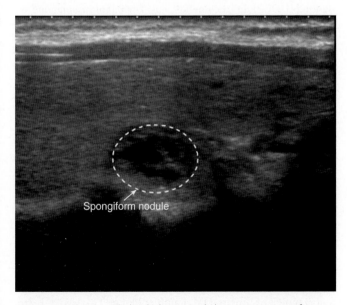

Figure 4-10. Longitudinal ultrasound showing a spongiform nodule. (Reprinted from Cozen N. Thyroid and parathyroid. In: *Clinical Ultrasound.* 3rd ed. Vol. 2. 2011: 867–889, with permission from Elsevier.)

Sagittal   Transverse

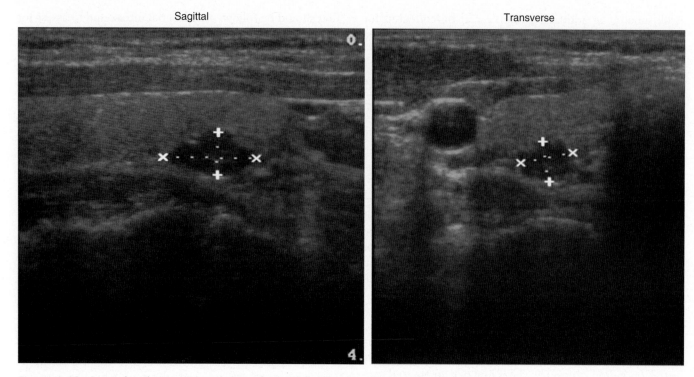

Figure 4-12. Sagittal and transverse imaging of the right neck with inferior parathyroid identified.

suspicious for metastatic thyroid cancer subsequently confirmed by FNAB. Real-time sonography allows the clinician to choose the appropriate operation for the patient (in this case, total thyroidectomy, central neck dissection, and left lateral neck dissection).

▶ Case 3

A 50-year-old woman was found on routine blood tests to have an elevated calcium. Her calcium level was 11 with a concomitant PTH of 100 and vitamin 25-D of 40. She denies a family history of endocrine disease or a personal history of radiation therapy. She does complain of fatigue and "brain fog." She had a recent bone density scan which demonstrated osteoporosis of the forearm. Ultrasound identified a 1.3 × 1 × 0.8 cm mass suspicious for parathyroid adenoma (Figure 4-12). The patient underwent a successful focused parathyroidectomy with intraoperative parathyroid hormone monitoring.

Discussion: After confirming a biochemical diagnosis, surgeon-directed ultrasound is a critical part of the localization process to identify diseased parathyroids. In general, normal parathyroid glands are very difficult to see on USG. However, parathyroid adenomas are readily identified on USG with a sensitivity of 80–90%. Parathyroid adenomas are classically tear-drop shaped and hypoechoic. USG may miss ectopically located parathyroid adenomas in the tracheoesophageal groove, mediastinum, and thyrothymic ligament. During the search for a diseased parathyroid, it is important to assess the thyroid sonographically as well, as up to 30% of patients may have concomitant thyroid disease that may require evaluation.

SUGGESTED READINGS

American Thyroid Association (ATA) Guidelines Taskforce on Thyroid Nodules and Differentiated Thyroid Cancer, Cooper DS, Doherty GM, Haugen BR, Kloos RT, Lee SL, Mandel SJ, Mazzaferri EL, McIver B, Pacini F, Schlumberger M, Sherman SI, Steward DL, Tuttle RM. Revised American Thyroid Association management guidelines for patients with thyroid nodules and differentiated thyroid cancer. *Thyroid.* 2009 Nov;19(11):1167–1214.

Baskin HJ, Duick DS, Levine RA, eds. *Thyroid ultrasound and ultrasound-guided FNA.* New York: Springer; 2008.

Cappelli C, Pirola I, Cumetti D, et al. Is the anteroposterior and transverse diameter ratio of nonpalpable thyroid nodules a sonographic criteria for recommending fine-needle aspiration cytology? *Clin Endocrinol (Oxf).* 2005;63(6):689–693.

Hoang JK, Lee WK, Lee M, Johnson D, Farrell S. US features of thyroid malignancy: pearls and pitfalls. *Radiographics.* 2007;27(3):847–860.

Leboulleux S, Girard E, Rose M, Travagli JP, Sabbah N, Caillou B, Hartl DM, Lassau N, Baudin E, Schlumberger M. Ultrasound criteria of malignancy for cervical lymph nodes in patients followed up for differentiated thyroid cancer. *J Clin Endocrinol Metab.* 2007;92:3590–3594.

Rago T, Vitto P. Role of thyroid ultrasound in the diagnostic evaluation of thyroid nodules. *Best Practice and Research J Clin Endocrinol Metab.* 2008;22(6):913–928.

Shimamoto K, Satake H, Sawaki A, Ishigaki T, Funahashi H, Imai T. Preoperative staging of thyroid papillary carcinoma with ultrasonography. *Eur J Radiol.* 1998;29:4–10.

Solorzano CC, Carneiro DM, Ramirez M, Lee TM, Irvin GL 3rd. Surgeon-performed ultrasound in the management of thyroid malignancy. *Am Surg.* 2004;70:576–580; discussion 580–582.

5

BREAST ULTRASOUND

AIMEE MACKEY & PREYA ANANTHAKRISHNAN

The role of ultrasound in breast care has expanded considerably over the past 30 years. While in its infancy, it was used mainly to distinguish cystic from solid masses, it has evolved to be an essential component of state-of-the-art breast care for the breast surgeon. Currently, it is essential for work-up of breast symptoms or mammographic abnormalities, and is the preferred modality for image-guided procedures. Breast ultrasound is unique from ultrasound of other areas in the body in that it requires correlation of ultrasound findings with mammogram and physical examination. Major advantages of ultrasound over other breast imaging modalities include lack of exposure to ionizing radiation as well as patient comfort.

CLINICAL INDICATIONS FOR ULTRASOUND

The American College of Radiology defines several indications for breast ultrasound (Table 5-1). Ultrasound is the modality of choice for work-up of a palpable mass in a woman less than age 30, due to density of the breast on mammography. Breast tissue becomes less dense and more fatty as a woman ages. Adipose or fatty tissue is visualized well on mammography, so mammographic screening is most effective in older women with fatty breasts. In younger patients with dense breasts, mammography is much less sensitive, since dense breast tissue appears opaque and less radiolucent, making it more difficult to identify masses or asymmetric densities that can be signs of malignancy. When performing breast ultrasound, density is not a factor that affects the sensitivity. In addition, it is the preferred test for a palpable mass in a pregnant woman. Ultrasound can also be used to evaluate findings seen on mammography. For mammographic abnormalities including a mass, developing focal asymmetric density, or area of architectural distortion, sonography can further characterize the area and guide biopsy.[1] Breast masses detected on self-examination or clinical examination in women over age 30, focal breast thickening, breast pain, or nipple

discharge should first be evaluated mammographically. A negative mammogram should be followed with ultrasound for a symptomatic area or region of clinical concern.[2] For any lesion of concern, image-guided biopsy is the standard of care for diagnosis as opposed to surgical excisional biopsy (if technically feasible).[3]

Breast ultrasound can be divided into two categories: targeted and nontargeted. Targeted ultrasound is used to identify a specific lesion or region in the breast, but does not scan the entire breast. Palpable superficial lesions may be better seen on ultrasound than on mammogram.[4] Nontargeted ultrasound is used to evaluate the entire breast in the presence of symptoms such as nipple discharge, silicone implant rupture, and known breast cancer or axillary metastasis in the presence of a negative mammogram.[5] Whole breast ultrasound is not routinely performed for breast cancer screening in the general population due to the low sensitivity; however, certain populations such as

TABLE 5-1
Indications for Breast Ultrasound
Evaluation of a palpable mass or other signs/symptoms in the breast
Evaluation of abnormalities on other imaging studies (such as mammography or MRI)
Initial imaging of a palpable mass in women under 30 (who are not at high risk for breast cancer) and in lactating/pregnant women
Evaluation of problems with breast implants
Evaluation of lesions suspicious for malignancy (microcalcifications or architectural distortion) in the setting of dense fibroglandular tissue
Guidance of breast biopsy or interventional procedure
Treatment planning for radiation therapy
Screening for occult cancer as a supplement to mammography in certain populations of women who are not candidates for MRI
Identification and biopsy of abnormal axillary lymph nodes

TABLE 5-2
Documentation of an Ultrasound Image
Facility name and location
Examination date
Patient's first and last name
Medical record number and/or date of birth
Designation of right or left breast
Anatomic location using clock face notation or a labeled diagram of the breast. Transducer orientation and distance from the nipple to the abnormality should be documented
Sonographer/physician's identification number, initials, or other symbols

women with dense fibroglandular breasts or high-risk groups may benefit from sonographic screening.[2]

In the setting of a known breast cancer, ultrasound can be helpful for complete characterization of a lesion for surgical planning and tumor staging. Ultrasound may also help to visualize multifocal or multicentric carcinoma, and is frequently used to scan the axilla to check for the presence of suspicious lymph nodes. As MRI is used more frequently in breast cancer patients as well as for screening in high-risk populations, post-MRI ultrasound often identifies lesions and facilitates biopsy under ultrasound guidance.[2]

Intraoperatively, ultrasound can be useful to guide surgery.[6] Several studies have suggested that use of intraoperative ultrasound decreases reexcision rates by guiding margin excision around a lesion at the time of surgery. Intraoperative wire localization under ultrasound guidance can be performed by the surgeon for nonpalpable lesions, which saves time and is more comfortable for the patient. Ultrasound can also guide minimally invasive therapeutic interventions such as cryotherapy and radiofrequency ablation.[7,8]

Clear documentation is necessary for many reasons including billing and compliance, as well as to ensure accurate duplication of the study if additional procedures will need to be performed. Correct documentation includes several components (Table 5-2).

NORMAL ANATOMY

The form and function of the breast change over time and depend on hormonal factors occurring during puberty, pregnancy, and menopause. During reproductive years, the mature breast consists of 15–20 lobes of branched ducts, which radiate from the nipple and divide peripherally into lobules. Each lobe has numerous lobules and small branch ducts that join together to form larger ducts, which then form a main subareolar duct that drains the whole lobe. The lobes are different sizes and sometimes overlap one another. The gland is surrounded by support structures made up of subcutaneous connective tissue, which forms septa between lobes and lobules.

The terminal ductolobular unit (TDLU) makes up the functional unit of the breast. It consists of a single lobule and the terminal duct. The number of TDLUs varies between patients, and also changes in a single patient's breast for reasons including age, parity, body habitus, and hormonal factors. During pregnancy and lactation, women often have very rapid proliferation of TDLUs.[2]

Anatomy of the breast from superficial to deep consists of skin, subcutaneous fat, anterior fascia, breast parenchyma (containing ductal and lobular structures), retromammary fascia, retromammary fat, pectoralis muscle, ribs, and pleura.[6] Cooper's ligaments are present within the breast parenchyma and subcutaneous fat layers. The tail of Spence (or axillary segment) of the breast extends toward the axilla. The nipple is not perfectly centered on the breast, but lies just medial and inferior to the center. This subsequently allows for the upper outer quadrant of the breast to contain more volume, which may account for the greater number of breast lesions seen in the upper outer quadrant. The nipple and areola are covered by pigmented epithelium and contain smooth muscle, which can contract and cause acoustic shadowing during ultrasound.[2]

Lymphatic drainage of the breast is extensive, and is the route by which most breast cancers spread. The breast first drains into superficial lymphatic channels, which travel from the subareolar plexus along the major ducts, then along efferent veins to adjacent nodal beds. The majority of the breast drains primarily to the axilla, including the external mammary, axillary, and central nodal groups within the axilla. More distal groups involved in advanced disease include the interpectoral nodes, subclavicular nodes, and supraclavicular nodes. The scapular and subclavicular nodes are also contained within the axilla. Medial lymphatics also drain directly into the internal mammary nodes. The presence, level, and number of axillary lymph nodes involved are important in prognosis, as well as treatment, of breast cancer. Intramammary lymph nodes may also be present, and are most commonly located in the axillary tail but may be located anywhere within the breast.

Blood supply to the breast comes from perforating branches of the internal mammary artery along the medial aspect of the breast, intercostal perforators, and lateral thoracic and thoracoabdominal branches of the axillary artery. Venous drainage is variable in the breast. The deep veins tend to run along the same course as the arterial supply. In general, the superficial veins do not have corresponding arteries; rather the venous drainage runs with the lymphatic drainage.[2]

NORMAL APPEARANCE OF ULTRASOUND

The skin appears as a hypoechoic line at the top of the image, which becomes thicker toward the nipple-areola complex. A bright hyperechoic linear echo can be seen between the dermis and subcutaneous fat planes. The skin appears as a 1- to 3-ml isoechoic to hyperechoic strip sitting on top of this echo. The skin can be thickened on ultrasound secondary to scarring, infection, radiation-induced dermatitis, and fat necrosis (Figure 5-1).[2,9]

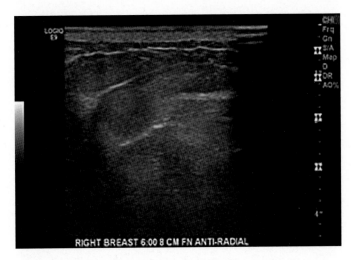

Figure 5-1. Skin thickening on ultrasound.

The subcutaneous zone lies between the skin and anterior mammary fascia. It includes subcutaneous fat, Cooper's ligaments, and blood vessels. The subcutaneous fat is between the skin and breast parenchyma. The amount of subcutaneous fat present in a breast varies with age, parity, and body habitus. The subcutaneous fat appears as a hypoechoic region below the skin, and thins out toward the nipple-areola complex. Cooper's ligaments are linear hyperechoic structures arising from the breast parenchyma, which can be seen throughout the glandular tissue as well as the subcutaneous fat. Blood vessels, ectopic ducts, and lobules may be present in the subcutaneous region as well. Most sonographic lesions seen in the subcutaneous zone arise from the skin or subcutaneous fat rather than breast tissue. These lesions are not specific to the breast, and include epidermal inclusion cysts, lipomas, hemangiomas, and sebaceous cysts.[2,10]

The mammary zone is also called the glandular region, and is composed of the actual breast tissue. The majority of breast abnormalities are seen in this region, which contains almost all of the ducts and TDLUs. The US appearance of this zone depends on the physiologic state of the breast as well as the patient's age. Within the ductal and lobular tissue, Cooper's ligaments extend from front to back and further subdivide the mammary zone unpredictably. In addition, fibrous tissue and fat lie within the mammary zone.[2]

There are four main parenchymal patterns evident on ultrasound of the breast: fibrous, premenopausal, postmenopausal, and pregnant. The juvenile or fibrous breast contains little fat, and therefore the glandular region in this pattern is hyperechoic. The premenopausal breast is usually partially involuted, with the glandular region containing more subcutaneous and retromammary fat with interspersed fatty lobules. The fatty lobules may have a spherical appearance in one projection, and tubular appearance when the probe is turned 90 degrees. With pregnancy and lactation, there is an increase in glandular tissue that appears more hyperechoic, and the ductal

structures are easily visualized. With this increase in glandular tissue comes compression of the subcutaneous and retromammary fat. The postmenopausal breast becomes fatty replaced, with the occasional presence of glandular elements.[11]

The nipple region contains dense connective tissue, which causes dramatic shadowing. This can make the resolution of structures immediately adjacent to the nipple difficult. The subareolar region is usually scanned at a tangential angle to avoid this shadowing.

The retromammary zone lies between the mammary zone and the pectoralis major muscle, and can be difficult to see on ultrasound. If seen, it usually appears as a narrow hypoechoic strip between the muscle and the glandular tissue. This zone contains mostly retromammary fat and some fibrous ligaments. Most pathologic processes that involve this zone do so secondarily, due to extension of malignancy or other processes from the mammary zone.[2]

When performing ultrasound on the breast, the premammary and retromammary fascia may be difficult to visualize. In older women, the breast has undergone fatty involution and the premammary fascia is not well seen, while in younger patients it can be dense (appearing as a well-defined thin line). The retromammary fascia is even more difficult to identify, and is often more readily seen on the lateral aspects of the breast where the breast is being pulled away from the chest wall.[10]

The chest wall is posterior to the retromammary zone. The most anterior structure seen in this region is the pectoralis major muscle, which appears as a hypo- or hyperechoic structure (depending on transducer angle) above the ribs. It has a striated appearance consistent with skeletal muscle. The pectoralis major muscle can serve as an orienting structure, since it is constant in location and relatively easy to identify. The intercostal and serratus anterior muscles are behind the pectoralis major muscle, followed by the ribs posteriorly. The ribs appear as hyperechoic crescents with posterior shadowing. The pleura and lung are seen deep to these structures, and the pleura can be seen moving with respiration.[2,10,11]

In describing a lesion on ultrasound, a standard or reference for echogenicity must be designated. Current practice is to use normal breast fat as the standard, since all women have fat in the subcutaneous zone regardless of the density of their breast tissue. Tissues that appear identical to the subcutaneous fat are considered isoechoic, tissues blacker than fat are hypoechoic, and those that are whiter than fat are hyperechoic. If a lesion lacks an internal echo, it is considered anechoic.[12]

Evaluating an entire duct is necessary because pathology can occur anywhere along its course. Generally, normal TDLUs that lie anterior to the main lobar ducts have longer extralobular terminal ducts than the posterior ones. This can result in the "taller than wide" appearance of cancers. The majority of TDLUs are in the mammary zone; however, they can extend into Cooper's ligaments as well as into the premammary zone. TDLUs are normally

1–2 mm in diameter; however, they can vary greatly in size. Larger TDLUs are more easily seen sonographically than smaller TDLUs.[5,11]

SCANNING TECHNIQUE FOR OBTAINING THESE IMAGES

Breast ultrasound is best performed with high-resolution equipment, and is highly operator-dependent. High-frequency linear array transducers are required due to the wider near field, which is especially important for US-guided procedures. The 2011 standards from the ACR suggest transducer frequencies of 10 MHz and preferably higher. The frequency should be appropriate for the size and depth of the abnormal area, using the highest frequency capable of penetrating to the depth of the lesion of interest. The power, time-gain-compensation (TGC) curve, and focal zone settings should also be optimized. The power is kept as low as possible such that the beam just penetrates the chest wall. The TGC should be set to allow even penetration of the entire field. Power and gain should not be so high as to create artifactual echoes within a simple cyst, causing it to appear solid. They also should not be so low as to miss real echoes in a solid mass. The focal zone is electronically adjustable, and should be set at a lesion's depth. Multiple focal zones are often needed to fully characterize a lesion.[7,11]

Proper positioning of the US machine, examiner, and patient is critical for a successful examination (Figure 5-2). The machine is usually placed to the patient's right, and the (right-handed) examiner scans with the right hand and operates the machine with the left hand. For an image-guided procedure, the machine is placed on the opposite side of the patient than the side of interest. The ultrasound machine is kept parallel to the examining table, with the control panel directly in front of the examiner. The screen should be easily visualized by the examiner. The room

should be warmed and the gel appropriately warmed to optimize patient comfort and facilitate the most successful examination.[12] The patient should be asked if there is an area of palpable concern.

A generous amount of warm gel should be placed on the breast, with the transducer face maintained perpendicular to the skin. Gentle continuous pressure should be applied to maintain transducer-skin contact. This contact can be difficult to maintain in the region of the nipple-areola complex due to the wrinkling of the areola; however, copious gel can help. Application of even pressure with the transducer can decrease reflective and refractive attenuation. Transducer pressure can be increased for greater penetration of the tissue as necessary, particularly in the subareolar region.

The patient is positioned supine with a pillow behind the shoulder and the ipsilateral arm raised above the head, which flattens the breast and minimizes tissue depth. The patient can be moved to optimize imaging based on location of the lesion. For medial lesions, the patient is best positioned supine with the ipsilateral arm raised above the head. Lateral lesions are visualized with the patient posterior oblique, and the ipsilateral arm over the head. The superior aspect of a pendulous breast is best examined with the patient sitting, and the ipsilateral arm over the head. The examiner should make sure the patient is comfortable before beginning the examination. Also, it is important to ask the patient if they can feel an abnormality in a particular position.[6,9,11]

Numerous scanning methods are described in the literature. The American Society of Breast Surgeons recommends a standard scanning protocol including a radial scan, transverse sweep, and a tangential scan of the nipple. The footplate is oriented with the nipple on the left side of the viewing screen, along the radius of the breast in that particular region. This lines up the probe and image with the ductal anatomy of the breast, allowing visualization along the entire length of a ductal system. The radial scan is performed in a clockwise fashion, using the nipple as a pivot for the transducer. A rocking motion is used to better visualize a particular region. This standard approach allows relocalization in the future, if a lesion is visualized. Each quadrant is imaged from the nipple region to the periphery of the breast. The number of radii needed to examine a breast depends on the volume of breast tissue present in a particular patient, and usually ranges from 12 to 30. It is important to ensure adequate overlap of the scanning areas, particularly at 12, 3, 6, and 9 o'clock positions.

The transverse sweep or scan involves rescanning the entire breast from top to bottom, with the transducer oriented transversely. This can be started either medially or laterally, and provides a second look of the same tissue that was examined in a radial direction.[9,11,12]

The nipple-areola region is difficult to evaluate because scanning the nipple directly from above can cause a dense shadowing, which obscures underlying anatomy.

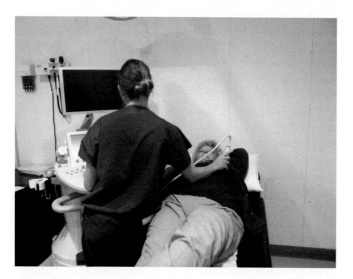

Figure 5-2. Positioning of patient, examiner, and machine.

The tissue behind the nipple is best evaluated by angling the probe tangentially. Applying pressure with the index finger of the opposite hand to the tissue on the opposite side of the nipple from the transducer improves visualization.[2] Alternatively, the compression technique can also be used to visualize the nipple, by placing the opposite hand on the lateral aspect of the breast and pushing medially. This allows the transducer to move toward the nipple to obtain better visualization. This region should be scanned from both above and below the nipple, allowing the entire ductal system of interest to be visualized within the nipple and into the breast.[11,12]

The axillary contents may be included in breast ultrasonography as well, and should be routinely evaluated in the setting of known malignancy. Scanning of the axilla is done in two planes. The axillary artery can be located by palpation, and is a useful guide for orienting the probe. Alternatively, the head of the humerus can be found with the probe and used as the superior most border of the axilla. The probe is then swept downwards through the axilla toward the tail of the breast. The longitudinal plane can be established by identifying the pectoralis major muscle and orienting the probe parallel to the muscle. Overlapping passes should be made in the axilla just as in the breast examination (Figure 5-3).[9,12]

Doppler examination can be utilized on the breast as well as the axilla, and may help distinguish between ducts and vessels within the breast.[13] The axillary vessels can be visualized and their proximity to lesions of interest noted within the axilla. Normal lymph nodes are often not visualized, and enlarged lymph nodes should be considered pathologic. Pathologic nodes may be reactive or malignant.

Once an abnormality is identified, a targeted approach is used. The lesion should be evaluated in multiple planes by turning the transducer, and must be visualized in at least two planes to confirm that it is in fact abnormal. Images should be captured and measurements taken. Documentation of a lesion should be done in a standard

TABLE 5-3
Documentation of a Lesion
Tumor size (widest diameter) Location (clock face position, distance from nipple) Shape Long tumor axis (horizontal vs. vertical) Margins (well-circumscribed, ill-defined, lobulated) Boundary Echo pattern Sound transmission (shadowing, enhancement) Elasticity (compressibility) Mobility Surrounding tissue changes

format, including the following information (Table 5-3). Differential diagnosis of a solid mass includes the following (Table 5-4).

COMMON FINDINGS/ABNORMALITIES

Both benign and malignant breast lesions can be identified on ultrasound.[14,15]

▶ Benign

Fibrocystic change (FCC)

This benign finding is often seen bilaterally, especially in women in their 30s and younger. FCC can also be seen in post-menopausal women depending on age-related degeneration of the glandular tissue. For women less than 30 with a palpable mass, ultrasound is the diagnostic test of choice. Mammography has decreased sensitivity in women with dense breasts, so ultrasound is commonly ordered on these patients as an adjunct to mammography. Commonly the breast parenchyma (mammary zone) is hyperechoic with prominent ductal anatomy. In a younger patient this may appear as "honeycombing".[16] In older patients, the increased reflexivity may make deeper structures difficult to identify. Of note, fibrocystic change can sometimes have focused hypoechoic areas containing ill-defined margins

TABLE 5-4
Differential Diagnosis of Hypoechoic Masses on Ultrasound
Fibroadenoma Carcinoma Abscess Cyst Fibrocystic change Intramammary lymph node Intraductal papilloma Phyllodes tumor Sebaceous cyst

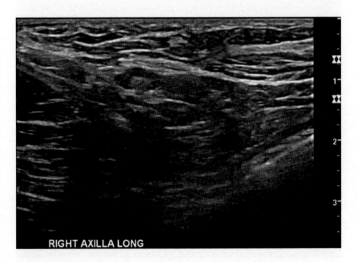

Figure 5-3. Axillary region-normal axillary nodes.

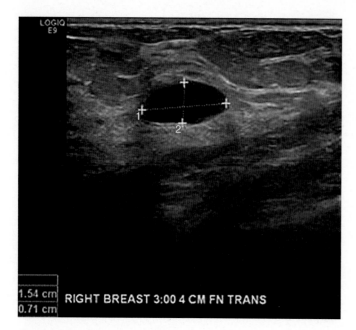

Figure 5-4. Simple cyst.

that sonographically mimic malignancy. Biopsy in this case may be indicated. If a benign result is found, it is essential to establish concordance with ultrasound, mammogram, and physical examination.

Cysts

Cysts are very commonly seen on ultrasound. Their size and location in the breast are variable, and they are typically round or oval in shape. Simple cysts are well circumscribed, anechoic, demonstrate posterior enhancement, and have thin edge shadows. They are mobile and do not cause any surrounding tissue changes. Simple cysts may be drained if symptomatic; however, intervention is not necessary for these lesions.[17] If all criteria for simple cysts are not met, the cyst is considered complex and aspiration or biopsy may be warranted as described below (Figures 5-4 and 5-5).[18]

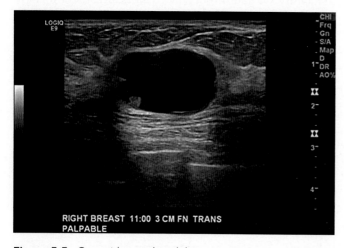

Figure 5-5. Cyst with mural nodule.

Intraductal papilloma

Papillomas sometimes present with symptoms including pathologic nipple discharge, which is unilateral, spontaneous, and often bloody. They may be visualized as a mass on mammography, usually as a small solid lesion within a duct near the nipple (although they may also be present more peripherally). The size of papillomas can vary; however, they may be as small as 1 or 2 mm. Papillomas are usually round in shape with a horizontal tumor axis, making them wider than tall, with well-circumscribed margins. Most papillomas are hypoechoic, moderately compressible, and mobile. Surrounding tissues may demonstrate ductal dilation and duct ectasia.[16] Core biopsy is usually warranted, although papillomas tend to fragment easily. Surgical excision may be recommended for smaller symptomatic lesions. Surgical excision is recommended for papillomas due to a 5–15% risk of malignancy on pathology from definitive excision (Figure 5-6).[19]

Fibroadenoma

This is the most common benign solid mass in the breast. Fibroadenomas usually present in 20- to 35-year-old females with a palpable mass. Physical examination characteristics include round or oval shape, rubbery texture, and mobility. Significant growth can be seen while on oral

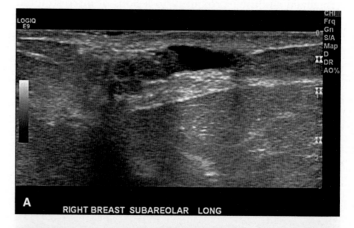

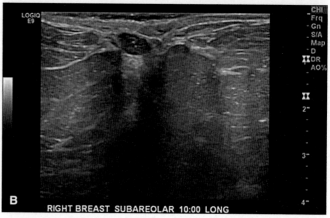

Figure 5-6. Intraductal papilloma.

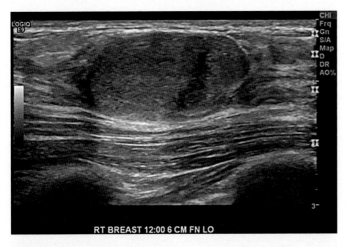

Figure 5-7. Fibroadenoma.

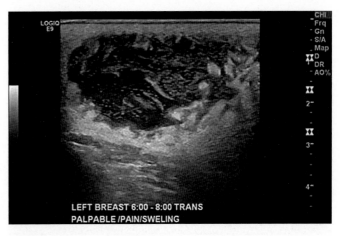

Figure 5-8. Breast abscess.

contraceptives or during pregnancy. Fibroadenomas are usually in the 10–30 mm size range and their location is variable.[10,16] They have a wider than tall appearance on US and a well-circumscribed margin; however, they can also appear lobulated. Fibroadenomas will appear hypoechoic on ultrasound with posterior enhancement, are not compressible, are easily mobile, have a clear interface with adjacent tissue, and are not associated with surrounding tissue changes. They can sometimes have double edge shadowing posteriorly (Figure 5-7).

Phyllodes tumor

Cystosarcoma phyllodes are rare breast tumors that have a sonographic appearance similar to fibroadenomas. They should be in the differential diagnosis of any fibroadenomatoid lesion, particularly in women in their 40s. They usually present with a rapidly enlarging breast mass over several weeks or months. Phyllodes are also usually larger than fibroadenomas at presentation.[16] Sonographic characteristics include round or oval shape, horizontal long tumor axis, well-circumscribed margin, abrupt interface with surrounding tissue, hypoechoic pattern which may contain anechoic or cystic components, posterior enhancement, not compressible, and moderate mobility. Surrounding tissue may appear hypervascular, sonographically. Wide local excision is recommended for benign as well as malignant lesions, since both can be locally aggressive. Lymph node evaluation is not indicated for evaluation of metastases, since the metastatic pattern is similar to sarcoma (to the lungs rather than the lymph nodes).

Mastitis

Infections of the breast can affect females of all ages. Mastitis may or may not be associated with systemic signs, and may be localized within the breast or involve the whole breast. It is most commonly associated with staphylococcal infections, and is divided into two categories: lactational and nonlactational mastitis. Lactational mastitis is directly associated with breast feeding and usually occurs within

days of instituting breast feeding. Nonlactational can be periareolar or peripherally located. Ultrasound can be very useful in differentiating mastitis from a discrete breast abscess. The ultrasound appearance of mastitis is skin thickening or edema, and edema may be present throughout the breast tissue. The margin of mastitis is indistinct and the boundary is poorly defined. Mastitis is likely to appear hypoechoic on sonography with moderate compressibility.[10] Sonography can also identify dilated lymphatics as well as enlarged axillary lymph nodes that are reactive in nature. Ultrasound, however, cannot differentiate mastitis from inflammatory breast cancer. If the breast does not clinically respond to antibiotics, a biopsy should be performed (Figure 5-8).

There are a number of other additional benign breast lesions that can be identified on ultrasound; however, these are much less common than those listed above. These include lactating adenomas in pregnant or lactating women, galactoceles, hamartomas, and breast lipomas (Figures 5-9 to 5-12).

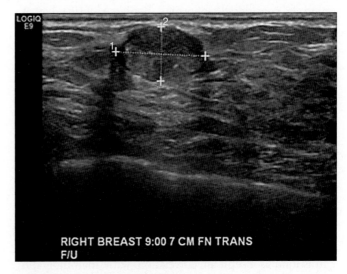

Figure 5-9. Lactating adenoma.

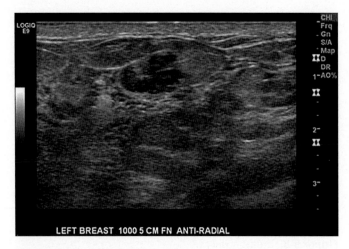

Figure 5-10. Galactocele.

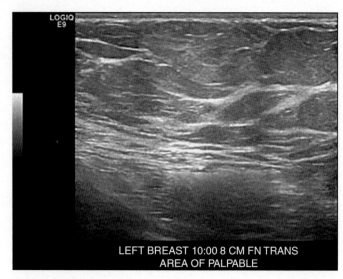

Figure 5-12. Lipoma.

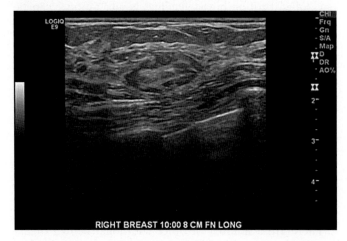

Figure 5-11. Hamartoma.

Lymphadenopathy

Intramammary lymph nodes can often be seen within the breast tissue. Enlargement on mammography and ultrasound is considered abnormal. Benign reactive lymphadenopathy is associated with central (hilar) hyperechoic preservation and symmetrical hypoechoic- surrounding cortex. Roundness, loss of hilar hyperechoicity, and eccentric cortical thickening, particularly in the presence of underlying malignancy, are suggestive of malignant involvement of the node.[7] If lymphoma is suspected, excisional biopsy is often performed to obtain enough tissue for hematopathology analysis (Figure 5-13).

▶ Malignant

Noninvasive carcinoma

Ductal carcinoma in situ (DCIS) is the most common noninvasive breast cancer. DCIS is usually identified on mammography as clustered, linear, or branching calcifications. Ultrasound is useful in correlation with mammography in DCIS, to identify whether a mammographically occult

mass is present. This would allow for ultrasound-guided biopsy as opposed to stereotactic biopsy.[20] In addition, if a mass is identified, biopsy may facilitate preoperative upstaging of the lesion. DCIS is treated as a cancer, with lumpectomy, radiation, and endocrine therapy as appropriate (Figure 5-14). Lobular carcinoma in situ is most often an incidental finding with variable sonographic appearance, indicating an increased risk of cancer in both breasts.[21]

Invasive ductal carcinoma

Invasive cancers can present as an imaging abnormality or as a palpable mass in the breast. The presence of any suspicious findings for malignancy warrants a biopsy for tissue diagnosis. Invasive ductal carcinoma is variable is size and location. Lesions usually have an irregular shape, with jagged edges and indistinct margins. They are hypoechoic masses that are taller than wide (with a lateral/anteroposterior ratio of less than 1). There is noted to be posterior shadowing (rather than enhancement) with poor

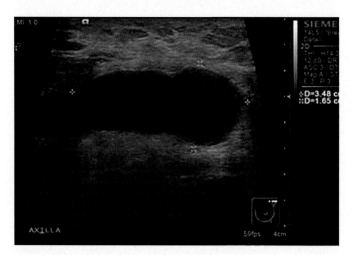

Figure 5-13. Suspicious axillary lymph node.

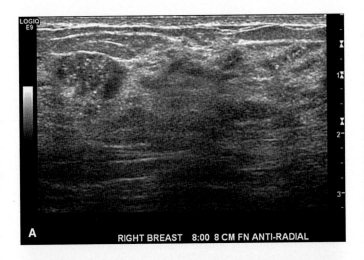

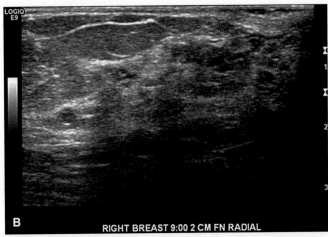

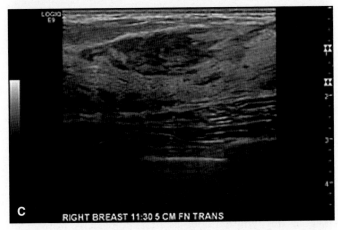

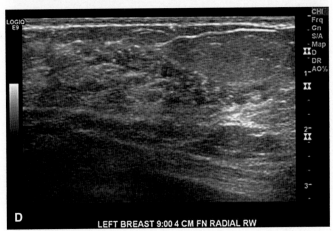

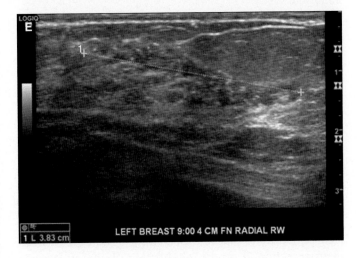

Figure 5-14. DCIS.

through-transmission. These lesions will be rigid with no compressibility. Most carcinomas will still be moderately mobile on examination and ultrasound. There is also noted to be architectural distortion in the surrounding tissue, disrupting the natural tissue planes (Figure 5-15).[10,16]

Invasive lobular carcinoma

Invasive lobular carcinomas are more difficult to identify on imaging and clinical examination. Lobular carcinomas display a wide spectrum of appearances on mammogram and ultrasound. Sonographically, ILC may appear as an irregular hypoechoic mass with spiculated margins and posterior acoustic shadowing. It can also appear as an ill-defined region of architectural distortion with no discrete mass visualized. Lobular carcinomas can also be difficult to identify on physical examination, as they may present with a "thickening" rather than a discrete mass. Histologically, these cancers have an "indian-file" orientation on histology,

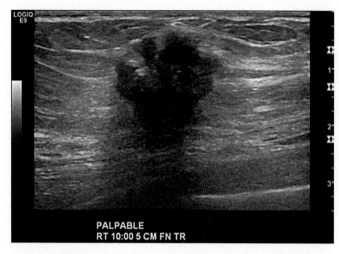

Figure 5-15. IDC.

with finger-like projections that can make it difficult to obtain clear margins surgically (Figure 5-16).[22]

▶ Lymph Node Metastasis

As discussed above, the lymph nodes in the axilla should be included in routine ultrasound in the setting of a known malignancy. Lymph node involvement affects medical treatment and surgical planning. To classify a lymph node as morphologically abnormal, the following criteria should be met:

Enlargement >10 mm in short axis (resulting in a "round" lymph node)
Loss of hilar hyperechoic center
Asymmetric focal hypoechoic cortical lobulation
Uniformly hypoechoic lymph node

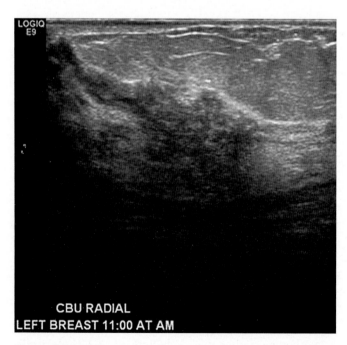

Figure 5-16. ILC.

If these criteria are met, a biopsy should be performed to rule out metastatic lymph node involvement.[23] If lymph node positivity is established preoperatively, then the sentinel lymph node procedure is not necessary at the time of surgery and axillary lymph node dissection is considered. In some instances, knowing that the lymph node is positive preoperatively may change the algorithm for the patient's cancer care in that neoadjuvant chemotherapy may be recommended prior to surgery.

Features suggestive of reactive lymphadenopathy include nodal matting and surrounding soft tissue edema, with prominent hilar vascularity on Doppler US. Doppler US features suggestive of malignancy include peripheral or capsular vascularity, avascular areas, displacement of vessels, and aberrant course of hilar vessels.[10]

INFLAMMATORY BREAST CANCER

Inflammatory breast cancer is defined by dermal lymphatic involvement with invasive carcinoma. It is often advanced at time of diagnosis, and it is treated initially with chemotherapy. Clinically, the breast examination can mimic mastitis; however, failure to improve on antibiotics should warrant further work-up, specifically skin biopsy. Ultrasound typically demonstrates marked skin thickening, thickening of Cooper's ligaments, and dilated superficial lymphatic channels. Both mastitis and inflammatory breast cancer can present with axillary lymphadenopathy and ultrasound can be useful to characterize the appearance of the lymph nodes as morphologically normal or abnormal.[10]

COMMON PITFALLS

Pitfalls are important to recognize in sonography of the breast, since they can lead to missing a cancer as well as unnecessary biopsy of a benign finding.[24] Failure to recognize normal anatomy can lead to diagnostic errors with ultrasound, and there are several lesions that can appear confusing. Misdiagnosis can also occur due to unique characteristics of sonography physics, improper setting of instrument controls, and the presence of air or foreign bodies in the breast.

The key to determining whether a lesion is real is visualizing it in multiple planes. The rib (particularly the cartilaginous portion) can be mistaken for a solid breast mass in cross section. It can be identified as rib by the location posterior to the pectoralis muscle, as well as its elongated shape when imaged in a longitudinal plane. Fat lobules are present within normal breast tissue, and can be mistaken for solid masses that are isoechoic to surrounding tissues. Rotation of the transducer in multiple planes will help to demonstrate that the lobule is in continuity with adjacent adipose tissue. The 15–20 lactiferous ducts present in the breast converge at the nipple. Normal caliber ducts imaged in cross-section can mimic cysts, and should be examined in a different plane.

Cysts are quite common in the breast, and simple cysts often require no intervention. Simple cysts are anechoic, well circumscribed, have a thin, echogenic outer wall, demonstrate posterior enhancement, and have thin edge shadows. If all criteria are not met, then a cyst is considered complex. The majority of complex cysts in the breasts are benign findings, and fall within the spectrum of fibrocystic change. Usually cysts are described as complex due to the presence of internal echoes. Causes of internal echoes include cell debris, protein globules, red blood cells, leukocytes, lymphocytes, epithelial cells, and apocrine cells.[24]

Internal echoes within a cyst can also be caused by solid masses, including papilloma and carcinoma. Stravros et al developed an algorithm to help differentiate between benign and malignant cystic lesions. First, a determination must be made whether the lesion is simple or complex. If complex, the next step in evaluation involves looking for suspicious findings including presence of thick isoechoic septations, mural nodules, presence of a fibrovascular stalk, or a microcystic microlobulated appearance. If any of these findings are identified, cytology with FNA alone is not adequate for diagnosis. A core biopsy should be performed and marking clip should be placed.

If no suspicious findings are seen, findings of inflammation or infection are then identified. These include uniform thickening of the cyst wall, hyperemia of the cyst wall, or a fluid-debris level. If these are seen, cyst aspiration with Gram stain and culture should be performed. An infected cyst should not be misdiagnosed as a breast abscess and the terms are not interchangeable. If no evidence of infection is identified, the area is examined for clusters of simple cysts, thin echogenic septations, milk of calcium (tiny stones in the dependent portion of the cyst), circumferential calcification of cyst wall, punctuate calcifications in cyst wall, lipid cysts, fat-fluid levels, mobile cholesterol crystals, and cysts of skin origin. Other features that may be seen include eccentric nonmobile concave wall thickening, diffuse low-level echoes filling entire cysts, and indeterminate cystic versus solid lesions. Close follow-up, cyst aspiration, or biopsy can be performed as appropriate.[4,18,24]

Acoustic shadowing is a sonographic feature that can be associated with malignancy; however, it is also associated with several benign conditions. Isolated acoustic shadowing without an associated mass can be seen along a normal Cooper's ligament. Usually this appears faint and narrow; however, it can be hypoechoic and wide enough to raise suspicion for a tumor. Slight increases in pressure of the transducer or changes in the angle can often resolve this shadowing. Postsurgical scar can also cause acoustic shadowing without an associated mass, which can be difficult to differentiate from tumor in a lumpectomy bed. Finally, poor contact between the transducer and skin can also cause acoustic shadowing. This is seen as echogenic lines present at fixed intervals from the skin to the acoustic shadowing (Figure 5-17).[24]

Edge shadowing is a thin line of shadowing only behind the peripheral edge of a mass, caused by absorption and

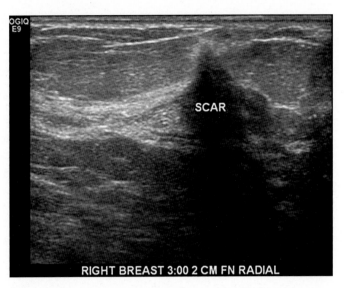

Figure 5-17. Postsurgical scar with acoustic shadowing.

refraction along the mass border. It is considered a nondiagnostic feature, as it can be seen with cysts and benign as well as malignant masses. Reverberation artifact can cause the appearance of debris or solid material along the nondependent wall of a cyst. It is perpendicular to the direction of the ultrasound beam, and moves position within the cyst when the angle of the transducer is changed.[24]

Improper setting of controls on the ultrasound can also lead to diagnostic error. Gray-scale gain sets the amplitude of the returning sonographic signal. If the gain is too high, a simple cyst can appear to be a complex cyst or a solid mass. Gray scale should be set so that fluid in a cyst appears black, while fat lobules vary from dark gray to light gray. Dynamic range settings that are set too low can cause the low-level echoes in a solid mass to be seen as black pixels, so that a solid mass appears to be a simple cyst. Setting the dynamic range too high causes an image with little contrast, so that it is difficult to differentiate a fat lobule from a subtle mass. The focal zone should be set to match the depth of the object being imaged, since resolution and beam depth are worse outside the focal zone. An incorrectly positioned focal zone can make it difficult to appreciate a subtle mass, cause sharp edges to appear hazy, and give the appearance of internal echoes in a simple cyst.[6,12,24]

Foreign bodies can have a variety of appearances on ultrasound. An extracapsular silicone implant rupture may mimic a cyst or a hypoechoic solid mass with posterior acoustic enhancement. The presence of short echogenic lines parallel to the back wall of the structure can confirm that it is an implant rupture.

Interventional procedures can lead to sonographic abnormalities in the breast. Percutaneous needle procedures introduce air along the path of the needle, which can obscure visualization of the needle and require reinsertion of the needle at a different site. This can be limited by removing all air from syringes and needles before administration of local anesthesia.[3,9] After a procedure, an

TABLE 5-5

Characteristics of Benign, Indeterminate, and Malignant Lesions

	Benign	Indeterminate	Malignant
Shape	Oval/round	Variable	Irregular/angular, spiculations
Lobulations	Gentle bi or trilobulations	Variable	Microlobulations
Margins	Sharp/smooth	Sharp/smooth or indistinct	Indistinct/jagged
Retrotumoral acoustic phenomena	Posterior enhancement Bilateral edge shadowing	No change	Posterior shadowing, unilateral edge shadowing
Echogenicity	Hyperechoic (can also be isoechoic, anechoic, or hypoechoic)	Isoechoic or hypoechoic	Hypoechoic
Internal echo pattern	Homogenous	Variable	Heterogenous, may contain calcification echoes
Lateral-anteroposterior diameter ratio	Lateral greater than anteroposterior (ratio of lateral to anteroposterior >1)	Variable	Anteroposterior diameter greater than lateral (ratio of lateral to anteroposterior <1)
Compressibility	Compressible	Variable	Noncompressible
Compression effect on internal echoes	Echoes swirl more homogenous	Variable	No change
Adjacent architecture	Unaffected	Usually unaffected	Disrupted

echogenic line caused by air along the needle tract can actually look like a needle remaining within the mass. If the needle is reinserted for further sampling, it can be differentiated from the air tract by rapidly moving the needle tip back and forth.

If a solid or hypoechoic mass is encountered, a decision must be made about whether imaging follow-up is adequate or biopsy is indicated. Stavros et al, in a prospective study of 750 sonographic solid masses of the breast, described a sonographic classification system to help guide management.[15] Lesions were described as benign, indeterminate, or malignant. Benign features included three categories: intense and uniform hyperechogenicity, ellipsoid shape with thin echogenic capsule, and gentle lobulations with thin echogenic capsule. Malignant features included spiculation, angular margins, hypoechogenicity, shadowing, calcification, duct extension, branch pattern, and microlobulation.[9] The presence of a single malignant feature excluded the lesion from the benign category. Indeterminate lesions did not fit into any of the benign categories, but did not have malignant features either. Malignant lesions required biopsy and establishment of concordance. This study described a sensitivity of breast ultrasound of 98% and a negative predictive value of 99.5% for malignancy.

CLINICAL PEARLS/TIPS

▶ **Benign Versus Malignant Characteristics**

Multiple criteria are used in evaluating breast lesions with ultrasonography as described above. Features that can help distinguish benign from malignant masses are listed in Table 5-5.

Therapeutic maneuvers—ultrasound guided procedures

Ultrasound has become the modality of choice for guiding interventional procedures, due to patient comfort as well as ease of biopsy when compared to mammography and MRI. With ultrasound, the linear transducer facilitates long-axis visualization of a needle into a sonographic abnormality. Proper needle position can be confirmed real time while performing the procedure. Cyst aspiration, core needle biopsy, and wire localization under ultrasound guidance can be done rapidly in experienced hands.[9] Necessary equipment is listed in Table 5-6.

The breast is first scanned for localization of the image. The lesion is scanned to the maximum diameter in any plane (longitudinal or transverse) and compared to the diagnostic ultrasound. Viewing and documentation should occur in at least two 90 degree views, and the lesion is measured in

TABLE 5-6

Equipment List for Ultrasound-Guided Procedures

Ultrasound machine with 7.5 MHz or greater linear array transducer

Needles for aspiration. FNA or cyst aspiration can be performed with a 22-gauge needle. An 18 gauge can be helpful for thicker aspirate. Core biopsy needles range from 10 to 14 gauge, and automated vacuum assisted core-needle biopsy needles can also be used

Needle-localization wires (usually 5 cm and 7.5 cm)

Specimen cup with formalin

Papanicolaou fixative, for FNA samples.

Local anesthesia, scalpel, prep/drape, gloves, gauze, and sterile gel

three dimensions. Painting, by scanning perpendicular to the long axis of the transducer, is done to find the widest point of the lesion. The needle or device is centered under the middle of the long axis of the transducer, and inserted parallel to the long axis of the transducer. Painting is again used to evaluate the relationship of the biopsy device to the lesion. Skiing, or moving the transducer along the breast parallel to the long axis, can be done to position the lesion on the monitor.

Cyst aspiration under ultrasound guidance allows direct visualization of the procedure, and should confirm that the cyst resolves (Figure 5-18). Cyst fluid that is clear or green is discarded. Lesions with an irregular cyst wall or bloody/turbid fluid, or those that do not resolve with aspiration are sent to cytopathology.[25]

FNA of solid masses can provide immediate cytologic diagnosis; however, it is unable to differentiate in situ from invasive cancer. A benign FNA alone is not adequate for diagnosis; it must be evaluated with the triple test of clinical features, imaging features, and cytology. Most FNAs revealing malignancy are followed with core biopsy for further characterization of a malignancy, including receptor status.

Core needle biopsy devices are 12- to 18-gauge spring-loaded devices, allowing multiple insertions. The probe is first placed on the unprepped skin to identify the lesion. The probe is maneuvered in two different ways. "Skiing" is employed to move the lesion from left to right on the screen or vice versa. "Painting" is used to move the lesion superior or inferior (90 degrees from the other view while "skiing"). By using both of these techniques, the view of the lesion is optimized and the surgeon is better oriented. Next, the skin is prepped and local anesthesia is injected. Following this, under ultrasound guidance, local anesthesia is injected

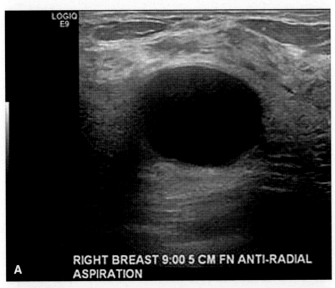

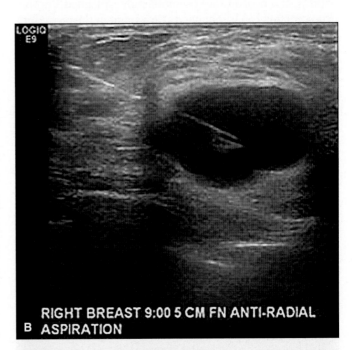

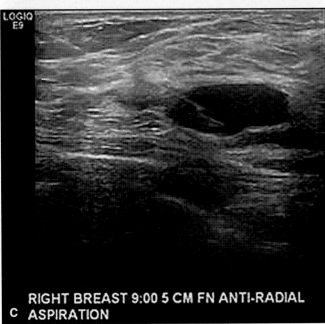

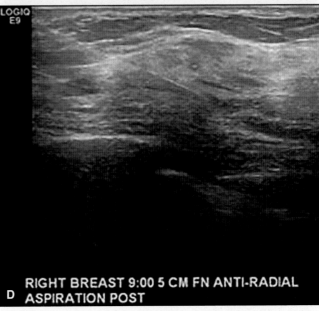

Figure 5-18. Cyst aspiration.

superior, inferior, anterior, and posterior to the lesion. Of note, the injectate can distort the sonographic appearance of the lesion and surrounding tissue. For core biopsy, a small nick in the skin is made using an #11 blade (not necessary for FNA.) The biopsy needle is inserted through the nick in the skin. The distance from the transducer edge depends on the device type and location of the lesion. The needle is then advanced to the edge of the lesion under ultrasound guidance, with the biopsy device or needle parallel to the transducer and parallel to the muscle. This sometimes requires "painting" the ultrasound probe to identify the needle on the screen. Once the needle is at the lesion in good position, the needle is fired and biopsy is taken. Before the needle is withdrawn, "painting" should again be performed to ensure that the lesion is identified on both sides of the needle. A marker or clip should be placed if the lesion is removed in its entirety, or if neoadjuvant chemotherapy is planned. Photodocumentation can be obtained at any point in the procedure. Three to five core biopsies are usually obtained to ensure adequate sampling of the lesion (Figures 5-19 and 5-20).

Vacuum or rotation-assisted device types are either single sample with multiple insertions, or single insertion devices that remove multiple samples. These vacuum or rotation-assisted devices provide larger contiguous tissue samples without removal of the probe, and can remove some smaller lesions in their entirety. Less precise

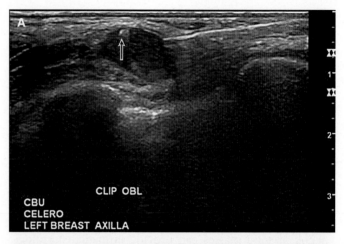

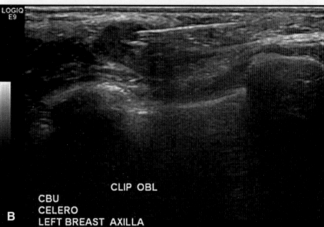

Figure 5-20. Core biopsy of a metastatic axillary lymph node.

targeting of the lesion is required, since the vacuum or rotation device assists by removing a larger amount of tissue in the area. This is a good option for lesions close to the chest wall or close to breast implants, since sampling occurs above the tip (the device is not fired forward).[3]

CASE STUDIES

1. Complex Cyst—A 43-year-old female presents to the Breast Surgery clinic after being referred by her gynecologist for left breast pain. She underwent diagnostic breast ultrasound for left breast pain. The patient is known to have a history of fibrocystic breast disease; however, on her most recent ultrasound, a 1.3-cm complex cyst with septations was noted at the 3 o'clock position of her left breast (Figure 5-21).

   She has no other significant past medical history; however, her mother was diagnosed with early-stage breast cancer at age 48. On physical examination, her right breast demonstrates fibrocystic changes; however, it has no palpable masses. Her left breast demonstrates fibrocystic change, with a palpable mass at 3 o'clock position corresponding to the ultrasound finding. Given the physical examination findings, along with the ultrasound, an ultrasound-guided biopsy is recommended of the complex cyst.

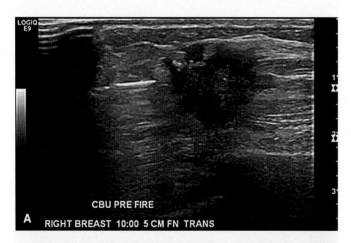

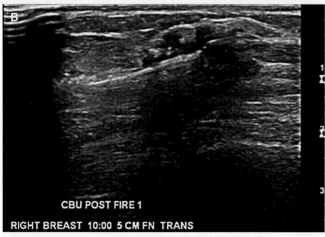

Figure 5-19. Core biopsy of a malignant lesion.

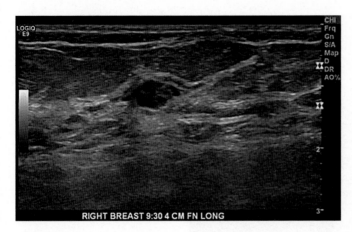

Figure 5-21. Complex cyst.

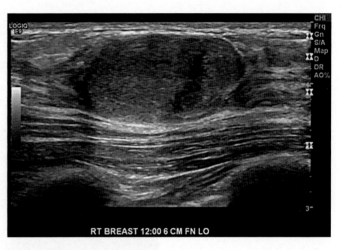

Figure 5-22. Fibroadenoma.

The patient underwent biopsy and pathology demonstrated ductal carcinoma in situ. The patient then opted to undergo breast-conserving surgery.

2. Fibroadenoma—A 28-year-old female presents to her gynecologist with a lump in her right breast. The patient reports that the mass has been there for 4 months. She does report occasional pain associated with it, mostly related to her menstrual cycle. She denies any prior breast complaints. Her gynecologist orders a targeted breast ultrasound, which demonstrates a 2.1-cm hypoechoic, well-defined oval mass that is not compressible. The patient is referred to Breast Surgery clinic for evaluation (Figure 5-22).

On physical examination, a 2-cm firm, mobile mass is palpable at 12:00, 6 cm from the nipple. Physical examination and ultrasound both suggest a fibroadenoma.

Given the size of the lesion, along with occasional pain, excisional biopsy is recommended. The patient underwent surgical right breast excisional biopsy and pathology confirms fibroadenoma.

3. Breast Cancer with Lymph Node Metastasis- A 39-year-old African American female presents for evaluation of a lump in her left axilla present for one month. She feels no breast masses, and has no family history of any breast or ovarian cancer. She underwent menarche at age 13, is nulliparous, and denies history of oral contraceptives or hormone replacement therapy. She undergoes diagnostic mammogram and left breast and axillary ultrasound (Figure 5-23).

Imaging shows a 3-cm mass in her left breast, as well as a 3-cm palpable lymph node in her axilla. Following imaging, the patient undergoes ultrasound-guided

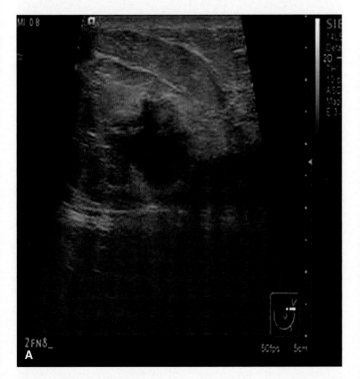

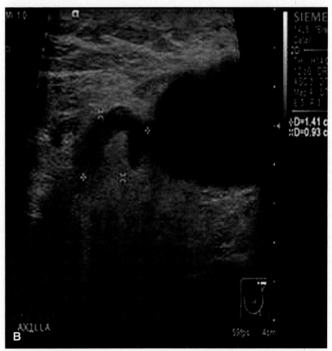

Figure 5-23. Breast cancer with axillary lymph node metastasis (u/s and mammogram images).

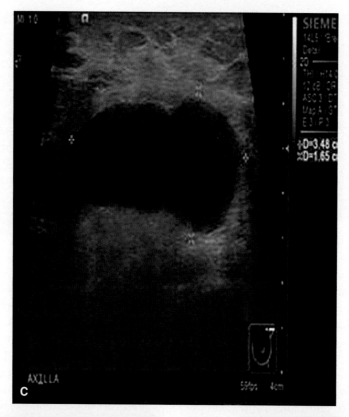

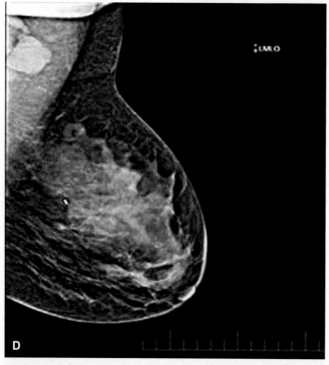

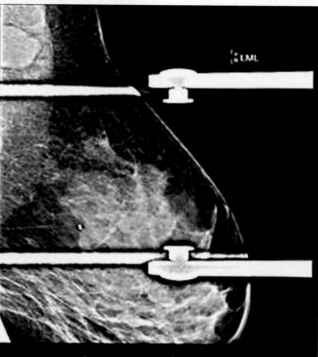

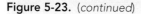

Figure 5-23. (continued)

biopsy of the breast mass and the lymph node. Both demonstrated infiltrating ductal carcinoma, poorly differentiated, estrogen receptor negative, progesterone receptor negative, and Her2Neu negative. The patient was referred to medical oncology and started on neoadjuvant chemotherapy.

CONCLUSION

Breast ultrasound has become an integral part of caring for patients with breast concerns. Through mastery of breast ultrasound, the surgeon takes the lead in both diagnosis and management of breast cancer. Ultrasound is also becoming an increasingly important tool in the armamentarium of

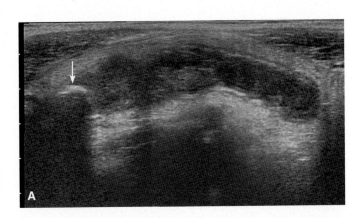

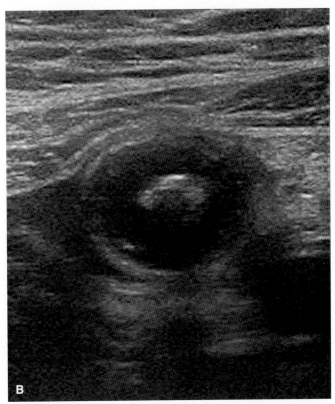

Figure 6-1. (**A**) Longitudinal view of acute appendicitis with thickened, noncompressible hypervascularized appendix and fecolith (arrow). (Used with permission from www.ultrasoundcases.info/Slide-View.aspx?cat=187&case=4773) ID: /32589-Afbeelding2.jpg; (**B**) Transverse view of a fluid-filled appendix and a large fecolith at the base with a "target sign" appearance. (Used with permission from www.ultrasoundcases.info/Slide-View.aspx?cat=187&case=4774) ID: /32594-Afbeelding2.jpg

An obstructed bowel appears distended, fluid-filled with thickened walls; there is an absence of peristalsis. Computed tomography is superior to ultrasonography at delineating the cause and location of an intestinal obstruction. Ultrasonography, however, is considered the method of choice for diagnosing intussusception. The findings on imagining are characterized by segmental pathologic target phenomena consisting of multiple concentric rings with demonstration of mechanical obstruction (Figure 6-2).[10,11]

The value of ultrasonography in the difficult diagnoses of mesenteric infarction is unclear. The images demonstrate hyperperistaltic bowel with mucosal edema, which are nonspecific findings. As the ischemia progresses, the bowel wall may appear thicker than 6 mm. Phillips and colleagues have reported the successful use of color Doppler imaging in certain cases of small bowel infarction of the proximal superior mesenteric artery or thrombosis of the superior mesenteric vein.[12]

Hernias and abdominal wall masses Transabdominal ultrasound can be used to identify and distinguish between hernias, seromas, abscesses, and other abdominal wall masses. Moreover, it can be used to guide aspiration or biopsy of such lesions with high accuracy and minimal morbidity or risk to the patient.

Abdominal aortic aneurysm Abdominal aortic aneurysm should be considered in any patient who presents with abdominal pain of unknown etiology. In patients who are unstable, CT scan is too time-consuming and may delay definitive treatment. Bedside transabdominal ultrasound can rapidly and accurately detect the presence and size of a ruptured or nonruptured AAA with a sensitivity that approaches 100%.[1]

With the patient lying supine, a 3.5 MHz convex transducer should be used to identify the aorta below the xiphoid. The normal aorta should be an anechoic tubular

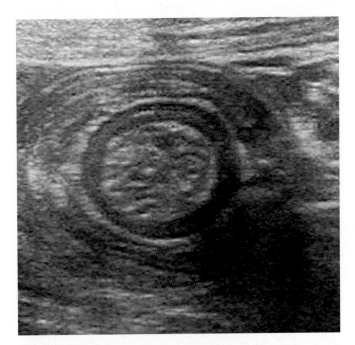

Figure 6-2. Small bowel intussusception with multiple concentric rings in transverse section. (Used with permission from www.ultrasoundcases.info/Slide-View.aspx?cat=185&case=4968) ID: /34565-Afbeelding3.jpg

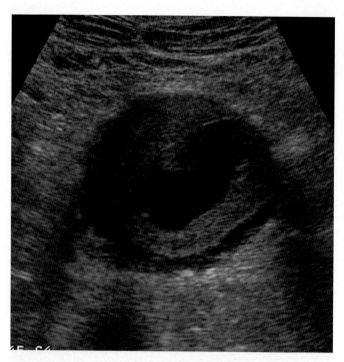

Figure 6-3. Transverse view of aortic aneurysm with intramural hemorrhage and dissecting thrombus. (Used with permission from www.ultrasoundcases.info/Slide-View. aspx?cat=205&case=616) ID: /3336.jpg

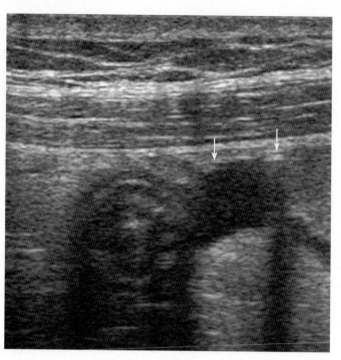

Figure 6-4. Inflamed, thickened small bowel with free fluid (arrow) and air in the peritoneal cavity. (Used with permission from www.ultrasoundcases.info/Slide-View. aspx?cat=194&case=3085) ID: /16168.jpg

structure with reflective walls that follows the curve of the lumbar spine and tapers off slightly at the inferior portion. The transducer should then be swept caudally toward the umbilicus in a transverse orientation to obtain measurements above and below the takeoff of the renal arteries. By orienting the transducer longitudinally, anteroposterior (AP) measurements can be obtained and the aorta assessed for the presence of a mural thrombus (Figure 6-3).

Ultrasonography can also be used to detect the presence of an aortic dissection. In the presence of an aortic dissection, a channel of blood will track down inside the tunica media and appear as a thin echogenic septum within the true lumen. An intimal flap can sometimes be seen on longitudinal view and the vascular channels delineated using color Doppler flow.

Intra-abdominal sepsis and ascites In patients that present with signs of sepsis, it is often difficult to elicit a complete history or obtain a reliable physical examination. In this situation, ultrasound can be used to examine the dependent portions of the abdomen for free fluid and bowel edema that would suggest peritonitis (Figure 6-4). It can also be used to look for reverberation artifacts in the epigastric region and right upper quadrant, which might indicate presence of pneumoperitoneum.

Solid organ injury Ultrasound has become an indispensable tool in the emergency room setting and care for the patient with acute trauma. First introduced into practice in the 1970s in European trauma rooms, it was adopted into routine use by North American emergency teams in

the 1990s. The focused assessment with sonography for trauma (FAST) is a limited ultrasound assessment with the sole objective of identifying the presence of free intraperitoneal or pericardial fluid. It is quick, can be performed at the bedside, and offers the option of repeat serial scans that may aid in the follow-up of a trauma patient who is managed nonoperatively. Ultrasound is less sensitive than DPL in detecting intraperitoneal blood and in estimating the blood volume that is free in the peritoneal cavity, but it does not involve any invasive intervention, which is required for DPL.

The accepted practice in emergency rooms is to screen all patients with blunt trauma and possible solid organ injury or hemoperitoneum with rapid ultrasound assessment (FAST). The patient may be monitored with repeat scans or taken for emergency surgical exploration depending on the findings and the clinical status of the patient.

Gallbladder and biliary tract pathology Transabdominal ultrasound is the initial diagnostic method of choice in cases of suspected cholecystitis and choledocholithiasis as the finding of cholelithiasis and bile duct stones will help guide further management. The normal gallbladder is typically an anechoic, oval-shaped, thin-walled structure that lies just under the right lobe of the liver, lateral to the portal vein. Occasionally it is enveloped within the liver parenchyma or is located more inferiorly toward the right iliac fossa. It is best visualized when the patient has been fasting. In the sagittal orientation, the probe should be swept horizontally from the right edge of the liver along its

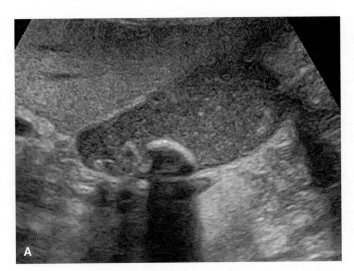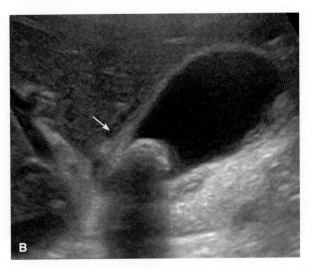

Figure 6-5. (**A**) Gallbladder filled with sludge and echogenic stones with posterior shadowing. (Used with permission from www.ultrasoundcases.info/Slide-View.aspx?cat=154&case=3705) *ID: /20500.jpg*; (**B**) Inflamed gallbladder with pericholecystic fluid (arrow) and stone in the gallbladder neck. (Used with permission from www.ultrasoundcases.info/*Slide-View. aspx?cat=161&case=6224) ID: /47219-Afbeelding2.jpg*;

inferior surface toward the portal vein until the gallbladder comes into view. Gallstones should produce acoustic shadows that differ from shadows caused by loops of bowel by their lack of echogenic streaks.

The cystic duct can be seen running posteromedially from the medial side of the gallbladder neck toward the common bile duct. The corkscrew-shaped spiral valve of Heister is located at the most superior aspect of the duct. The common bile duct can be seen anterolateral to the portal vein. Unlike the branches of the portal vein, the intrahepatic bile ducts arising from the CBD have brightly echogenic walls. The CBD should be imaged in the transverse plane and traced through the head of the pancreas to the medial aspect of the duodenum. A curvilinear transducer with large footprint can help to minimize shadowing from overlying bowel gas and help to better visualize the duct.

The use of ultrasound in assisting in the diagnosis of gallbladder disease is well established. The patient is usually required to fast and is maintained in the supine position. The gallbladder is approached with the probe in the right lateral longitudinal and intercostal planes. Gallstones will appear as round, mobile echogenic foci within the lumen of the gallbladder. Stones larger than 1 mm will often cast a posterior shadow. The typical findings of acute cholecystitis include gallbladder wall thickening greater than 4 mm, hypoechogenic thickening of the tissues around the gallbladder, pericholecystic fluid, and localized pain while imaging the gallbladder with mild compression which is referred to as a "sonographic Murphy sign" (Figure 6-5).[13,14] The presence of gallbladder wall stranding or layering echogenic gas within the lumen are suggestive of gangrenous and emphysematous cholecystitis, respectively. Chronic cholecystitis can be distinguished from acute cholecystitis by the pattern of mural calcification on ultrasonography (porcelain gallbladder) with or without obliteration of the gallbladder lumen.

Ultrasound can also be utilized to detect other pathologic findings in the gallbladder and biliary tree, including adenomyomatosis, polyps, malignant neoplasms, and choledocholithiasis with biliary obstruction. Adenomyomatosis is a benign condition due to hyperplasia and invagination of the epithelium and muscular layers of the gallbladder. It most typically presents as small echogenic intramural diverticula or as a polypoid lesion located in the gallbladder fundus. Gallbladder carcinoma can appear as diffuse wall thickening (especially if greater than 1 cm) or a heterogeneous, vascular mass that obscures the normal plane between the gallbladder and liver.

Ultrasonography has a sensitivity of 75% for the detection of stones within the common bile duct.[15] The normal extrahepatic bile duct should be less than 6 mm at the level of the crossing right hepatic artery. A dilated duct in the presence of obstructive symptoms is highly suggestive of choledocholithiasis and can be confirmed by the presence of echogenic stones with distal acoustic shadows on ultrasonography. Dilated common bile ducts within the porta hepatis with tapering of the CBD and surrounding mass are suggestive of a cholangiocarcinoma. This intra- or extrahepatic malignancy can either spread outward from the CBD (exophytic), be contained within the wall of the duct (infiltrative), or appear as a polyp-like mass within the duct (polypoid) (Figure 6-6).

Liver pathology The normal liver has a homogeneous pattern that is more echogenic than the renal cortex, but less echogenic than the spleen. It is anatomically divided into eight segments based on the branching of the portal structures and hepatic veins that appear as sonolucent tubular structures within the liver parenchyma. The three hepatic veins typically run in an oblique direction from the upper end of the IVC to the right, middle, and left portions of the liver.

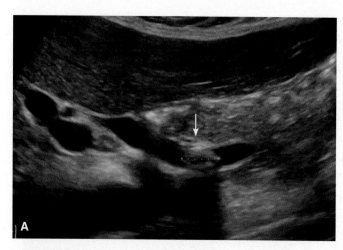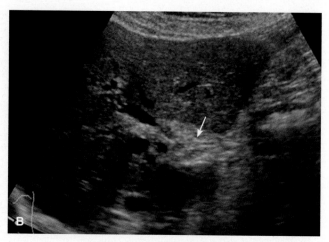

Figure 6-6. (**A**) Longitudinal view of stones in the distal common bile duct. (Used with permission from www.ultrasoundcases.info/Slide-View.aspx?cat=154&case=5664) *ID: /41318-Afbeelding1.jpg;* (**B**) Cholangiocarcinoma with an intraductal mass (arrow) and dilated intrahepatic ducts. (Used with permission from www.ultrasoundcases.info/Slide-View.aspx?cat=156&case=3421) *ID: /18694.jpg*

The liver is best evaluated with the patients turned slightly on their left side, which allows the liver to slide downward into a better view. The patient should hold his or her breath, which depresses the diaphragm. The probe is placed in a sagittal orientation in the right anterior axillary line and swept horizontally from right to left until the far edge of the left lobe is visualized. The probe is then rotated and oriented axially under the right ribs and angled upward until the top of the liver comes into view. It is then swept vertically from the cranial to caudal direction. If the liver is obscured by the lower ribs, the probe can be rotated until it lies along the intercostal space. In order to visualize the hepatic veins, the probe should be oriented axially under the xiphoid and tilted cranially to bring the junction of the IVC with the right atrium into view. The hepatic veins should then be visualized running into the IVC.

The portal vein runs in a horizontal orientation from the inferior surface of the liver along the right lobe. The portal vein has a more reflective wall than the hepatic veins and is therefore more echogenic. It is best visualized by placing the probe in the midclavicular line, where it is rotated counter-clockwise from the sagittal orientation until it points toward the right shoulder, and is then tilted medially toward the aorta. The portal vein can then be followed down to where it joins the superior mesenteric and splenic veins.

Transabdominal ultrasound is often used to detect and localize benign or malignant neoplasms, metastases, cysts, hemangiomas and abscesses within the liver (Figure 6-7). Hepatic adenomas typically appear as well-demarcated, isolated lesions with variable echogenicity on ultrasound. Focal nodular hyperplasia is difficult to distinguish from an adenoma, but is more often isoechoic with characteristic "spoke wheel" or "stellate" vascularity on color Doppler. Hepatic metastases have a variable appearance depending on their origin and there are no features that routinely distinguish them from primary hepatocellular carcinoma. Tumors arising from the gastrointestinal tract are more

likely to be multifocal, hyperechoic, and have a hypoechoic rim creating a "bull's-eye" or "target" appearance on ultrasound. Hepatocellular carcinoma is more often hypoechoic in relation to the surrounding liver parenchyma, with posterior echo enhancement or "halo" effect. Portal or hepatic vein invasion is also more suggestive of hepatocellular carcinoma than metastatic disease.

Ultrasound can localize benign and malignant lesions based on the liver segments involved and the distance of the lesion from the hepatic and portal veins. The proximity to the vessels also helps determine resectability and to plan the operative approach. Transabdominal ultrasound is also useful for following focal hepatic lesions over time and for monitoring patients' response to therapy. Ultrasound with Doppler capability can be used to assess hepatic arterial and portal venous flow after hepatectomy or liver transplantation. When neoplasms are deemed unresectable, ultrasound is a useful adjunct to alternative ablative procedures such as radiofrequency thermal ablation or cryoablation.

Pancreatic pathology Unlike children in whom the liver appears brighter than the pancreas on ultrasound, in adults, the pancreas is brighter than the liver and lies posterior to the antrum of the stomach. Occasionally it is obscured by the transverse colon. With the patient lying supine, a 3.5 MHz transducer should be placed over the xiphoid and aimed downward. Images should be obtained in both longitudinal and transverse planes in order to best identify the pancreas in relation to the surrounding vasculature. The pancreas will appear as an inverted "U" inferior to the splenic vein. The head and neck of the pancreas should be seen wrapping around the echogenic fat pad at the origin of the SMA, while the tail runs superiorly toward the left axilla. The tail can best be seen by rotating the probe counterclockwise until it points toward the left axilla or by turning the patient on his/her right side and visualizing it through the spleen.

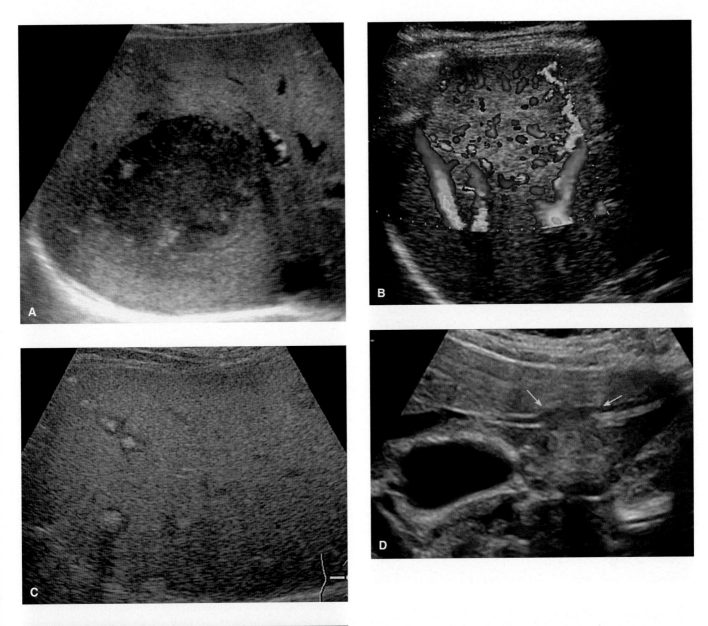

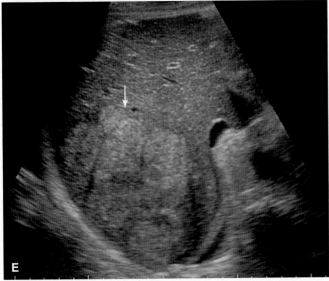

Figure 6-7. (**A**) Amebic liver abscess. (Used with permission from www.ultrasoundcases.info/Slide-View. aspx?cat=141&case=3082) *ID: /16124.jpg;* (**B**) Large focal nodular hyperplasia characterized by isoechoic mass and color Doppler demonstrating "spoke wheel" vascularity. (Used with permission from www.ultrasoundcases.info/Slide-View.aspx?cat=129&case=3141) *ID: /16595.jpg;* (**C**) Multiple hyperechoic calcified liver metastases with hypoechoic halo in a patient with breast carcinoma. (Used with permission from www.ultrasoundcases.info/Slide-View.aspx?cat=144&case=8) *ID: /129.jpg;* (**D**) Liver metastasis with invasion and stenosis of a left portal vein. (Used with permission from www. ultrasoundcases.info/Slide-View.aspx?cat=144&case=3597) *ID: /19900.jpg;* (**E**) Large hepatocellular carcinoma (arrow) in a cirrhotic, nonhomogenous liver. (Used with permission from www.ultrasoundcases.info/Slide-View. aspx?cat=142&case=3144) *ID: /16631.jpg*

Transabdominal ultrasound is often the first imaging study done for suspected pancreatitis and can identify peripancreatic edema, fluid collections and pseudocysts in advanced disease (Figure 6-8). The first sign of acute pancreatitis is often an increase in pancreatic volume on ultrasound; as the disease progresses, pancreatic necrosis and edema will give the pancreas a nonhomogenous and hypoechoic appearance. Pancreatic pseudocysts are usually round, well-defined anechoic structures with acoustic enhancement on ultrasound, while hemorrhagic or infected pseudocysts may have a more complex appearance with septations and internal echoes.

Transabdominal ultrasound can also be used to identify pancreatic malignancies, especially in the head of the pancreas. Even in the absence of a discrete mass on imaging,

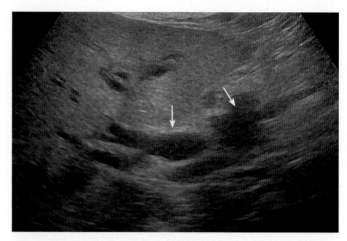

Figure 6-9. Pancreatic head carcinoma with tumor obstructing the common bile duct and a "double duct" sign (arrows). (Used with permission from www.ultrasoundcases.info/Slide-View.aspx?cat=168&case=5371) ID: /38493-Afbeelding1.jpg

the finding of common bile duct and pancreatic duct dilatation due to obstruction is highly suggestive of a malignancy. This characteristic finding is called the "double duct" sign (Figure 6-9).

Splenic pathology The spleen is often obscured by the lower ribs in the left mid-axillary line. It will appear kidney shaped with a homogeneous gray echo-texture. The small acoustic window between the ribs often limits the scope of view. By flattening out the swept gain control, the spleen may appear more uniform. The patient should be turned onto his/her right side and the probe aligned along the 9th-11th intercostal spaces. By having the patient hold his or her breath, the spleen may be pushed down into a better view. The splenic artery and vein run from the middle of the deep surface of the spleen.

Transabdominal ultrasound can be used to identify cysts, abscesses, and infarcts as well as to distinguish benign from malignant mass lesions of the spleen (Figure 6-10). A simple splenic cyst will usually appear as a thin-walled, anechoic, homogeneous structure within the parenchyma. More complex cysts or those with an infectious etiology can have septations, echogenic wall calcifications, or irregular wall thickening. There is often mixed echogenicity within the parenchyma due to tribeculation or hemorrhage. A common benign lesion found within the spleen is the hemangioma. These are most often small, solitary vascular lesions with a variety of ultrasound patterns depending on the type of hemangioma. Capillary hemangiomas are usually hyperechoic while the cavernous type is hypoechoic with a heterogeneous pattern and calcifications.

Renal tract pathology An adult kidney is between 8 and 13 cm long and 5 cm wide, surrounded by a renal capsule that appears as a dense linear echo at the periphery. The gray echogenic parenchyma of the cortex surrounds the hypoechoic renal pyramids in the medulla. The renal

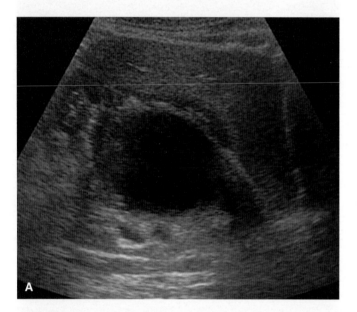

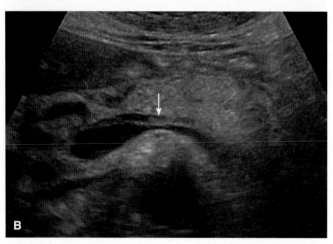

Figure 6-8. (A) Large pseudocyst in the body of the pancreas. (Used with permission from www.ultrasoundcases.info/Slide-View.aspx?cat=173&case=2679) ID: /13024.jpg; **(B)** Acute pancreatitis with edema between the pancreas and splenic vein (arrow) and a small peripancreatic effusion. (Used with permission from www.ultrasoundcases.info/Slide-View.aspx?cat=172&case=5563) ID: /40317-Afbeelding1.jpg

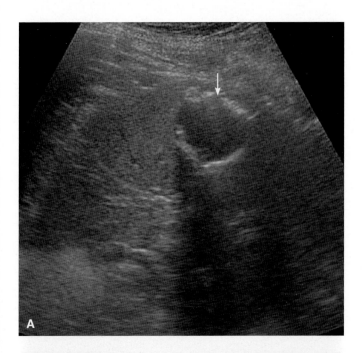

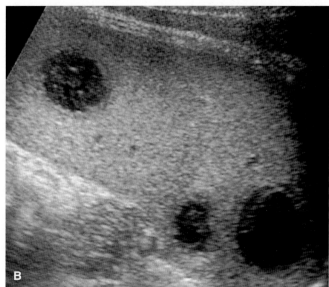

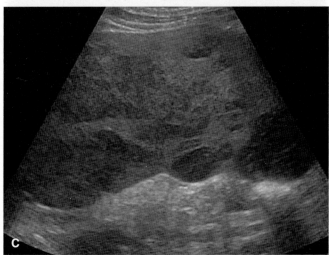

Figure 6-10. (**A**) Calcified splenic cyst (arrow). (Used with permission from www.ultrasoundcases.info/Slide-View. aspx?cat=176&case=3843) *ID: /21505.jpg;* (**B**) Multiple splenic abscesses. (Used with permission from www.ultrasoundcases. info/Slide-View.aspx?cat=176&case=3743) *ID: /20788. jpg;* (**C**) Malignant lymphoma with multiple vascularized hypoechoic splenic lesions and lymphadenopathy. (Used with permission from www.ultrasoundcases.info/Slide-View. aspx?cat=180&case=4069) *ID: /23400.jpg*

calyces and renal pelvis that comprise the renal sinus appear as central dense hyperechoic complexes (Figure 6-11).

The patient should be positioned in the anterior oblique or lateral position. Coronal images are obtained by placing the probe at the flank and sliding it posteriorly until the kidney comes into view. The liver can be used as an acoustic window on the right and the spleen on the left, moving the probe intercostally until the entire kidney is visualized. Kidney measurements can best be obtained with the patients lying prone. A cross-section of the kidney is obtained at the hilum to determine the width and depth. The dimension from the hilum to the posterior aspect of the kidney is obtained and the maximum dimension is determined at right angles to this.

Normal ureters are small and in a retroperitoneal location making them difficult to visualize using ultrasonography. Nondilated distal ureters can sometimes be seen as two small projections in the trigone, on either side of the midline of the posterior wall of the bladder. The lumen of the bladder is best seen when the bladder is distended, and should be scanned longitudinally and transversely by rocking the probe side to side to visualize the dome, the base, and the sidewalls. The bladder wall in adults is typically 3 mm thick when distended versus 5 mm when empty. The volume of the bladder can be estimated as can the degree of emptying by measuring the residual volume in the bladder.

Ultrasound techniques can be used to identify a number of pathologic conditions involving the urinary tract, including renal cysts, benign tumors of the bladder and kidney, renal and transitional cell carcinoma, nephrocalcinosis and nephrolithiasis (Figure 6-12). Kidneys that are obstructed by a mass or stone will have echo-free areas within the white, hyperechoic center, compressed renal parenchyma, and thinned renal pyramids. Renal or ureteral stones will appear as bright objects that cast shadows within the

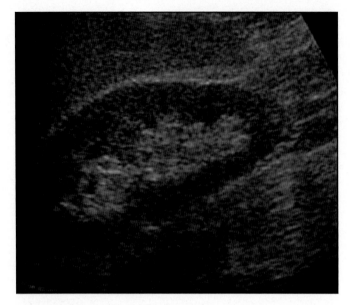

Figure 6-11. Longitudinal view of normal right kidney. (Used with permission from www.ultrasoundcases.info/Slide-View. aspx?cat=598&case=736) *ID: /3916.jpg*

kidney or dilated ureter. Renal cysts will often be single or multiple, smooth, well circumscribed, hypoechoic regions usually found at the periphery of the kidney (which differentiates them from hydronephrosis).

Advances in transabdominal ultrasound

Despite the considerable advances in ultrasound technique over the past decade, conventional B-mode ultrasound has a limited ability to detect blood flow at the tissue level. Over the past several years, contrast-enhanced ultrasound (CEUS) has emerged as a specialized imaging technique that enables dynamic, real-time evaluation of tissue perfusion. Utilizing microbubble contrast agents that enhance the Doppler signal within the bloodstream, CEUS can detect solid and hollow organ lesions that would otherwise be missed using conventional ultrasound.

CEUS has been most widely used throughout Europe and Asia for characterizing liver lesions and is shown to have 92% sensitivity and 86.7% specificity for detecting hepatocellular carcinoma.[16] CEUS can evaluate lesions in the arterial, portal-venous and late contrast phases and is comparable to CT or MRI for detecting isolated hepatic metastases (Figure 6-13). It can detect smaller masses than those typically seen on conventional ultrasound and can therefore provide a more accurate and timely diagnosis of metastatic disease.

Other advantages of CEUS include its ease of use and its relative safety compared to other imaging techniques. It is noninvasive, utilizes no ionizing radiation, and can be safely used in pregnant women, children, and patients with renal insufficiency. The use of CEUS will undoubtedly continue to expand and improve our accuracy for detecting pancreatic, kidney, splenic, breast, and lymph node pathology in the near future.

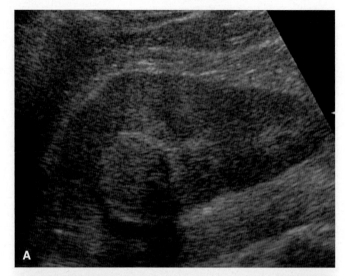

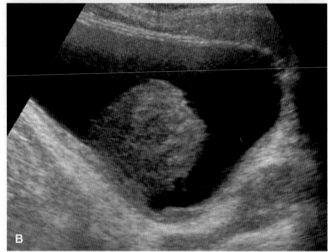

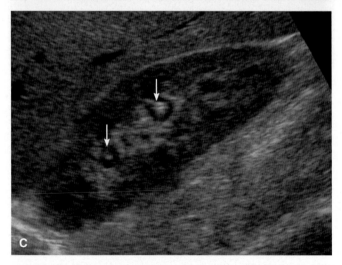

Figure 6-12. (**A**) Longitudinal view of renal cyst with multiple internal echos and calcified wall. (Used with permission from www.ultrasoundcases.info/*Slide-View.aspx?cat=238&case=694*) *ID: /3656.jpg;* (**B**) Large bladder carcinoma with bladder wall invasion (Used with permission from www.ultrasoundcases. info/*Slide-View.aspx?cat=245&case=3528*) *ID: /19504. jpg;* (**C**) Calyceal stones and ureteric stone (arrows) causing dilatation of the collecting system of the right kidney (Used with permission from www.ultrasoundcases.info/*Slide-View. aspx?cat=598&case=2780*) *ID: /13816.jpg*

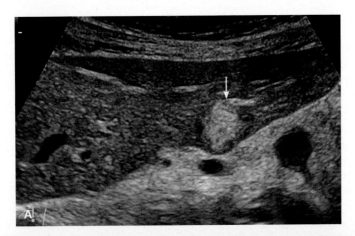

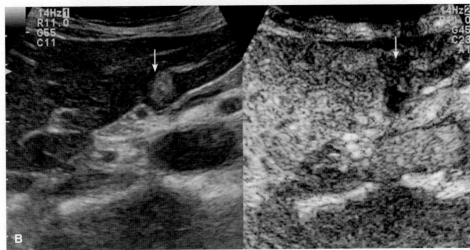

Figure 6-13. (**A**) Liver metastasis from a colon carcinoma with a hyperechoic lesion in the left lobe (arrow) (*Used with permission from www.ultrasoundcases.info/Slide-View. aspx?cat=144&case=3746*) *ID: /20808.jpg*; (**B**) Contrast-enhanced ultrasound image of same lesion shows it to be hypoechoic in the late phase, consistent with metastases (*Used with permission from www.ultrasoundcases.info/Slide-View.aspx?cat=144&case=3746*) *ID: /20812.jpg*

Advantages and limitations to transabdominal ultrasound

- A disease process that causes only microscopic changes in an organ structure will not be visible on ultrasound.
- Diagnostic accuracy can be affected by incorrect gain settings or image processing.
- False negative or false positive findings may be found when the patient is inadequately positioned or poor technique is employed.

▶ Intraoperative Ultrasound

Overview of intraoperative ultrasound

The first attempt at intraoperative ultrasound for identifying bile duct calculi occurred in the early 1960s utilizing A-mode ultrasound. Due to the difficulty in obtaining and interpreting the images, the technique did not gain widespread acceptance until the late 1970s when IOUS with real-time B-mode imaging was developed.[17] In 1977, the initial use of electronic linear array transducers for

intraoperative ultrasound examination of the liver and pancreas, together with real-time B-mode sector and linear IOUS, were introduced for a wide range of surgical procedures.[17] Hepatobiliary and pancreatic surgery in particular have benefitted from the introduction of IOUS, as it is one of the few ways to assess the liver parenchyma during surgery. This development has significantly influenced the operative decisions and therefore has had a major impact on the outcomes of surgery. Color Doppler imaging and laparoscopic ultrasound were incorporated into IOUS in the 1990s and further helped to guide intraoperative decision-making.

Intraoperative ultrasound provides real-time images without subjecting patients to unnecessary radiation. It quickly distinguishes between cystic and solid lesions and accurately assesses blood flow within solid organs. IOUS is also useful for obtaining biopsies of suspicious lesions by facilitating the placement of biopsy needles in the correct and safe plane. IOUS continues to be an indispensable method for diagnosing and staging of malignancies. It is gradually being introduced into the training curriculum of surgical residents.

General instrumentation and technique

Intraoperative ultrasound is best performed using B-mode ultrasound with high frequency linear-array or sector transducers. Transducer frequencies for IOUS range from 5 to 10 MHz, with 7.5 MHz being the most common.[18] A 5–10 MHz transducer penetrates less deeply than transducers at lower frequencies, but obtains greater resolution images, and can detect calculi and vascular lesions as small as 1mm.[18] Unlike the transabdominal approach, IOUS is applied directly to the surface of the organ being evaluated and does not need to penetrate the abdominal wall. Therefore, a higher frequency transducer with a depth of penetration of 6–8 cm is adequate during surgery.

For side-viewing of large, flat organs such as liver and pancreas, a flat T- or I-shaped probe is often used. End-viewing is best done using a small cylindrical probe that can scan small vessels and ductal structures. Intra-abdominal organs should be examined from both longitudinal and transverse planes, thereby eliminating the potential artifact from refraction and differentiating the organ of interest from nearby surfaces.

In order to examine deeper lesions within the parenchyma of an organ, the probe should be applied directly on the surface of the organ being evaluated (contact scanning) in a dry field.[1] A small amount of saline can be added for acoustic coupling between the probe and the tissue. For more superficial lesions or organ surfaces, the probe can be completely immersed in saline and positioned several centimeters away from the structure being examined (probe-standoff technique), placing the structure of interest at the focal distance of the transducer.[18] Compression scanning is another technique employed in IOUS whereby the probe is used to compress the tissue being examined in order to eliminate any air between the tissue and the transducer. This technique can be used when gas in the bowel obscures the view of other structures, or when it is necessary to distinguish between veins and arteries.

The area of interest should be scanned systematically, and a combination of longitudinal, transverse, and oblique views of the target lesion must be obtained. The longitudinal view is parallel to the long axis of any given structure, while the transverse view is at a right angle to the long axis. Lateral movement, rotation and angulation of the probe are various scanning maneuvers used to obtain real-time three-dimensional images.[1]

Indications for intraoperative ultrasound

Intraoperative ultrasound is a safe and rapid way to obtain information that cannot otherwise be obtained using standard preoperative imaging techniques or routine exploration. It can aid in localizing suspected lesions that are not visible on the CT scan or on the MRI; it is therefore useful for detecting occult metastases and determining the extent of tumor invasion. Intraoperative ultrasound is also a useful adjunct to intraoperative angiography during biliary and vascular surgery, with even higher accuracy for detecting ductal

calculi, intimal flaps, or thrombi. IOUS can also be used to confirm complete resection of tumors or lesions and to assess the patency of vascular reconstructions or anastomoses. In addition, IOUS can help guide diagnostic and therapeutic procedures such as biopsies, fine needle aspirations, and cannula placements for ablative procedures.

Typical appearance on intraoperative ultrasound

Although tumor appearance varies widely depending on its histology, size, and vascularity, tumors, in general, can have a hypochoic, hyperechoic, or mixed appearance. Even though intraoperative ultrasound cannot reliably distinguish between benign and malignant lesions, smaller malignancies are more often hypoechoic compared to the surrounding parenchyma and they can sometimes appear as target lesions, especially in solid organs such as liver.

Calculous lesions are characteristically echogenic with an anechoic posterior shadow caused by a difference in acoustic impedance from surrounding bile. Gallbladder calculi are usually mobile, while pancreatic and renal stones are often fixed. Simple cystic lesions are usually thin walled, anechoic, and demonstrate posterior enhancement due to an artifact from surrounding tissue.[19] A simple cyst with these features is most likely benign. Complex cysts can be associated with abscesses, hemorrhage or tumors, and typically appear septated, with irregular, thickened walls. They may or may not contain debris and should be aspirated or evaluated with other imaging modalities to rule out malignancy.

Evaluation of specific organ systems

Stomach and spleen Gastrointestinal tumors such as adenocarcinoma and lymphoma should be evaluated by high-frequency IOUS that demonstrates a layered appearance of the abdominal wall and can accurately detect the depth and lateral extent of tumor invasion. Surrounding structures including regional lymph nodes can be assessed for metastatic involvement and this information is used to help determine resectability and to guide in further management. When a splenic lesion is known or suspected based on preoperative imaging, IOUS can be used to determine whether it is solid or cystic, and to guide aspiration or biopsy of the lesion. When splenectomy is performed for malignancy, IOUS provides useful staging information and can help localize accessory spleens that are not otherwise visible or palpable intraoperatively.

Liver Makuuchi et al was the first to describe the use of intraoperative ultrasound for determining the resectability of hepatic tumors.[18] Unlike other diagnostic modalities such as CT scan and MRI, IOUS can detect smaller lesions within a cirrhotic liver, both prior to surgery and, most importantly, intraoperatively. It can further accurately determine the extent of tumor involvement and can therefore help define the extent of anatomic resection and provide the information on the best chance for negative margins. Detection of location and of tumor metastases is routinely practiced prior to resection or cryoablation to identify intrahepatic tumor deposits and to delineate the extent of resection or ablation that is required. Even though IOUS is less sensitive for detection of superficial lesions smaller than 1 cm in diameter, IOUS can assist surgeons to detect 35% more lesions than is achieved by liver palpation alone. When IOUS is combined with palpation, it further improves the accuracy for detection of hepatic lesions.[18]

More than 12% of patients with colorectal cancer that metastasized to the liver have lesions that are so small that they are only detectable on intraoperative ultrasound.[20,21] Although not used routinely in all colorectal cancer patients, IOUS is an excellent screening test, since it has a 90% sensitivity and specificity for detecting colorectal metastases.[20] The use of IOUS is currently limited to patients with locally advanced tumors, lymph node involvement, or recurrent colorectal cancer.

Intraoperative ultrasound of the liver is best performed using a T-shaped transducer that can access the lateral segments. Starting with the probe in a transverse orientation, each lobe is scanned carefully beginning with the left medial segment, looking for any intraparenchymal lesions or abnormalities. The normal parenchyma appears homogenous with echolucent holes representing the hepatic veins that join the vena cava. Colorectal, pancreatic, and gastric carcinomas metastatic to the liver often appear as well-defined hyperechoic lesions with a hypoechoic periphery that lacks the homogeneous ground-glass appearance of the liver parenchyma. The major hepatic veins and two major branches of the portal vein should also be visualized in order to define the lobar anatomy and to detect any tumor thrombus within the lumen. Submerging the porta hepatis in saline helps visualization of the biliary tree, including the common bile duct.

Biopsies or aspirations of intraparenchymal liver lesions can also be accomplished using intraoperative ultrasound. Ultrasound-guided radiofrequency ablation is increasingly being used in patients with unresectable primary, metastatic, or recurrent liver tumors to provide local control.[22] It is less invasive, safer, and has fewer complications than either surgical resection or cryoablation techniques.

Biliary system Evaluation of the biliary tree during laparoscopic cholecystectomy was among the first uses of laparoscopic ultrasound. Even though this is the most widely studied application of IOUS, it can also be used to determine the extent of biliary or gallbladder tumor invasion into the liver or surrounding vascular structures, as well as to guide biopsies of these structures to help determine resectability. End-viewing transducers are best used for visualization of the biliary tree due to the minimal contact required with ductal structures to obtain high-resolution images.

IOUS can accurately diagnose small biliary calculi with a sensitivity of 90–95% and a specificity of 98–99%, making it comparable to intraoperative cholangiography.[23] This is clearly an adequate and almost required screening method for choledocholithiasis.[18,23] The gallbladder is first imaged to visualize cholelithiasis and to adjust the ultrasound settings as necessary. The transducer is then positioned to obtain a transverse view of the portal triad at the level of the cystic duct. Ducts and vessels in this region have a distinct ultrasound appearance and anatomic relationship, enabling IOUS to identify aberrant or obscured ductal anatomy, guide dissection, and help to avoid iatrogenic injury to the ducts and surrounding structures during surgery.

Within the porta hepatis, the normal common bile duct appears as a thin walled structure with anechoic lumen that is located in an anterolateral position. The portal vein is posteromedial and displays a venous signal on Doppler flow detection. The hepatic artery is often interposed between the vein and common duct in an anteromedial position and appears pulsatile and noncompressible. Stones within the bile duct have an echogenic surface with posterior shadowing that point away from the ultrasound transducer. A common duct that contains stones may have a thickened wall and exhibit distal tapering before it enters the duodenum.

Disadvantages of IOUS include its inability to display the entire biliary tree at once. It is also less sensitive for evaluating bile duct strictures, fistulae, and injuries. In the setting of more complex biliary disease or equivocal IOUS results, intraoperative cholangiogram should also be performed in conjunction with IOUS.

Pancreas Intraoperative ultrasound can provide helpful information during the evaluation of a complicated pancreatitis, as well as localization of pancreatic neoplasm and of endocrine nodules such as islet cell tumors and can, thus, guide pancreatic procedures. Patients with pancreatitis can progress to develop pseudocysts, dilated pancreatic ducts, pancreatic abscesses, and splenic vein thrombosis. The diagnosis of these complications is facilitated by the use of IOUS, which can detect small lesions or subtle abnormalities, otherwise missed on preoperative imaging. IOUS can also be used to guide needle placement for cyst drainage procedures or biopsies, or for opening of small pseudocysts.

IOUS is particularly useful in assessing the extent of tumor invasion to the liver, portal system, and lymphatics, and for determining pancreatic tumor resectability during laparotomy.[18] In fact, IOUS can detect nonpalpable liver metastases and is more accurate than CT for detecting portal vein involvement.[18] The pancreas can be evaluated either transgastrically (if the stomach is decompressed), or directly by opening the lesser sac and placing the ultrasound probe directly on the pancreas. Any lesions within the parenchyma as well as the major vessels that course beneath it can be visualized.

Intraoperative ultrasound can also help localize small primary endocrine neoplasms that are often not seen on preoperative CT scan or MRI. Combining open exploration and palpation with intraoperative ultrasonography allows exact localization of tumors that have been regionalized preoperatively by intra-arterial calcium stimulation with hepatic venous sampling. Islet cell tumors appear hypoechoic on IOUS, making it possible to detect lesions as small as 3 mm that are not palpable or visible to the naked eye. In fact, IOUS has been found to detect and localize insulinomas and intrapancreatic gastrinomas with a sensitivity of 83–100%, and 95%, respectively, which is superior to that of preoperative angiography.[18,24] This is especially true for insulinomas located in the body and tail of the pancreas.

Advantages and limitations

- IOUS should be accomplished using a small flat or cylindrical probe with high-frequency linear array or convex transducers.
- IOUS provides multiplanar images from multiple locations providing more imaging information than conventional radiography.
- IOUS is more accurate than other preoperative imaging studies such as CT and MRI in detecting locoregional metastases and deep, nonpalpable lesions.
- IOUS can be accomplished rapidly with greater accuracy than conventional radiography and yields immediate results.
- IOUS can be used to guide diagnostic and therapeutic procedures and therefore has a wider applicability than intraoperative contrast radiography.
- The use of color or power Doppler imaging with IOUS facilitates image interpretation by clarifying vascular anatomy in relation to the lesion of interest.
- IOUS is less reliable for smaller lesions and will not detect lesions smaller than 3–5 mm.
- IOUS cannot detect tumors that are isoechoic to surrounding tissue.[16]
- IOUS is unable to display an entire ductal system or vascular tree in one image.
- IOUS should not be used in lieu of other intraoperative techniques, but as an adjunct to surgical exploration, palpation, and other appropriate radiographic modalities.

Future developments in intraoperative ultrasound

With ongoing advances in technology, the clinical applications of IOUS will continue to expand. Improved resolution and tissue penetration of IOUS will support its routine use in a wider range of surgical procedures. Despite ongoing improvements in the sensitivity of ultrasound, Doppler-based techniques cannot yet accurately detect low-velocity blood flow in smaller vessels. The future use of harmonic imaging with contrast agents will hopefully improve the use of color or power Doppler imaging to detect arterial enhancement of metastases. In fact, studies already show that intraoperative ultrasound with contrast is the most sensitive imaging modality for detection of deeper lesions as well as those that are smaller than 1 cm and are not visualized on CT or MRI.[25] Harmonic imaging with contrast is

already being used to provide angiography-like images of intracranial vascular pathology.

Further advances in three-dimensional (3D) imaging, including the use of contrast, will facilitate IOUS-guided tumor ablation and resection by providing better anatomical information. 3D imaging with contrast can further guide needle placement for radiofrequency ablation procedures and for biopsies, and improve the visualization of active lesions.

▶ Laparoscopic Ultrasound
Overview of laparoscopic ultrasound

Laparoscopic ultrasound (LUS) using an A-mode rigid probe to define the extent of a liver tumor was first reported in 1958.[26] Fukada et al first documented the use of real-time two-dimensional imaging for localizing intrahepatic lesions in 1984.[26] But it wasn't until laparoscopic cholecystectomy became popular in the early 1990s that laparoscopic ultrasonography began to evolve and be accepted. At the time, it was most commonly used for the evaluation of the biliary tract for stones and for masses during laparoscopic cholecystectomy. Its use has now been expanded to include staging of hepatic and pancreatic tumors during diagnostic laparoscopy and multiple other applications in gastric and hepatopancreaticobiliary surgery. The development of laparoscopic color Doppler imaging has also made it possible to rapidly differentiate between bile ducts and vascular structures and to determine the extent of vascular invasion by tumor, or the presence of tumor thrombus within a vessel.

General instrumentation and technique

Most current laparoscopic ultrasound devices consist of linear array 6–10 MHz transducers that are mounted on flexible or rigid probes and are connected to compact, real-time B-mode scanners. The probes must measure less than 10 mm to fit through a laparoscopic port and must range from 35 to 50 cm in length. Flexible probes can be bi- or quad-directional and are most often used for visualizing the liver, pancreas, and other retroperitoneal structures, while rigid probes are best used for examining the bile ducts. Rigid probes can also be used for transgastric imaging of the pancreas and for ultrasound-guided biopsies that require parallel alignment of the aspirating needle with the beam of the ultrasound waves.

During LUS, the transducer is apposed directly to the structure being imaged and the scanner can usually be controlled from the sterile field. Higher-frequency probes (10 MHz) are used to image structures closer to the transducer, while lower-frequency probes (7.5 MHz) are ideal for evaluating the liver, kidney, and other solid organs. Instruments that are capable of Doppler flow are ideal and usually include audible flow signals or flow wave patterns displayed on a screen. Color Doppler imaging was introduced in the 1990s and provides color-coded images of blood flow within vascular structures.

Indications for laparoscopic ultrasound

Although best known for its use in diagnosing choledo-cholithiasis, laparoscopic ultrasound can also be used to identify anatomic variations in the biliary tree and to help guide dissection during laparoscopic cholecystectomy. It can also aid in the detection of gastrointestinal tumors, guide biopsies of lesions, and help determine the extent of local neoplastic spread and invasion.

Evaluation of specific organ systems

Stomach and esophagus Laparoscopic ultrasound is currently part of the routine staging of upper GI malignancies. It is more accurate than CT or endoscopic ultrasound for assessing tumor stage, and for detecting carcinomatosis and metastatic lesions in the liver. It has been found to be useful in determining resection margins for primary gastric cancer, although it is less sensitive when recurrent cancer or gastric lymphomas are involved. Laparoscopic ultrasound can accurately detect metastatic disease and nodal involvement, and prevent unnecessary laparotomy in a significant number of patients, especially when combined with diagnostic laparoscopy. However, it can also downstage more advanced tumors by excluding the presence of direct invasion. Apart from adding no additional risk to diagnostic laparoscopy, it can be done quickly and does not increase patient morbidity.

The placement of three ports is generally required for adequate assessment of gastric malignancies, including a 10-mm port at the umbilicus, a 10- to 12-mm port in the right upper quadrant and a 5-mm port in the left upper quadrant. The anterior gastric wall is usually examined by placing the probe directly on the stomach and instilling saline for acoustic coupling. By compressing the stomach or filling the stomach with saline, the posterior wall can be visualized and assessed for masses or for posterior invasion of the pancreas. Tumors usually appear as hypoechoic masses that arise from the mucosa. A probe with a flexible tip is used to examine the liver parenchyma, celiac axis area, and hepatoduodenal ligament for metastases. It is also used to evaluate the presence of perigastric nodes, including those around the celiac trunk, splenic hilum, and aorta, to determine local invasion and to confirm resectability.

Liver and biliary tree Laparoscopic ultrasound is primarily used for staging of hepatocellular and metastatic colon cancer. It has also been found to effectively detect gallbladder carcinoma, cystic diseases, and other benign tumors of the liver, as well as tumors of the proximal common bile duct. Studies have also found LUS to be equivalent or superior to intraoperative cholangiography for diagnosing choledocholithiasis with a sensitivity of 90–96% and a specificity of 100%.[27,28] Compared to laparoscopic intraoperative cholangiography (IOC), laparoscopic ultrasound is less sensitive for detecting intrapancreatic common bile duct stones and identifying abnormal ductal anatomy. However, it can be done more rapidly and requires less dissection than is needed for IOC.

When laparoscopic ultrasonography and diagnostic laparoscopy are combined, the sensitivity and specificity for staging of hepatocellular carcinoma are reported to be 80–100% and 75–90%, respectively; this combination identifies almost 50% more liver lesions when compared to preoperative CT scan alone.[1,29,30] Even without diagnostic laparoscopy, laparoscopic ultrasound can provide additional staging information and thereby alter the management of liver tumors in more than 40% of cases.[30]

Laparoscopic ultrasound of the liver is best accomplished with a 6 MHz flexible probe introduced through ports at the umbilicus and right abdominal wall, in order to gain access to the anterior and superior surfaces of the liver.[1] The left lateral segment can be visualized via an additional left-sided port or by placing the transducer obliquely against the falciform ligament. The appearance of the liver and any other lesions is similar to that seen on open intraoperative ultrasound.

For laparoscopic ultrasound of the biliary tree the port placement is similar to that used during laparoscopic cholecystectomy. This usually requires placement of a 10-mm port below the xiphoid or subcostally between the mid- and anterior axillary line in order to obtain transverse imaging of the porta hepatis. The junction of the cystic duct and common duct can be seen by sweeping the probe along the lateral edge of the hepatoduodenal ligament. The transducer can also be placed directly over the bile duct following retraction of the liver, superiorly. Orienting the probe transversely in the middle of the CBD produces a cross-sectional image of the hepatic artery, portal vein, and common duct that has a very characteristic appearance (Figure 6-14).[31] The portal vein is the largest, most posteriorly located structure within the portal triad. The hepatic artery lies anterior and to the left of the portal vein, while on cross-sectional imaging, the common bile duct lies anterior to the portal vein and to the left of the proper hepatic artery.

To obtain longitudinal images the flexible probe can also placed through an umbilical port. This permits scanning of the liver and visualization of the common bile duct medial to the gallbladder. This view also facilitates imaging of the proximal intrahepatic ducts and of the porta hepatis from a posterior position.

Pancreas Despite extensive diagnostic workup, the majority of patients with pancreatic cancer are found to have unresectable disease at the time of surgery. Even with advanced preoperative imaging techniques, 20–70% of patients will undergo nontherapeutic laparotomy.[32] Diagnostic laparoscopy has therefore become an important tool in the accurate staging of pancreatic cancer. Laparoscopic ultrasound can improve the results of staging by compensating for the lack of tactile information that laparoscopy alone can provide. A recent meta-analysis demonstrated that the routine combined use of laparoscopy with laparoscopic ultrasound can prevent up to 50% of unnecessary laparotomies, thereby expediting the commencement of alternative treatments following a low risk, minimally invasive procedure.[32]

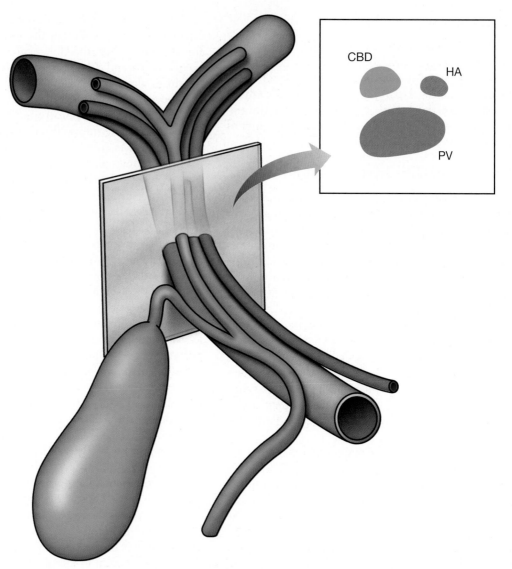

Figure 6-14. Schematic view of the hepatoduodenal ligament showing characteristic appearance of the portal triad during laparoscopic ultrasound (CBD = common hepatic duct; HA = hepatic artery; PV = portal vein). (Adapted from Holzheimer RG, Mannick JA. *Surgical Treatment: Evidence Based and Problem-Oriented.* W. Zuckschwerdt Verlag GmbH; 2001.)

Pancreatic cancer is considered unresectable when there is metastatic tumor in the liver, or if there is involvement of celiac lymph nodes or invasion of the celiac, hepatic, or superior mesenteric arteries. With the use of color Doppler signals, laparoscopic ultrasound can identify occult metastatic disease and predict tumor resectability with an accuracy of 98%.[33] LUS has also been found to identify unresectable disease in up to 28% of patients whose lesions were missed on diagnostic laparoscopy alone, with less than 10% false negative rate.[30] One report found that diagnostic laparoscopy combined with laparoscopic ultrasound is more sensitive than many other diagnostic modalities for the detection of liver and peritoneal metastases.[34] Compared to diagnostic laparoscopy, laparoscopic ultrasound is better for assessing tumor size and for detecting small liver metastases that are missed on inspection and other imaging studies alone.[34]

Laparoscopic ultrasound assessment of the pancreas usually requires a single port placement in the umbilical region or right lateral abdominal wall. The body and tail of the pancreas can be visualized by placing the probe on the anterior wall of the stomach. The head of the pancreas is best seen directly via the lesser sac by opening the gastrocolic ligament and placing the probe on the surface of the pancreas. Alternatively, the head can be seen by compressing the walls of the duodenum with the probe. The normal pancreas appears homogeneous with a ground-glass appearance, while most pancreatic lesions appear as ill-defined hypoechoic masses.[1] If a thorough inspection reveals no metastatic disease, a more detailed examination is performed to inspect the liver parenchyma, portal vein, mesenteric vessels, celiac trunk, hepatic artery, peripancreatic, and periportal lymph nodes. For intraoperative localization of pancreatic insulinomas thought to be located at the head or neck of the pancreas, a laparoscopic Kocher maneuver can be performed allowing positioning of the probe posterior to the uncinate process.

The morbidity of LUS for the evaluation of pancreatic cancer ranges from 0% to 4% and is primarily related to the risk of wound infection and port-site bleeding. This is often balanced by the shorter hospital length of stay associated with laparoscopic staging and LUS compared to open exploration.[30]

Kidney and adrenal Laparoscopic ultrasound can help localize and guide the intraoperative drainage and decortication of renal cysts as well as lymphoceles after kidney transplantation. It has also been used to help guide radiofrequency ablation of renal tumors. LUS can identify deeper structures not seen on inspection or laparoscopy alone and thereby decrease the incidence of iatrogenic injury to the kidney and surrounding structures. It can lead to a decrease in length of hospital stay and local infections of the fluid collections compared to open drainage of lymphoceles and renal cysts, as well as a decrease in postoperative pain.

Laparoscopic ultrasound can also be used to localize the adrenal gland (which can be difficult to visualize in the adipose tissue of the retroperitoneum) and surrounding vasculature during laparoscopic adrenalectomy. The use of laparoscopic ultrasound during adrenal surgery requires a 12-mm camera port to allow passage of the flexible ultrasound probe. Retracting the liver anteriorly and dividing the posterior peritoneal attachments of the liver exposes the superior portion of the right adrenal gland, while the left adrenal can be visualized after medial rotation of the spleen. Neoplastic lesions of the adrenal gland appear hypoechoic relative to other structures and they have a hyperechoic rim.

Advantages and limitations

- LUS combined with staging laparoscopy has a higher success in diagnosing patients with locally advanced pancreatic cancer compared to other types of periampullary tumors.

- The advantages of laparoscopic ultrasound include the ability to accurately determine the extent of tumor invasion and to plan the operative approach on the basis of this information.

- Even though laparoscopic ultrasound can help guide appropriate treatment for locally advanced disease, false negative studies may lead to unnecessary laparotomies and therefore increased morbidity and cost to the patient.

- The diagnostic yield of LUS is operator-dependent and has a steep learning curve; it is also influenced by tumor histology, size, and location.

REFERENCES

1. Machi J, Sigel B. *Ultrasound for Surgeons*. New York: Igaku-Shoin; 1997.
2. Puylaert JBCM. *Ultrasound of Appendicitis and Its Differential Diagnoses*. Berlin and Heidelberg: Springer;1990.
3. Imaging Signs in Diagnostic Radiology. Available at: http://imagingsign.wordpress.com. Accessed on 2012 May 30.
4. Lim HK, Lee WJ, Kim TH, Namgung S, Lee SJ, Lim JH. Appendicitis: usefulness of color Doppler US. *Radiology*. 1996;201(1):221–225.
5. Quillin SP, Siegel MJ. Appendicitis: efficacy of color Doppler sonography. *Radiology*. 1994; 191(2):557–560.
6. Walker S, Haun W, Clark J. The value of limited computer tomography with rectal contrast in the diagnosis of acute appendicitis. *Am J Surg*. 2000;180:450–455.
7. Horton MD, Counter SF, Florence MG. A prospective trial of computed tomography and ultrasonography for diagnosing appendicitis in the atypical patient. *Am J Surg*. 2000;179:379–381.
8. Morris KT, Kavanagh M, Hansen P. The rational use of computed tomography scans in the diagnosis of appendicitis. *Am J Surg*. 2002;183:547–550.
9. Meiser G. Gastrointestinale Ultrasschalldiagnostik: Chirurgische Bedeutung fassbarer Befunde. *Ultraschall Klin Prax*. 1987;2:137–145.
10. Holt S, Samuel E. Multiple concentric ring sign in the ultrasonographic diagnosis of intussusception. *Gastrointest Radiol*. 1978;3:307–309.
11. Radiologyinfo.org. Available at: http://www.radiologyinfo.org/en/photocat/gallery3.cfm?image=bowel-us-intussusception.jpg&pg=intussusception. Accessed on 2012 May 30.
12. Phillips G, Dimitrievea Z. Sonographic diagnosis of thrombosis of the superior mesenteric vein and small bowel infarction. *J Ultrasound Med*. 1985;4:565–571.
13. McGahan JP, Lindfors KK. Percutaneous cholecystostomy. An alternative to surgical cholecystectomy in acute cholecystitis? *Radiology*. 1989;136:725–728.
14. Gutman H, Landau O, Deutsch AA. Acute calculous cholecystitis versus acute acalculous cholecystitis: Review 1970-1988. *Digestive Surgery*. 1989; 9:121–132.
15. Rubens D. Ultasound imaging of the biliary tract. *Ultrasound Clin*. 2007;2:391–413.
16. Wilson S, Greenbaum L, Goldberg B. Contrast-enhanced ultrasound: what is the evidence and what are the obstacles? *AJR*. 2009;193:55–60.
17. Makuuchi M., et al. History of intraoperative ultrasound. *Ultrasound in Medicine and Biology*. 1998;24:1229–1242.
18. Machi J, et al. Intraoperative ultrasound. *Surg Clin N Am*. 2004;84:1085–1111.
19. Harness JK, Wisher DB. *Ultrasound in Surgical Practice: Basic Principles and Clinical Applications*. New York: Wiley-Liss, Inc.; 2001.
20. Kulig J, Popiela T, Kłęk S, Milanowski W, Kołodziejczyk P, Szybiński P. Intraoperative ultrasonography in detecting and assessment of colorectal liver metastases. *Scandin J Surg*. 2007;96:51–55.
21. Goletti O, Celona G, Galatioto C, Viaggi B, Lippolis PV, Pieri L, Cavina E. Is laparoscopic sonography a reliable and sensitive procedure for staging colorectal cancer? *Surg Endosc*. 1998;12:1236–1241.
22. Machi J, et al. Ultrasound-guided radiofrequency thermal ablation of liver tumors: percutaneous, laparoscopic, and open surgical approaches. *J Gastrointest Surg*. 2001;5: 477–489.
23. Sigel B, et al. Comparative accuracy of operative ultrasonography and cholangiography in detecting common bile duct calculi. *Surgery*. 1983;94:715–720.

24. Lo CY, Lo CM, Fan ST. Role of laparoscopic ultrasonography in intraoperative localization of pancreatic insulinoma. *Surg Endosc.* 2000;14(12):1131–1135.

25. Leen, E et al. Potential value of contrast enhanced intraoperative ultrasonography during partial hepatectomy for metastases: an essential investigation before resection? *Ann Surg.* 2006;243(2):236–240.

26. Machi J, et al. Operative ultrasound in general surgery. *Am J Surgery.* 1996;172:15–20.

27. Tranter SE, Thompson MH. A prospective single-blinded controlled study comparing laparoscopic ultrasound of the common bile duct with operative cholangiography. *Surg Endosc.* 2003;17(2):216-219.

28. Ohtani T, Kawai C, Shirai Y, Kawakami K, Yoshida K, Hatakeyama K. Intraoperative ultrasonography versus cholangiography during laparoscopic cholecystectomy: a prospective comparative study. *J Am Coll Surg.* 1997;185:274–282.

29. Santambrogio R, et al. Survival and intra-hepatic recurrences after laparoscopic radiofrequency of hepatocellular carcinoma in patients with liver cirrhosis. *J Surg Oncol.* 2005;89(4):218–225.

30. Society of American Gastrointestinal and Endoscopic Surgeons (SAGES). "Guidelines for the Use of Laparoscopic Ultrasound." Publ Mar 2009. Available at: http://www.sages.org/publication/id/36/. Accessed 2012 June.

31. Schirmer BD. Intra-operative and laparoscopic ultrasound. In: Holzheimer RG, Mannick JA, eds. *Surgical Treatment: Evidence-Based and Problem-Oriented.* Munich: Zuckschwerdt; 2001.

32. Hariharan D, et al. The role of laparoscopy and laparoscopic ultrasound in the preoperative staging of pancreatico-biliary cancers – a meta-analysis. *EJSO.* 2010;36:941–948.

33. Patel AC, Arregui ME. Current status of laparoscopic ultrasound. *Surg Technol Int.* 2006;15:23–31.

34. Catheline JM, et al. The use of diagnostic laparoscopy supported by laparoscopic ultrasonography in the assessment of pancreatic cancer. *Surg Endosc.* 1999;13(3):239–245.

HEPATOBILIARY ULTRASOUND

MICHAEL R. MARVIN, CHRISTOPHER M. JONES, JEROME A. BYAM, & DAVID A. IANNITTI

Ultrasound (US) plays a critical role in the evaluation and management of patients with hepatobiliary disorders. Diagnostically, US is able to identify common illnesses related to cholelithiasis, including acute cholecystitis and choledocholithiasis. It is the optimal test for detection of biliary dilation, and is also a mainstay of screening for hepatobiliary malignancies and other liver masses (eg, cystic vs. solid lesions). US also plays a vital role in therapy for hepatic disorders, particularly in guiding surgical resection and ablational therapies. Because of its widespread applicability, facility and familiarity with US are important to all physicians involved in the management of hepatobiliary disease. Indications, technique, normal and abnormal findings, and therapeutic maneuvers applicable to US will be discussed in the following pages.

CLINICAL INDICATIONS FOR ULTRASOUND

a. Investigation of right upper quadrant pain, particularly when there is suspicion for symptomatic cholelithiasis

b. Investigation of abnormal liver function tests. Specifically, US may demonstrate dilation of the bile ducts in the setting of extrahepatic biliary obstruction, or can identify the stigmata of chronic liver disease

c. Screening for hepatocellular carcinoma in cirrhotic patients

d. Assessment of hepatic vasculature to aid in the planning of liver resection

e. Guidance (either transcutaneous or intraoperative) for ablative therapy or biopsy

f. Intraoperative assessment of tumor anatomy with respect to vasculature

g. Detection of venous or hepatic arterial thrombosis after liver transplantation

h. Identification of intraperitoneal hemorrhage in cases of suspected hepatic trauma (Focused Assessment with Sonography in Trauma, FAST)

i. Assessment of portal hypertension

NORMAL ANATOMY

► Segmental Anatomy of the Hepatic Parenchyma

An understanding of the segmental anatomy of the liver is fundamental to modern radiological investigation and surgical management of hepatic malignancy (Figure 7-1). The classification was first described in 1957 by the French surgical anatomist Couinaud, and later popularized by Bismuth and is globally recognized.[1] The eight hepatic segments are divided into those constituting the right hemiliver (segments V–VIII), the left hemiliver (segments II–IV), and the caudate lobe (segment I). The right and left hemilivers are separated in the functional midline by the plane of the principal fissure between the gallbladder fossa and the inferior vena cava (IVC) (Cantlie Line). This plane is defined by the course of the middle hepatic vein, and has no external markings. In the left lobe of the liver, the plane formed by the umbilical fissure divides the left lateral sector (segments II and III) from the left medial sector (segment IV). The medial sector is divided into segments IVA superiorly and IVB inferiorly. In the right lobe of the liver the plane formed by the right hepatic vein and the IVC divides the right anterior sector (segments V and VIII) from the right posterior sector (segments VI and VII).

► Vascular Anatomy

The inferior vena cava courses to the right of the aorta in the retroperitoneum. Prior to ascending posterior to the liver, the IVC lies posterior and lateral to the duodenum

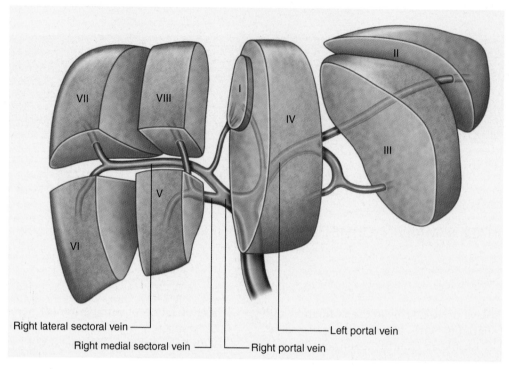

Figure 7-1. The segmental anatomy of the liver with the tributaries of the portal vein. (Ellis H. Anatomy of the liver. *Surgery (Oxford).* 2011;29(12):589–592.)

and head of the pancreas. The retrohepatic portion of the IVC lies on the posterior surface of the right lobe of the liver, and ascends to the central tendon of the diaphragm behind the bare area of the liver, prior to entering the right atrium. There are three major hepatic veins that enter directly into the inferior vena cava at the superior surface of the posterior liver (Figure 7-2). The right hepatic vein is the shortest of these and lies in the plane dividing the right hemiliver into the anterior and posterior sectors. The length of the right hepatic vein is

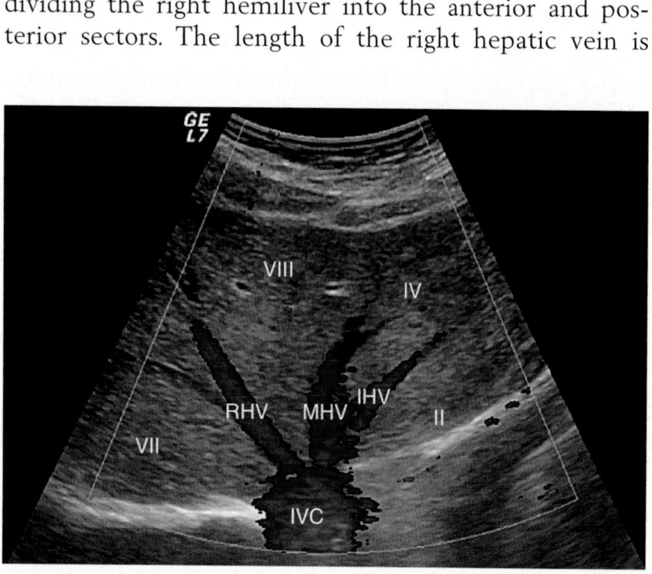

Figure 7-2. Hepatic veins. Transverse diagram of the liver shows the right hepatic vein (RHV), middle hepatic vein (MHV), and left hepatic vein (LHV) draining into the retrohepatic inferior vena cava (IVC). The hepatic veins divide the liver into Couinaud system segments as indicated.

typically only 1 cm. The middle hepatic vein lies in the plane separating the liver into the right and left lobes (aka, portal fissure, Cantlie line), and commonly joins the left hepatic vein outside the liver parenchyma to enter the IVC as a common trunk, although it may drain directly into the vena cava.[1] The left hepatic vein lies in the umbilical fissure separating the left liver into segment IV and the left lateral sector (segments II and III) and has a relatively long extrahepatic course. As described above, the left hepatic vein typically, though not always, joins the middle hepatic vein prior to entering the vena cava.

The proper hepatic artery arises from the common hepatic artery after branching of the gastroduodenal artery and ascends superiorly toward the liver in the lateral free edge of the lesser omentum with the common bile duct and portal vein, the portal triad. Typically the hepatic artery lies anterior to the portal vein and medial to the bile duct in this region. The hepatic artery then divides into branches that supply the right and left liver at the level of the hepatic hilum. The right hepatic artery typically follows a very short extrahepatic course before entering the hepatic parenchyma, where it further divides into right anterior and posterior sectoral branches. The cystic artery supplying the gallbladder arises from the right hepatic artery. The left hepatic artery follows a longer extrahepatic course where it runs to the base of the umbilical fissure. The left hepatic artery then gives off a branch to segment IV known as the middle hepatic artery, and then enters the left lateral segment to supply segments II and III. The caudate lobe (segment I) is also typically supplied by branches of the left hepatic artery.

There are several common anatomic variants of hepatic arterial anatomy that are worth noting. The right hepatic artery may arise directly from the superior mesenteric artery, in which case it is described as being a replaced right hepatic artery. Alternatively, an accessory right hepatic artery may arise from the same location. A replaced right hepatic artery can be identified as a pulsatile structure ascending to the right of, and posterior to, the common bile duct within the portal triad. Similarly, a replaced or accessory left hepatic artery may arise from the left gastric artery and run through the gastrohepatic ligament to supply the left lobe of the liver. Anomalous right hepatic arterial anatomy is present in 10–20% of patients, while anomalies in the course of the left hepatic artery are present in 7–18% of patients.[2]

The portal vein arises from the union of the superior mesenteric and splenic veins posterior to the neck of the pancreas. The portal vein then ascends toward the liver as the most posterior structure of the portal triad. The portal vein branches into segments supplying the left and right lobes of the liver at the hilum. The course of the portal vein follows that of the hepatic arteries within the liver, and the branch points of the portal triads within the liver define the hepatic segments.

▶ Biliary Anatomy

Within the liver, the bile ducts follow the course of the hepatic arterial and portal venous branches within portal triads. The extrahepatic right and left ducts join at the hepatic hilum to form the common hepatic duct. The common hepatic duct descends to the right of the hepatic artery and anterior to the portal vein. Typically, the right hepatic artery passes posterior to the common hepatic duct, but an important variant is passage of the right hepatic artery anterior to the duct. The common hepatic duct is joined by the cystic duct, which drains the gallbladder, at which point it is known as the common bile duct. The level of union between the cystic and common hepatic ducts can be highly variable. While the classic anatomy is for the cystic duct to enter the common duct obliquely on the right, common variants include a cystic duct that runs parallel to the common duct for a variable course prior to union, and a cystic duct that spirals posteriorly to the common duct before entering on the left. Inferiorly, the common bile duct passes posterior to the pancreas where it is joined by the pancreatic duct to form a common channel draining into the duodenum. The blood supply to the common bile duct is via the hepatic artery and typically courses in the 9 o'clock and 3 o'clock positions. It should be noted that anomalies from the "typical" pattern described above are frequent and must always be considered during surgical dissection.

▶ Gallbladder

The gallbladder lies in a fossa on the inferior surface of the liver between segments IV and V. Typically, the gallbladder is completely extrahepatic with a fibrous attachment to the liver bed known as the cystic plate. The gallbladder may occasionally be intrahepatic, that is, surrounded by varying degrees of hepatic parenchyma, or it may be attached to a longer gallbladder mesentery. The gallbladder comprises the fundus most superiorly, body, and neck (or infundibulum). The cystic duct arises from the gallbladder neck and courses medially to join the common hepatic duct, most commonly in an angle to the lateral surface of the hepatic duct. The cystic duct may run parallel to the common hepatic duct before joining, however, and it may spiral around the hepatic duct, prior to entering. There are less common variants in which the cystic duct may enter the hepatic ductal confluence, or into branches of the right or left hepatic ducts. The blood supply to the gallbladder is the cystic artery, which is typically a branch of the right hepatic artery. The typical location for the cystic artery is within the triangle of Calot, the borders of which are the cystic duct inferiorly, the liver bed superiorly, and the common hepatic duct medially.

NORMAL APPEARANCE OF US

The normal liver is homogeneous in appearance. The echogenicity of the liver should be slightly greater than that of the cortex of the right kidney.[3] Distinguishing portal veins from hepatic veins within the liver parenchyma may be somewhat of a challenge to the novice ultrasonographer. The distinction can be made by the echogenicity of the vessel walls (Figure 7-3). Portal veins typically have hyperechoic walls (as they are invested by Glisson capsule), and thus appear bright, while hepatic veins do not have reflective walls.[4] Once the hepatic and portal veins are identified, the ultrasonographer can define the various segments of the liver as defined by their relation to the hepatic venous and portal venous structures as described above.

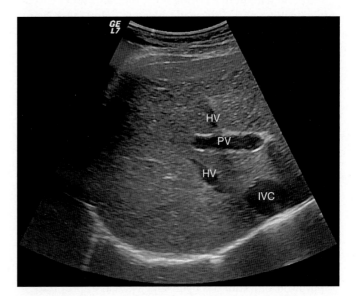

Figure 7-3. Hepatic veins (HV) and inferior vena cava (IVC) are anechoic structures with very thin walls. The portal vein (PV) has echogenic walls that appear brighter on sonographic examination.

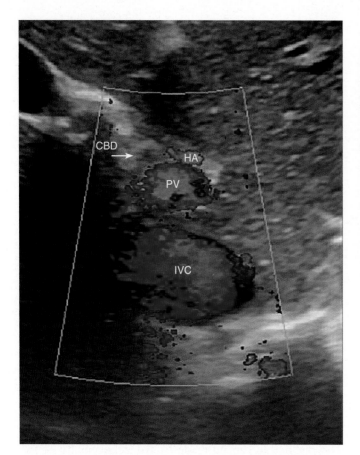

Figure 7-4. The "mickey mouse" sign is made up of the three portal structures. The left ear is the hepatic artery (HA), the right ear (at the arrow tip) is the common bile duct (CBD), and the portal vein is the face.

Intrahepatic ducts, when normal in diameter, are not visualized on transcutaneous US.

With the patient in a fasting state, the gallbladder is typically anechoic with thin walls. Normal gallbladder diameter is typically 3–4 cm, with length up to 10 cm.[3] An anatomic aid in identifying the gallbladder includes the main lobar fissure of the liver, which appears as a linear echogenic structure and points toward the gallbladder neck. In addition, the hepatic artery can sometimes be seen anteromedial to the portal vein with the common bile duct anterolateral to the portal vein, forming the so called "Mickey Mouse" sign (see Figure 7-4).[5] The normal thickness of the gallbladder wall in the fasting state is less than 3 mm.[6,7] If the patient is not in the fasting state; however, the gallbladder will be contracted, which may appear as wall thickening. The normal size of the common bile duct is dependent upon the patient's age, as the CBD is known to dilate over time.[8] Normal CBD diameter is considered to be up to 6 mm, although this figure may need to be revised upward in the elderly (Figure 7-5). An upper limit of 8 mm has been suggested as appropriate in patients over 50.[9] Another important consideration is the postcholecystectomy patient as the CBD typically dilates after cholecystectomy.[10,11] A diameter of up to 10 mm

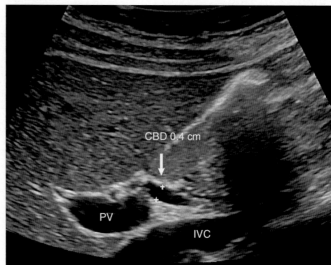

Figure 7-5. Long axis view of the portal vein (PV) demonstrates the normal common bile duct (CBD). The PV can be seen coursing toward the porta hepatis with a portion of the nondistended CBD above. The inferior vena cava (IVC) is seen immediately below.

has been suggested as appropriate in the postcholecystectomy setting,[9] but larger diameters can be seen in the absence of other pathology (Figure 7-6).

SCANNING TECHNIQUES

▶ Transabdominal US

Transabdominal US of the liver, gallbladder, and biliary tree is typically performed with a 2.5–5.0 MHz sector or

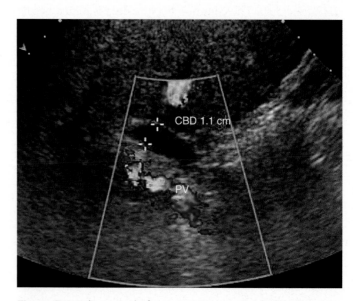

Figure 7-6. Ultrasound of a patient 1 year postcholecystectomy. The common bile duct is dilated to compensate for an absent gallbladder. This is a normal duct variant postcholecystectomy. Dilated ducts are also seen in older patients without a cholecystectomy.

convex probe. Ideally the patient will be fasting to minimize bowel gas and insure a physiologically distended gallbladder. The scan should begin with the probe placed longitudinally along the right costal margin, so that the posterior right lobe of the liver and the right kidney can be visualized. The depth of penetration of ultrasound waves can be adjusted and should be such that the posterior right lobe is at the bottom of the screen.[12] The probe is then placed in a transverse plane below the xiphoid process. The patient is asked to hold his breath, to allow the diaphragm to push the liver down toward the probe, and the probe is angled cephalad to visualize the superior portion of the liver. The junction of the hepatic veins with the inferior vena cava can be seen only through this window. The probe is then moved caudally, while remaining in the transverse configuration. At this point the left portal vein can be visualized as a tubular anechoic structure with hyperechoic walls. The left portal vein should be the only tubular structure visualized within the liver on this view. The presence of other structures suggests intrahepatic biliary dilatation. The probe is then moved further in the caudal direction along the right costal margin. The portal vein as it enters the liver can now be seen, and again should be the only tubular structure visualized. The presence of another tubular structure, the so-called "shotgun" sign,[13,14] indicates extrahepatic biliary ductal dilatation. The probe is then moved further along the costal margin of the ribs until the gallbladder can be visualized, which will appear as an anechoic round structure inferior to the portal vein, and then along the costal margin past the gallbladder to examine the right posterior sector.

After the right posterior sector has been examined, the probe is returned to the subxiphoid position, this time in the longitudinal configuration. The probe is slid caudally along the costal margin as described above. This sweep of the probe will allow visualization of the right, left, and caudate lobes, the aorta, and the inferior vena cava. The scan should progress from the xiphoid until the image has moved past the liver to the right kidney.

After examination of the liver has been completed, attention is then turned to the gallbladder, which is seen in the longitudinal plane at the level of the supine patient's elbow just below the costal margin. The gallbladder will appear as an anechoic, ovoid structure with a tapering neck (Figure 7-7). After thoroughly examining the gallbladder in the longitudinal plane, the probe is rotated to the transverse position without losing contact with the patient's skin. After passing the probe through the gallbladder several times, the patient is placed in the left lateral decubitus position and the gallbladder is reimaged using the technique above. Decubitus positioning of the patient will cause stones to move into the gallbladder fundus, aiding in visualization.

Visualization of the common hepatic duct is aided by having the patient in a 45 degree, right side up position. The probe is placed halfway down the costal margin in the transverse plane. After identification of the portal vein, the

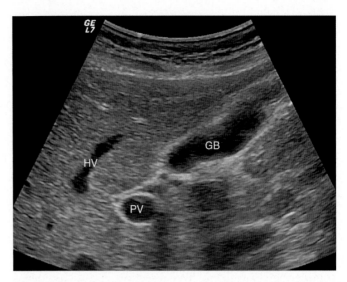

Figure 7-7. Long axis view of normal gallbladder (GB). The main lobar fissure is seen between the GB neck and the right portal vein (PV).

probe is rotated to the transverse position, again without losing contact with the patient's skin. The portal vein will change from a horizontal structure to a circle as the probe rotates. The common hepatic duct will come into view as a tubular structure anterior to the portal vein. Measurement of the common hepatic duct should be from inside wall to inside wall (Figure 7-8).[3]

THERAPEUTIC MANEUVERS

Intraoperative US plays a pivotal role in hepatic surgery, including detection and localization of lesions and planning of hepatic resection. Ultrasound is essential when performing liver-directed therapy for resection or ablation. Although modern cross-sectional imaging such as

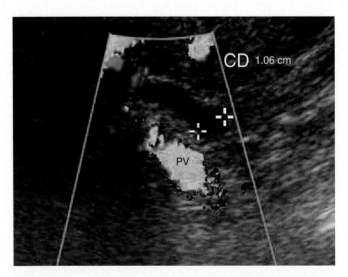

Figure 7-8. Common hepatic duct is seen here as a tubular structure anterior to the portal vein (PV). The common duct diameter is measured from inside wall to inside wall.

CT scans and MRIs are highly sensitive, there is still an incidence of additional lesions found by intraoperative ultrasound that are not visualized by preoperative imaging. This incidence can range up to 20% of patients.

IOUS allows evaluation of the relationship between tumor and the hepatic veins, thus allowing for determination of the amount of liver parenchyma that must be resected. Such determination is particularly important in patients with cirrhosis, in whom it is critical to leave an adequate liver remnant postoperatively. In this setting, IOUS allows greater use of segmental resection rather than formal anatomic lobectomy.[42,43] The value of IOUS in operative planning has been demonstrated by reports that have revealed changes in surgical management of hepatic tumors due to sonographic findings in 30% to 50% of operations.[17,44-47] Facility with IOUS is particularly crucial when considering laparoscopic liver resection, and is considered a mandatory part of the surgeon's skill set prior to starting a laparoscopic liver program. In addition to aiding in planning for hepatic resection, IOUS may also detect occult hepatic metastases during colorectal surgery in 5–10% of operations.[17,48]

US is also widely used for guidance in the ablation of hepatic tumors. Thermal ablation, either with radiofrequency (RF) or with microwave (MW) energy has become an important part of the treatment algorithm for patients with unresectable tumors. These procedures may be performed percutaneously, laparoscopically, or at the time of laparotomy. US has become the ideal method for proper localization of the ablation probes, as it gives real-time information on proper placement. Typically, lesions will become hyperechoic as ablation progresses, although assessment of ablation margins by US is limited. These approaches are highly operator dependent, and require a high degree of facility with US on the part of the surgeon.[49]

▶ Intraoperative Ultrasound

Intraoperative US (IOUS) of the hepatobiliary tree can be performed either laparoscopically or via an open approach. The transducers used for IOUS may vary depending on the technique and are typically of higher frequency than employed for transcutaneous ultrasound, generally in the range of 7–8 MHz (Figure 7-9).[15-17] The use of such high-frequency probes allows for visualization of subcentimeter lesions. Probes for IOUS are typically either flat or cylindrical. The flat probes provide a wide field of view and are particularly well suited for imaging the liver. Probes with a flexible tip that can be articulated or flexed and extended to allow the user to maintain contact on the curved liver surface for optimal visualization are also particularly useful, especially in the laparoscopic setting.

There are two basic techniques utilized. One is the "lawn mower" technique (Figure 7-10) where the ultrasound transducer is swept back and forth across each sector of the liver in a systematic fashion. The second is the "pedicle tracking" technique (Figure 7-11) where the transducer

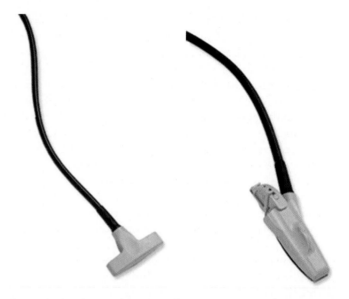

Figure 7-9. Ultrasound probes for intraoperative ultrasound.

is used to identify the main portal pedicle and then the left and right branches of the portal venous system are followed out through their sectoral and segmental branching points. Ultrasound is then used to map out the location of the hepatic veins as they track and drain into the inferior vena cava. Rotation of the probe in clockwise or counterclockwise direction, along with superior and inferior angulation ("rocking"), allows for structures to be followed and masses outlined with precision.

US imaging of the gallbladder and extrahepatic biliary tree is best performed by a saline immersion technique. In this method, the subhepatic space is filled with saline solution. A 7.5 MHz probe is utilized for optimal resolution.

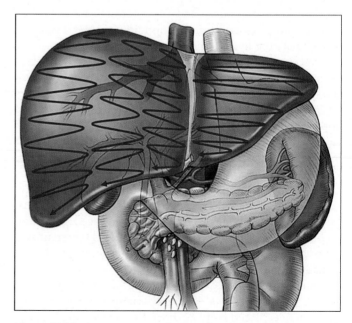

Figure 7-10. Lawnmower technique for ultrasound imaging of the liver.

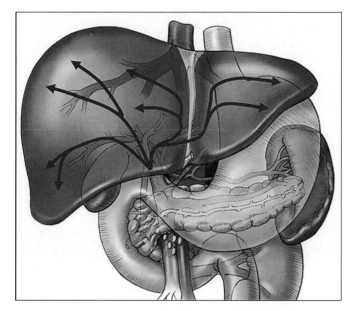

Figure 7-11. Pedicle tracking technique for intraoperative ultrasound.

The gallbladder is imaged from the fundus to the infundibulum. Imaging of a normal cystic duct and common bile duct can be challenging by US. Use of the color flow Doppler assists in distinguishing between bile ducts and blood vessels. The presence of dilated ducts is also helpful to the sonographer as it may permit visualization of the cystic duct to its junction with the common bile duct. If this is the case, the ducts are best visualized with the probe and the hepatoduodenal ligament in parallel, allowing the duct to be seen in longitudinal section. The duct can be followed medially to the ampulla of Vater. Compression of the first part of duodenum may be necessary to avoid interference of bowel gas. The common bile duct is seen in either oblique or transverse section coursing through the pancreatic head.

Ultrasound for hepatic resections

When planning a hepatic resection, intraoperative ultrasound can be used to determine the intrahepatic vascular anatomy and its relationship to the lesion or region of the liver that is undergoing planned resection. The inflow vessels should be tracked and identified, and the outflow vessels that are planned to be preserved or resected can also be mapped (Figure 7-12). The liver capsule can then be scored along the planned transsection line with an electrosurgical device and the ultrasound transducer can be tracked along the score line. An acoustic shadow from the cautery mark will be visualized on the ultrasound screen as a trajectory of the transsection plane, and this can then be correlated with the intrahepatic vascular anatomy, so that the appropriate vessels can be resected or preserved within that transsection plane and margins of the resection can be anticipated.

Case report: HCC in patient with nonalcoholic steatohepatitis (NASH)

The patient is a 55-year-old man with a long history of diabetes, obesity, and hyperlipidemia, s/p coronary artery bypass grafting who was found to have abnormal liver enzymes upon routine physical examination by his primary care physician. An ultrasound was then performed, which revealed a markedly fatty liver and the presence of a 2-cm hypoechoic mass in the right lobe of the liver. Follow-up triple phase CT scanning confirmed a hypervascular lesion on late arterial phase with "washout" in the portal venous phase of imaging. This was diagnostic for hepatocellular carcinoma. Additional findings included a normal-sized spleen and no evidence of portal hypertension.

Several treatment options were possible. A cardiac work-up revealed that the patient had an ejection fraction of 40% with areas of hypokinesis of the left ventricle.

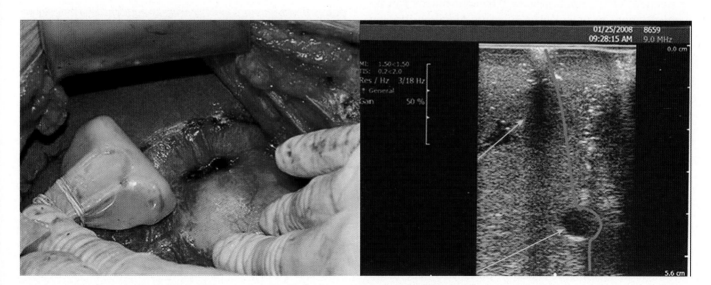

Figure 7-12. Scored liver capsule results in acoustic shadow of planned transection line. Here medial margin of the tumor was preablated, left lobectomy with preservation of middle vein.

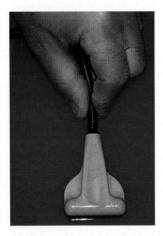
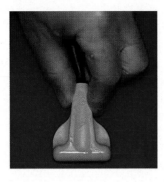

Figure 7-13. Holding the transducer cable or back of the transducer leads to less haptic feedback.

The patient was cleared for ablative therapies, but not for major surgical resection or transplantation.

The patient underwent laparoscopic radiofrequency ablation of the centrally located HCC under laparoscopic ultrasound guidance. The patient was able to be discharged in postoperative day one after the ablation.

Targeting

Hepatic lesions are often targeted for either biopsy or treatment with radiofrequency, microwave, or other ablation devices, and intraoperative ultrasound is essential for most accurate targeting. Multiple variables need to be considered when performing real-time targeting with intraoperative ultrasound. These variables include transducer-positioning, hand-positioning, as well as angle of approach. Following identification of a lesion to be targeted, the transducer is usually placed over the lesion and the applicator is then aligned in line with the transducer plane so that it can be followed accurately into the target. It is important to align the transducer in an angle that allows for maximum degree of freedom of the applicator so that adjustments can be made for more accuracy of the puncture. Hand-positioning on the transducer in an open or hand-assisted case is also important. Not only is visual feedback important for the operator in terms of targeting, but haptic senses are as well (Figure 7-13). If one's hand is placed on the transducer cable or on the back end of the transducer itself, there can be loss of the haptic sense. It is our recommendation that the operator's fingers are placed directly over the transducer so that the target can then be positioned between the operator's fingers or over a specific finger to utilize the operator's haptic sense in addition to visual feedback for more accurate placement of an applicator or biopsy needle.

When performing a laparoscopic targeting procedure, the operator must fuse input from his haptic sense as well as visual input from the laparoscopic and ultrasound images to form a mental model in three-dimensional space to carry out targeting. It is also important to understand the angles of approach, since during a laparoscopic procedure the abdominal wall as well as the liver represents

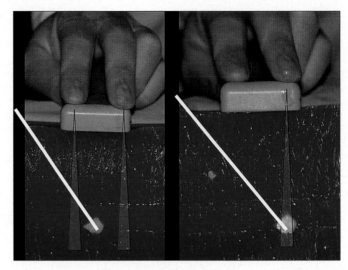

Figure 7-14. Fingers on transducer allow for improved haptic sense and more accurate targeting.

two fixed points along a line, and opportunities to readjust are limited. Thus, the initial angle of approach needs to be as accurate as possible when placing a biopsy needle or ablation applicator. As the target is approached it is usually easiest to approach the lesion in-plane with the ultrasound transducer, so that the applicator can be seen in its longitudinal access; however, this may not always be technically possible (Figures 7-14 and 7-15). Frequently the operator is forced to approach the lesion out-of-plane, and the more out-of-plane the ultrasound transducer is to the applicator, the less the visualization of the applicator. If the transducer is perpendicular to the plane of the applicator, only a single dot will be seen and the loss of depth and the angle of approach can be compromised. With experience an operator can be able to place applicators safely and accurately out-of-plane.

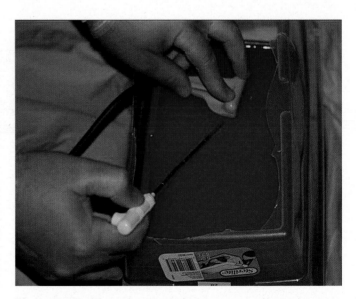

Figure 7-15. When obtaining a biopsy approaching a lesion in line with the transducer provides more accurate targeting.

In order to facilitate targeting of lesions, several advanced image-guidance systems have been developed. These systems have the ability to merge cross-sectional imaging data with real-time mapping of the surface of the liver as well as fusing with ultrasound to give the operator a three-dimensional real-time view of the target and the applicator for ease of approach.

COMMON FINDINGS/ABNORMALITIES

▶ Acute Cholecystitis

Suspected acute cholecystitis is probably the most common indication for right upper quadrant US. The accuracy of US in making the diagnosis of acute cholecystitis has been reported to be 88% to 95%, making it the first-line test of choice.[18-20] The presence or absence of gallstones is the primary sonographic criteria for acute cholecystitis,[6] as 95% to 99% of patients with acute cholecystitis will have stones present within the gallbladder,[18] although it should be noted that up to 10% of patients will have acalculous cholecystitis.[21] Gallstones on US appear as an echogenic mass with posterior acoustic shadowing. Positioning of the patient in the left lateral recumbent position will aid in identification by causing stones to settle in the dependent position.[5] Stones less than 3 mm may not cast a shadow.[6] Gallbladder wall-thickening greater than 3 mm is an adjunctive sign in making the diagnosis of acute cholecystitis (Figure 7-16). The mean gallbladder wall thickness in cases of acute cholecystitis has been reported to be 9 mm.[22] Gallbladder wall-thickening in the presence of gallstones has a positive predictive value of greater than 90%.[18] However, the presence of ascites can lead to increased wall-thickening on US in the absence of cholecystitis.

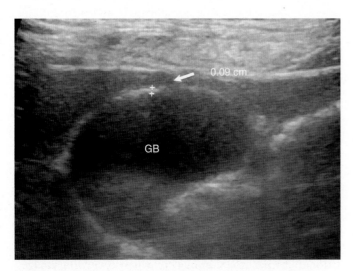

Figure 7-16. Transverse view of a gallbladder (GB) with abnormal thickening of the wall. Wall thickness should be measured while in transverse on the anterior wall. <3 mm is normal (in a contracted GB, the wall may appear thickened.) It will usually be >5 mm in chronic and >9 mm in acute cholecystitis.

Gallbladder distention (due to either obstruction or dysmotility) is the initiating event in the sequence of gallbladder inflammation. Traditionally, gallbladder width greater than 4 cm is considered to be the threshold for a gallbladder to be diagnosed as distended;[23] however, variation in gallbladder morphology from patient to patient makes such objective evaluation somewhat limited.[21] More subjective evaluation of distention involves assessment of the gallbladder contour. A nondistended gallbladder has concave walls, which straighten and then assume a convex contour as distention progresses.[21] A study of cases of overcalled cholecystitis demonstrated that the gallbladder was nondistended in all overcalled cases.[24] Thus, although evaluation of gallbladder distention is highly subjective, its absence calls into question the diagnosis of acute cholecystitis.

The final two sonographic signs of acute cholecystitis are the presence of pericholecystic fluid and the sonographic Murphy sign. Pericholecystic fluid appears as a hypoechoic stripe around the gallbladder wall, and it has a high specificity for gallbladder disease.[22] Sonographic Murphy sign is present when maximal abdominal tenderness is elicited by pressure of the US probe over the gallbladder. Sensitivity of this sign has been reported up to 85%,[25] with specificity ranging from 35% to 95%.[18,25] Thus, a positive sonographic Murphy sign may be highly useful in securing the diagnosis of acute cholecystitis, although its absence should not be used to rule out the disease. For cases of suspected choledocholithiasis, measurement of the common bile duct diameter may be useful. As noted previously, the normal common bile duct diameter is 6 mm, although this figure needs to be revised upward in the elderly.

▶ Hepatocellular Carcinoma

Hepatocellular carcinoma (HCC) is the most common primary liver malignancy, and most often occurs in the setting of cirrhosis. HCC is the fifth most common solid tumor in the world and the third most common cause of cancer-related death.[26-28] Since less than 30% of patients with HCC are diagnosed at a stage where the tumor is amenable to resection or transplantation, early diagnosis is critical.[29] The most typical surveillance protocol for HCC in the setting of cirrhosis involves hepatic US and +/− determination of serum AFP levels every six months.[30] When compared to the presence of disease in explanted liver specimens, the sensitivity of US in detecting HCC has been reported to range from 33% to 72%,[30-32] and is greatly influenced by the size of the lesion with lower sensitivity for smaller lesions (<2 cm). Ultrasonographically, HCC may appear as round or ovoid lesions, with small lesions typically having smooth or sharp margins.[30] The cirrhotic liver has increased echogenicity compared to the nondiseased liver owing to diffuse fatty infiltration. HCC, especially small lesions, will typically appear hypoechoic.[33] The use of Doppler US may be a useful aid in diagnosis, with arterial flow visualized within the lesion. This technique, however, is limited for small lesions. Typical arterial flow pattern within the tumor is detected in less than half of all nodules.[34] The primary utility of US in diagnosing HCC is to identify hepatic nodules in the background of cirrhosis. US is also helpful in assessing the status of portal vein branches in proximity to HCC. HCC-related thrombosis of the portal vein is a contraindication to transplant. US findings typically lack the specificity to make the diagnosis on their own, however, and confirmation with triple phase CT, or gadolinium-enhanced MRI, is required. Given the advances in CT and MRI-imaging of HCCs, biopsy is uncommonly indicated in that if imaging clearly demonstrates late arterial hypervascularity and delayed images demonstrate "washout," biopsy is unnecessary and exposes patients to unwarranted risk of bleeding and tumor spread. Patients can be listed for transplantation solely based on imaging characteristics without a biopsy. Only when imaging is nondiagnostic for HCC should biopsy be considered.

▶ Other Focal Liver Lesions

Focal nodular hyperplasia (FNH) is generally thought to begin as a hyperplastic proliferation of cells arising from an arterial malformation. On US, FNH is typically isoechoic to the liver parenchyma.[35] Doppler US will often demonstrate a "spoke and wheel" pattern of internal vascularity.[36] Hepatic lipomas appear as well circumscribed, uniformly hyperechoic lesions, and are exceedingly rare. The sonographic appearance of hepatic adenoma is nonspecific, and can be hypoechoic, isoechoic, hyperechoic, or of mixed echogenicity.[37] On the whole, while US is able to identify many hepatic masses, there is sufficient variation in sonographic appearance to prevent specific diagnosis from being made on noncontrast enhanced US. In this respect, the primary use of US is to inexpensively, and without the radiation inherent in CT scanning, detect the presence of lesions that may warrant further evaluation.

▶ Blunt Trauma

Focused assessment for the sonographic examination of the trauma patient (FAST) has become an important adjunct in the initial evaluation of the unstable blunt trauma patient. The examination is typically performed with a 3.5 MHz probe and involves views of the pericardium, Morrison pouch, the splenorenal recess, and the pelvis.[38] The goal of this examination is to detect fluid in the pericardium or peritoneum, which will appear as an anechoic stripe. In a prospective study, FAST has demonstrated 79% sensitivity and 95.6% specificity for clinically significant injuries.[39] FAST has virtually replaced bedside diagnostic peritoneal lavage for evaluation of the majority of trauma patients.

▶ Portal Hypertension

Normal direction of blood flow through the portal vein is toward the liver (hepatopetal flow), which may be reversed in cirrhosis (hepatofugal flow) because of the resistance to flow induced by the fibrotic liver. Because of resistance to

hepatopetal flow in cirrhosis, patients often develop portosystemic collaterals, which may manifest as varices. Classically, measurement of the pressure gradient between the hepatic and portal veins (hepatic venous portal gradient, HVPG), is the gold standard for determining the degree of portal hypertension. However, as determining the HVPG is an invasive procedure, there have been efforts to develop Doppler US indices as appropriate substitutes. Indices that have been investigated include portal and splenic blood flow and velocity, and the arterial resistance index of the hepatic, superior mesenteric, and renal arteries. All of these have been demonstrated to be inadequate as substitutes for direct HVPG determination due to lack of sensitivity.[40] Doppler US assessment of the hepatic veins, on the other hand, has shown more promise. The normal hepatic venous waveform is triphasic in noncirrhotic patients, while it becomes biphasic or even monophasic in the presence of cirrhosis. As HVPG increases, Baik has demonstrated progressive flattening of the hepatic venous waveform, although this measure is limited by its subjective nature.[40] The dampening index (DI) is a quantitative measure of the degree of hepatic venous waveform flattening, and is calculated by dividing the minimum velocity of the hepatic venous waveform by the maximum velocity. Kim has demonstrated that DI >0.6 has sensitivity of 75.9% and specificity of 81.8% for the prediction of severe portal hypertension.[41] This measurement thus appears to be the most promising sonographic index for the assessment of portal hypertension.

COMMON PITFALLS

Ultrasonography is very user-dependent. Varying levels of skill can lead to different, potentially care-altering decisions. For surgeons who are first learning how to use intraoperative ultrasound to guide ablations and/or resections, it is crucial to have an experienced user present in the operating room to help guide therapy. Poorly placed ablation probes can lead to unwarranted biliary and vascular complications. Moreover, inaccurate ablation targeting can lead to larger hepatocellular loss, which, in patients with cirrhosis, can lead to hepatic failure and death.

CLINICAL PEARLS/TIPS

Ultrasonography is widely accepted as the modality of choice for the initial evaluation of right upper quadrant abdominal pain and suspected hepatobiliary disease. The sonographic diagnosis of hepatobiliary pathology is often straightforward; however, this simplicity can cause practitioners to become complacent when reviewing images. Careful attention to the smallest detail is important and rescanning may be required in certain situations. Although US has less diagnostic accuracy in detecting hepatic lesions than contrast-enhanced CT and MRI,[50-52] there are helpful clues that may be used to raise suspicion

TABLE 7-1

Summary of Pearls in Hepatic US

	Focal Disease	Diffuse Disease
Grayscale mode	Pleural effusion and/or right lower lobe atelectasis may be a sign of an underlying lesion in the liver Refractive shadowing may help demarcate an otherwise sonographically invisible mass Distortion or absence of normal veinous landmarks may be a sign of an infiltrating mass Sonographic appearance of hepatic abscess varies depending on the etiology Focal fatty sparing typically appears as a hypoechoic, pyramid-shaped area around the gallbladder or the hilum	Further imaging with CT or MRI to evaluate for masses is often indicated when the liver shows markedly heterogeneous texture In diffuse fatty infiltration, the liver is hyperechoic with poor delineation of intrahepatic vessels and increased posterior sound wave attenuation Course, heterogeneous, and increased echotextures: surface nodularity; atrophy of the right lobe; hypertrophy of the caudate lobe; and signs of portal hypertension suggest cirrhosis Nodularity of the cirrhotic liver may be more prominent on the deep surfaces than on the anterior surfaces
Color Doppler imaging	Portal vein thrombosis is a common finding in hepatic malignancy and can be detected at color Doppler interrogation. Tumor thrombus may have visible internal flow Hepatofugal flow (away from the liver) in the protal veins suggests portal hypertension, a common manifestation of cirrhosis	
Spectral Doppler interrogation	Waveform of the hepatic vein may become monophasic owing to compression by an obstructing mass or secondary to diffuse parenchymal disease	

for underlying pathological processes. Shin et al[53] has summarized (Table 7-1) many of the important subtleties practitioners should consider when performing hepatobiliary US.

▶ **Case**

RC is a 57-year-old gentleman who presented to his primary care physician complaining of new-onset hematochezia. A diagnostic work-up was performed, which revealed a rectal cancer and an isolated hepatic metastasis to segment IVB. A low anterior resection was performed prior to commencing prehepatectomy chemotherapy. His treatment regimen consisted of five cycles of FOLFOX and Avastin. A partial response was noted. The image in Figure 7-17 shows his tumor postchemotherapy.

The patient was taken to the operating room for a planned segmental resection. Intraoperative US (IOUS) was performed, which demonstrated a 1-cm metastatic lesion in segment II near the left hepatic vein that was previously unrecognized (Figure 7-18). The operative plan was changed to a left hepatic lobectomy. The patient tolerated the operation and did well postoperatively.

▶ **Discussion**

Up to 50% of patients with a diagnosis of colorectal carcinoma will, at some stage, develop liver metastases with profound implications for survival.[54] Although synchronous liver metastases discovered at the time of the primary colorectal operation have been reported with an incidence of 15–20%,[54,55] a further group of patients are known to harbor "occult" liver metastases that may not be apparent until their metachronous discovery in the

postoperative period.[56] Early detection of occult liver metastases is therefore important for informed decisions regarding the appropriateness of additional regional or systemic adjuvant therapies.

Preoperative investigations contribute little to the detection of colorectal liver metastases in patients for whom an exploratory laparotomy is already inevitable. Prior prospective comparative studies evaluating the diagnostic accuracy of liver function tests, serum tumor markers, transabdominal US, abdominal CT, and/or MRI have shown little benefit over intraoperative assessment in

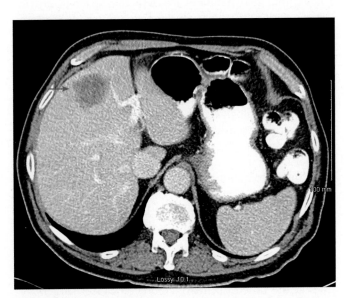

Figure 7-17. Computerized tomography demonstrates an isolated segment IVB rectal metastasis postchemotherapy.

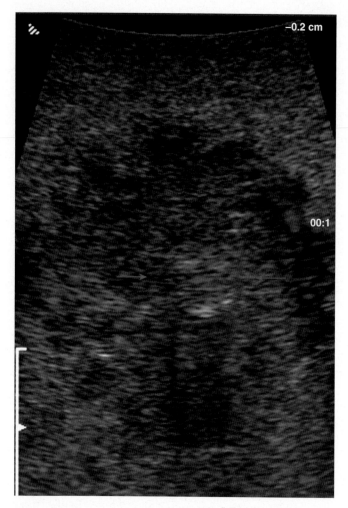

Figure 7-18. Intraoperative US demonstrates a 1-cm metastatic lesion in segment II.

detecting hepatic metastases in advance of exploratory laparotomy.[57-59] Despite technological advances in imaging quality, the 'gold standard' for detecting space-occupying lesions within the liver during exploratory laparotomy remains the combination of careful bimanual palpation of the organ and intraoperative US.

Careful bimanual palpation of the liver during exploratory laparotomy was the only method available for the detection of hepatic metastases prior to the development of modern radiological techniques.[60] Although this method was remarkably sensitive, the concept of occult liver metastases stimulated the search for more sensitive screening methods. The most effective aid for surgical planning and real-time information affecting surgical decision-making is IOUS.

IOUS, using high-resolution, linear-array, contact US probes in direct apposition with the smooth moist capsule of the liver, yields images of exceptional resolution and quality. Studies have demonstrated that IOUS is the most sensitive available method for the detection of liver metastases at the time of primary colorectal cancer surgery.[61-63] Also, IOUS has been reported to be the only method sensitive enough to detect nonpalpable lesions in 14–24% of

patients.[64-66] Intraoperative US has been shown to change the clinical management in up to 50% of patients undergoing hepatic resection for malignancy,[67-69] detecting more lesions than the preoperative conventional B-mode US, CT or angiography.[70]

SUGGESTED READINGS

Blumgart LH, Hann LE. Surgical and radiologic anatomy of the liver, biliary tract, and pancreas. In: Blumgart LH, Belghiti J, Jarnagin W, DeMatteo R, Chapman W, Buchler M, et al, eds. *Surgery of the Liver, Biliary Tract, and Pancreas.* Philadelphia: Saunders; 2007:3.

Brook OR, Kane RA, Tyagi G, Siewert B, Kruskal JB. Lessons learned from quality assurance: errors in the diagnosis of acute cholecystitis on US and CT. *AJR Am J Roentgenol.* 2011;196(3):597–604.

Hagen-Ansert S. The liver. In: Hagen-Ansert S, ed. *Textbook of Diagnostic Ultrasonography.* St. Louis: Mosby; 2006:142.

Larcos G, Sorokopud H, Berry G, Farrell GC. Sonographic screening for hepatocellular carcinoma in patients with chronic hepatitis or cirrhosis: an evaluation. *AJR Am J Roentgenol.* 1998;171(2):433–435.

Luck AJ, Maddern GJ. Intraoperative abdominal ultrasonography. *Br J Surg.* 1999;86(1):5–16.

Machi J, Oishi AJ, Furumoto NL, Oishi RH. Intraoperative US. *Surg Clin North Am.* 2004;84(4):1085–108i.

Raghavendra BN, Feiner HD, Subramanyam BR, et al. Acute cholecystitis: sonographic-pathologic analysis. *AJR Am J Roentgenol.* 1981;137(2):327–332.

Rifkin MD, Rosato FE, Branch HM, et al. Intraoperative US of the liver. An important adjunctive tool for decision making in the operating room. *Ann Surg.* 1987;205(5):466–472.

Rozycki GS, Ochsner MG, Jaffin JH, Champion HR. Prospective evaluation of surgeons' use of US in the evaluation of trauma patients. *J Trauma.* 1993;34(4):516–526.

Wisher D. Abdominal ultrasouhd: the basic principles. In: Harness J, Jarnagin W, eds. *US in Surgical Practice.* New York: Wiley-Liss; 2001:33.

REFERENCES

1. Blumgart LH, Hann LE. Surgical and radiologic anatomy of the liver, biliary tract, and pancreas. In: Blumgart LH, Belghiti J, Jarnagin W, DeMatteo R, Chapman W, Buchler M, et al, eds. *Surgery of the Liver, Biliary Tract, and Pancreas.* Philadelphia: Saunders; 2007:3.
2. D'Angelica M, Fong Y. The liver. In: Beauchamp D, Evers M, Mattox K, eds. *Sabison's Textbook of Surgery.* 18th ed. Philadelphia: Saunders; 2008.
3. Wisher D. Abdominal ultrasouhd: the basic principles. In: Harness J, Jarnagin W, eds. *US in Surgical Practice.* New York: Wiley-Liss; 2001:33.
4. Wachsberg RH, Angyal EA, Klein KM, Kuo HR, Lambert WC. Echogenicity of hepatic versus portal vein walls revisited with histologic correlation. *J US Med.* 1997;16(12):807–810.
5. Shah K, Wolfe RE. Hepatobiliary US. *Emerg Med Clin North Am.* 2004;22(3):661–73, viii.
6. Cooperberg PL, Gibney RG. Imaging of the gallbladder, 1987. *Radiology.* 1987;163(3):605–613.

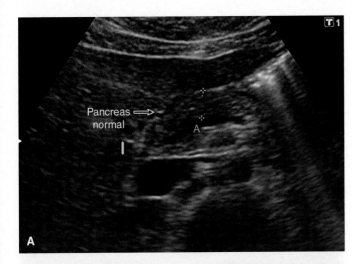

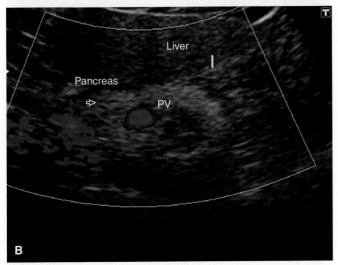

Figure 8-3. **(A)** Sonographic appearance of healthy pancreatic tissue. Note the uniformity of the gland, and its similarity in echotexture to the left lobe of the liver overlying it. **(B)** A fatty pancreas appears brighter than liver.

usually be visualized on transverse imaging in cross section in the head of the pancreas, where it normally measures below 4 mm. The hepatic artery is generally anteromedial to the bile duct, depending on the region imaged. The gastroduodenal artery can often be seen in cross section along the right anterior aspect of the pancreatic head. The neck of the pancreas is defined as it courses anterior to the superior mesenteric-splenic-portal venous confluence. The superior mesenteric artery lies medial to that in cross section, and often the left renal vein can be seen coursing between the superior mesenteric artery and aorta as it empties into the inferior vena cava.

SCANNING TECHNIQUE FOR OBTAINING THESE IMAGES

The pancreas is distinguished on ultrasound by its uniquely glandular parenchyma; however, since its echogenicity varies with age and disease process, it is most useful to rely on the adjacent anatomic structures as landmarks when tracing the gland in the transverse and longitudinal orientations. Of particular help in its identification is its relation to the aorta and splenic vein, which are both easily and consistently identified. In the transverse scan the splenic vein serves as the most useful landmark, whereas in the longitudinal/sagittal scan the aorta and its main branches are more helpful.

Using the left lobe of the liver as a starting point, in the transverse scan the pancreas is identified anterior to the splenic vein, which in turn lies anterior to the superior mesenteric artery and aorta. From there the transducer is moved upward and toward the left to scan the tail, which takes a posterior direction and often must be seen through the spleen. Next, to visualize the head of the pancreas in the transverse orientation, the transducer is returned to the midline starting position and then moved to the right and slightly downward. Helpful landmarks here are the superior mesenteric and splenic vein confluence and the left renal vein as it enters the inferior vena cava.

To view the pancreas longitudinally, it is helpful to assume the transverse starting position as mentioned above, and locate the aorta. Then, while keeping the gland in view, rotate the transducer toward a longitudinal orientation, maintaining the aorta in the center of the field, so that it lies in parallel to the aorta. Structures that serve as useful longitudinal landmarks are the aorta, celiac trunk, superior mesenteric artery, and the inferior vena cava.

Intraoperative imaging has the advantage of removing the abdominal wall from the ultrasound field; thus, higher frequencies may be used for greater resolution. Contemporary laparoscopic probes articulate in two directions, so that the pancreas may be comfortably and completely imaged from anywhere in the upper abdomen through an appropriately sized transducer. The pancreas may be imaged through the stomach, duodenum, or left lobe of the liver, although for target localization purposes, the lesser sac is opened, exposing the surface of the pancreas, so resection or biopsy may rely on surface landmarks. The uncinate and head of the gland may also be imaged through the duodenum.

As the pancreas abuts the stomach and duodenum, upper endoscopic ultrasound is an ideal modality for precise investigation of the gland. Expertise with this technique requires exquisite familiarity of the anatomy and transducer position, and further guidance on these techniques can be found elsewhere in this text.

COMMON FINDINGS/ABNORMALITIES

Ultrasound is often utilized to characterize cysts or tumors in the pancreas. There are several prognostic features definable on ultrasound, including size, borders, echotexture, or presence and type of internal architecture in cysts. Fluid aspirate and tissue biopsies are easily obtained via EUS-guided fine needle aspiration.

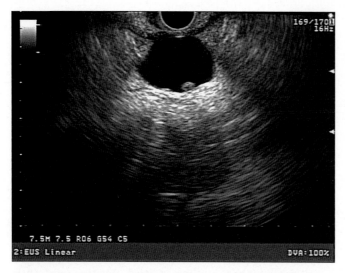

Figure 8-4. Mucinous cystic neoplasm in the head of the pancreas with a mural nodule. (Reprinted with permission from Schaberg FJ, Doyle MBM, Chapman WC, Vollmer CM, Zalieckas JM, Birkett DH, Miner TJ, Mazzaglia PJ. Incidental findings at surgery—Part 1. *Curr Prob Surg.* 2008 May;45(5): 325–374.)

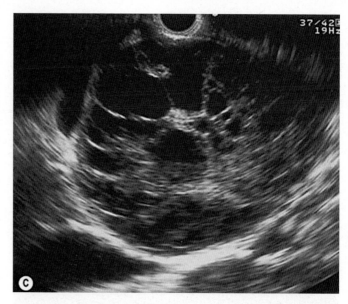

Figure 8-5. Serous cystadenoma on endoscopic ultrasound image with honeycomb appearance. (Reprinted with permission from Amin Z. Pancreas. In: *Clinical Ultrasound.* 3rd ed. Edinburgh;2011:285–323.)

Widespread use of cross-sectional imaging has led to an increased reported incidence of asymptomatic cystic lesions of the pancreas, both benign and malignant. Many of these incidental findings, if not already neoplastic, have the potential for malignant transformation, and it is important to characterize the lesions as fully as possible upon initial diagnosis. Imaging characteristics such as the size of the cyst, complexity of its borders, and presence or absence of internal architecture such as nodules or papillary projections all contribute to risk stratification.

International consensus guidelines ("Sendai criteria") suggest that for cysts with diameter greater than 30 mm surgical resection be considered (Tanaka et al, 2006); others (Jang, 2008, Rodriguez et al, 2007) have argued for a lower size criterion. A simple, anechoic cyst with one chamber usually predicts a benign neoplasm. Internal echoes, papillary projections, septae or mural nodules within the cyst can raise concern for occult or impending malignancy (Figure 8-4). Serous cystadenoma, a generally benign condition, has a characteristic microcystic or honeycomb appearance on imaging (Figure 8-5). Intraductal papillary mucinous neoplasm (IPMN) is a disorder of mucin secretion, leading to pancreatic ductal dilation. Considered a premalignant condition, up to 60% already harbor malignancy at the time of discovery. The thick mucinous secretions can also lead to acute or chronic pancreatitis. When malignancy is identified, or only a segment of the gland is affected, partial pancreatectomy is performed; in this scenario, though, it is imperative to maintain close, regular surveillance of the remainder of the gland. Endoscopic ultrasound has proven invaluable in the characterization of cystic lesions, with highly sensitive architecture description as well as the capability for sampling of cyst fluid, and potential for reliable, repeatable follow-up examinations.

Solid tumors of the pancreas can be primary neoplasms of the pancreas (adenocarcinoma, neuroendocrine tumors), metastases (renal cell carcinoma), or rarer entities such as pancreatic lymphoma or sarcoma. Similar to cystic lesions, ultrasound is invaluable in the characterization, biopsy, and treatment plan of solid pancreatic lesions. Most if not all solid masses will need a biopsy prior to surgery. Those with irregular borders are more concerning for adenocarcinoma (Figure 8-6), whereas lesions with a smooth, regular border

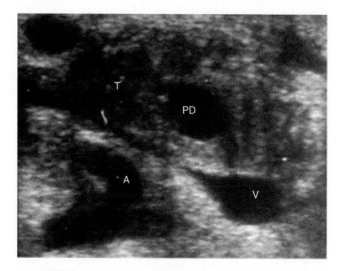

Figure 8-6. Intraoperative ultrasound scan of the head of the pancreas, showing a hypoechoic tumor (T) adjacent to a dilated pancreatic duct (PD). The splenic vein (V) and celiac trunk (A) are visible and clearly free of tumor. (Reprinted with permission from Long EE, Van Dam J, Weinstein S, Jeffrey B, Desser T, Norton JA. Computed tomography, endoscopic, laparoscopic, and intra-operative sonography for assessing resectability of pancreatic cancer. *Surg Oncol.* 2005 Aug;14(2):105–113.)

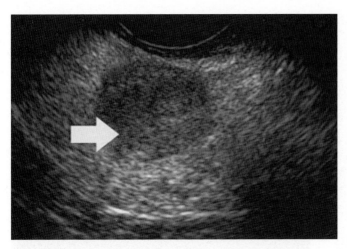

Figure 8-7. EUS image of a hypoechoic mass with a well-defined border, the typical appearance of a neuroendocrine tumor. (Reprinted with permission from McAuley G, Delaney H, Colville J, Lyburn I, Worsley D, Govender P, Torreggiani WC. Multimodality preoperative imaging of pancreatic insulinomas. *Clin Radiol.* 2005 Oct;60(10):1039–1050.)

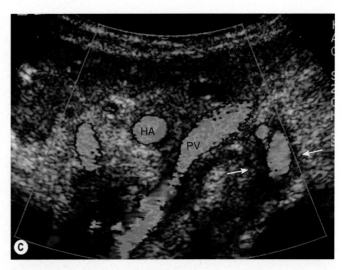

Figure 8-9. Doppler aids identification of tumor invasion by showing narrowing or even obstruction of vessel (Reprinted with permission Amin Z. *Clinical Ultrasound.* 3rd ed. Edinburgh; 2011.)

are more typical of a neuroendocrine tumor (Figure 8-7). Extremely relevant to the treatment plan is the assessment of the tumor for vascular involvement, as the retroperitoneal pancreas is essentially draped over numerous major abdominal blood vessels. Figure 8-8 shows a hypoechoic tumor abutting the superior mesenteric vein, with loss of the interface between the two, suggesting invasion. Doppler ultrasound can help delineate blood vessels and identify narrowing or the vessel or thrombosis, consistent with tumor invasion (Figure 8-9). As with cystic lesions, endoscopic ultrasound is invaluable for image-guided biopsy of solid pancreatic masses for tissue diagnosis (Figure 8-10).

Ultrasound, particularly intraoperative and endoscopic, is also important in the diagnosis and management of pancreatitis, in both its acute and chronic forms. Severe early acute pancreatitis is marked by peripancreatic edema, which often obscures details on imaging. However, as the disease progresses, ultrasound is useful in assessing complications such as pseudocyst formation (Figure 8-11) or abscesses, both of which can be managed with ultrasound-guided procedures.

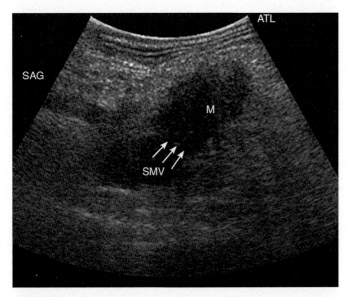

Figure 8-8. Intraoperative ultrasound demonstrating vascular invasion. M marks a hypoechoic solid tumor, SMV is the superior mesenteric vein, and the arrows show loss of the interface between the two, highly suggestive of tumor invasion. (Reprinted with permission from Brennan DD, Kruskal JB, Kane RA. Intraoperative ultrasound of the pancreas. *Ultrasound Clin.* 2006 July;1(3):533–545.)

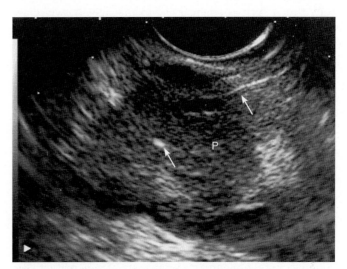

Figure 8-10. EUS-guided FNA of a solid tumor in the head of the pancreas. (Reprinted with permission from Chang KJ, Nguyen P, Erickson RA, Durbin TE, Katz KD. The clinical utility of endoscopic ultrasound-guided fine-needle aspiration in the diagnosis and staging of pancreatic carcinoma. *Gastrointest Endosc.* 1997 May;45(5):387–393.)

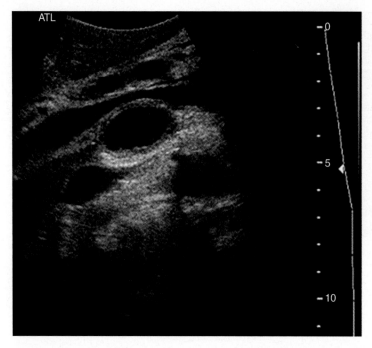
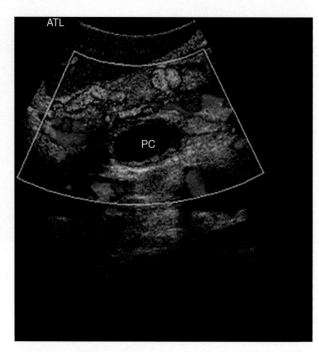

Figure 8-11. Identification of pseudocyst aided by Doppler. The image on the right reveals the pseudocyst, with the other structures seen on the gray-scale image on the left now identified a vessels. (Reprinted with permission from Brennan DD, Kruskal JB, Kane RA. Intraoperative ultrasound of the pancreas. *Ultrasound Clin.* 2006 July;1(3):533–545.)

Chronic pancreatitis is classically marked by progressive atrophy of the gland, often with accompanying ductal dilation, parenchymal calcifications, or intraductal calculi (Figure 8-12). Disease flares or clinical changes can be monitored with ultrasound; as often these patients require frequent imaging throughout their lifetimes, ultrasound is advantageous to minimize as much as possible the lifetime dose of ionizing radiation (CT), and the currently much greater expense of MRI.

Congenital anomalies are often discovered at inopportune times, such as when trying to manage a newly diagnosed solid tumor. A replaced right hepatic artery, for example, can make an otherwise resectable lesion a surgical challenge (Figure 8-13). Annular pancreas is a congenital abnormality where pancreatic tissue completely encircles the second portion of the duodenum. Embryologically this is thought to arise from a failure of the ventral pancreatic bud to rotate with the gut from right to left (where it would then normally fuse with the dorsal bud), thus encircling the duodenum. An alternative explanation is that the ventral bud, which is bifid early in fetal development, fails to fuse and thus encircles the duodenum. This condition can present in utero as maternal polyhydramnios, or more commonly as gastric outlet obstruction in the newborn, or in cases of an incomplete annulus, it may remain aymptomatic throughout life. Figure 8-14 shows a fetal ultrasound examination where a bright ring of pancreatic tissue is seen encircling the fluid-filled, anechoic duodenum.

Embryologic failure of normal ductal anatomy may result in a condition known as pancreas divisum, whereby the ductal systems of the ventral (Wirsung) and dorsal (Santorini) buds fail to fuse. It is generally agreed that this

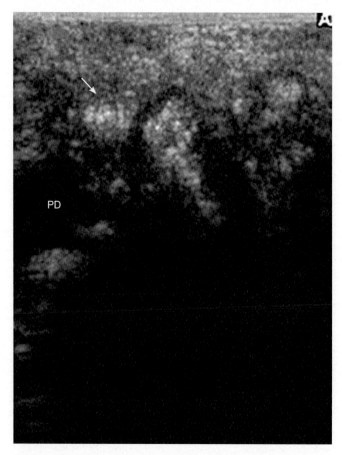

Figure 8-12. Intraoperative ultrasound of a patient with chronic pancreatitis showing an intraductal calcification. (Reprinted with permission from Brennan DD, Kruskal JB, Kane RA. Intraoperative ultrasound of the pancreas. *Ultrasound Clin.* 2006 July;1(3):533–545.)

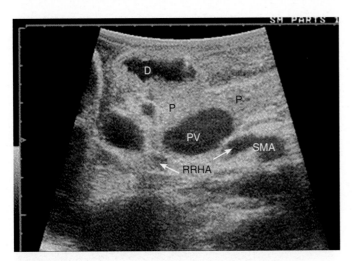

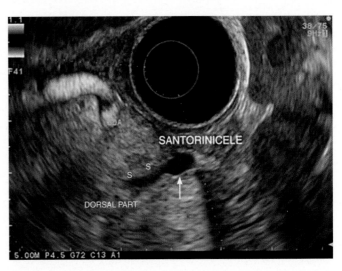

Figure 8-13. Intraoperative scan revealing replaced right hepatic artery off the SMA. D = duodenum; RRHA = replaced right hepatic artery; SMA = superior mesenteric artery; PV = portal vein; P = pancreas. (Reprinted with permission from Machi J, Oishi AJ, Furumoto NL, Oishi RH. Intraoperative ultrasound. *Surg Clin North Am.* 2004 Aug;84(4):1085–1111, vi–i.)

Figure 8-15. EUS of pancreas divisum with dilated minor duct of Santorini (Santorinicele). (Reprinted with permission from Amin Z. Pancreas. In: *Clinical Ultrasound.* 3rd ed. Edinburgh;2011:285–323.)

is present in about 7% of the population, but is asymptomatic for the vast majority (~90%). Symptoms that lead to the discovery of pancreas divisum and can be attributable to it include pain and pancreatitis. Although it can be diagnosed with ERCP and MRCP, pancreas divisum can also be detected with EUS, which of course saves a patient

exposure to ionizing radiation. Figure 8-15 shows an EUS image of pancreas divisum made apparent by a dilated minor duct of Santorini. The administration of secretin during imaging can dilate small ducts, enhancing their visibility.

COMMON PITFALLS

There are certain anatomic challenges when imaging the pancreas. A skilled sonographer will navigate surrounding confounders such as gas in the stomach and intestine, distinguish the borders of a fatty pancreas from surrounding fat, and appreciate a mass of matching echodensity by appreciating differential echotexture. An excellent sonographer will, however, recognize the limitations of the ultrasound examination in front of him or her. Ultrasound has appeal to interventionalists in that it offers real-time guidance for imaging; all physicians understand that there are many pieces to the puzzle.

Interventionalists face unique challenges beyond obtaining a good image, and have different priorities than a diagnostic sonographer. Although transducers for intraoperative applications may be sterilized, often for various reasons (sterilization technique, time limitations) the probes are simply covered with a sterile bag or probe cover. Improper preparation of the probe can result in unacceptable artifacts and poor image quality, if the transducer face is inadequately coupled to the interior of the cover. In the case of a loose bag, a generous amount of coupling gel should be placed between the transducer face and the interior of the bag, and any air bubbles should be squeezed away from the probe. Laparoscopic ultrasound transducers are often placed in a tight-fitting sterile sheath, into which a generous amount of coupling oil is placed at the tip of the receptacle where the active element lies.

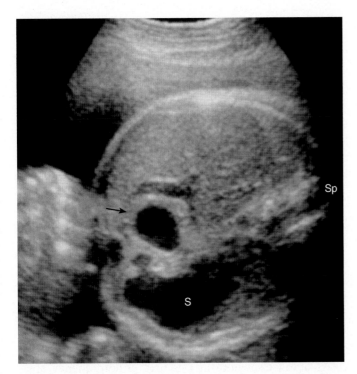

Figure 8-14. Fetal ultrasound demonstrating annular pancreas (arrow). S = stomach; Sp = spine. (Reprinted with permission from Etienne D, John A, Menias CO, Ward R, Tubbs RS, Loukas M. Annular pancreas: a review of its molecular embryology, genetic basis and clinical considerations. *Ann Anat.* 2012 Sep;194(5):422–428.)

In busy or large ORs, ultrasound equipment is often shared across multiple disciplines. An educated glance at the machine settings can save frustration and false information, as even the same type of examination on a different patient may necessitate altering default settings. For example, if power or gain settings were set very high for an obese patient, it could artifactually make a cystic lesion appear solid. In this case, a glance distally for posterior enhancement could confirm a cyst, even if noise in the system (caused by too high gain or power settings) shows echoes within the cyst.

Endoscopic ultrasound provides a view of the pancreas that has different perspective from traditional cross-sectional imaging, and has unique considerations. Details of EUS technique are found in detail elsewhere in this text.

CLINICAL PEARLS/TIPS

Because its midline retroperitoneal location leads it to be obscured by stomach and bowel gas, the pancreas is best examined in a fasting patient. Additionally, starting the abdominal examination with the pancreas may reduce the interference from overlying bowel gas that may become worse with the patient's deep inspiratory maneuvers as the examination progresses. Variable patient positioning maneuvers, such as placing the patient upright, or left and right decubitus, may also serve to displace stomach and bowel gas that would otherwise cause interference in the supine position. Furthermore, if positional maneuvers fail to improve the view, then having the patient drink 500 mL of water may augment visualization by creating an acoustic medium through the water-filled stomach (Figure 8-16). It has also been reported that the combination of simethicone with water further dissolved intraluminal gas, and with patient repositioning maneuvers, is particularly helpful in visualization of the tail region (Abu-Yousef et al, 2008).

Although direct application of the probe to the surface of the pancreas has its advantages in terms of resolution, lesions close to the surface of the gland may be lost in the near field of the transducer. In this case acoustic stand-offs may be employed. This can be as simple as a saline bath, or a sterile glove filled with saline. In using these techniques the operator must take care to minimize bubbles in the fluid. Alternatively, the left lobe of the liver or the foregut hollow viscera may serve as a standoff; for the later, gentle compression to coapt the opposing walls of the organ is necessary to eliminate gas or other artifact from the lumen.

Needle biopsy, particularly with the autofire-type biopsy systems, can be hazardous, given the relatively small size of the organ and its delicate location amongst large blood vessels. In-plane biopsy technique, where the entire needle is visualized in the ultrasound image at all times, is particularly important for safe practice. Since the "throw" of such systems may exceed the width of certain parts of the pancreas, familiarity with manual needle biopsy technique is also beneficial.

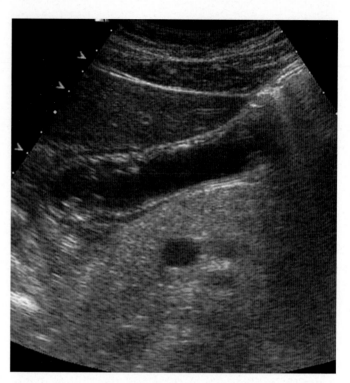

Figure 8-16. Transabdominal ultrasound image showing the appearance of water in the stomach, a technique effective to displace overlying gas in the stomach and allow penetration of the acoustic energy to the pancreas. (Reprinted with permission from Amin Z. Pancreas. In: *Clinical Ultrasound.* 3rd ed. Edinburgh;2011:285–323.)

THERAPEUTIC MANEUVERS

It is clear that image-guided biopsy offers the greatest opportunity for successful diagnosis. It is also clear that ultrasound is an excellent modality in terms of safety and ease of use. In the operating room real-time ultrasound insures preciseness and adequacy of resection, particularly for small lesions that are not easily palpated (or in laparoscopy, where tactile feedback is limited). In nontumor applications, such as endoscopic or surgical pseudocyst drainage, or duct localization for drainage procedures such as the Puestow procedure (Figure 8-17), ultrasound is easily employed in the surgeon's hands at the time of operation.

As a significant number of pancreatic tumors are locally unresectable, or the patient is a poor operative candidate for such complex surgery, local ablative therapies are becoming more widely utilized. Cysts of indeterminate significance or deemed high risk for malignant transformation may be treated with ablative therapies, such as ethanol injection directly into the cyst, to eradicate the epithelial lining and thus the malignant potential (Brugge, 2007).

As noted elsewhere in this text, radiofrequency ablation is a proven technique for local treatment of solid tumors, in the liver for example. Unfortunately because the technique relies on thermal energy, effectiveness of treatment is questionable near large vascular structures (because of a heat sink effect) and potential for thermal

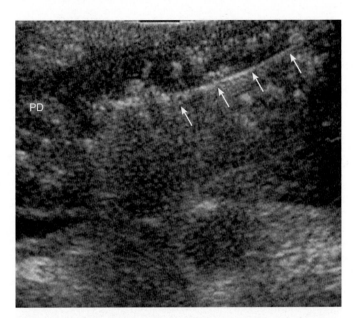

Figure 8-17. Intraoperative ultrasound image demonstrating a needle in an enlarged pancreatic duct, prior to incising the pancreas in preparation for longitudinal pancreaticojejunostomy. (Reprinted with permission from Brennan DD, Kruskal JB, Kane RA. Intraoperative ultrasound of the pancreas. *Ultrasound Clin.* 2006 July;1(3):533–545.)

damage to surrounding structures limits the application of this technique in the pancreas. Irreversible electroporation is a recently developed technique for local treatment of solid pancreatic tumors that are not resectable, or for those where resection margin may be close or positive. In this procedure an electrical field is applied precisely between two electrodes, causing an increase in permeability across the cell membrane and ultimately cell death.

This is a nonthermal and highly localizable method for tissue destruction. In addition to allowing precise application of electrodes for treatment, ultrasound imaging is employed to monitor the progress of tissue death, which has characteristic imaging features. Figure 8-18 shows sequential static images acquired during treatment of lesions in a swine liver (Kee et al, 2007).

CASE STUDIES

▶ Case 1

A 58-year-old man with a 42-pack-year smoking history presents with a 3-month history of progressive dull epigastric discomfort and 28-lb weight. Physical examination revealed scleral icterus and a palpable gallbladder. Ultrasound evaluation reveals a large mass in the head of the pancreas (Figure 8-19), a double duct sign (dilation of common bile duct and pancreatic duct), as well as a distended gallbladder filled with sludge (Figure 8-20) and dilation of the intrahepatic bile ducts (Figure 8-21). He was referred for endoscopic ultrasound, which showed effacement of the tumor/superior mesenteric vein interface as well as periportal lymphadenopathy. FNA biopsy of the pancreatic mass revealed malignant cells consistent with adenocarcinoma. He was referred for neoadjuvant chemotherapy, with consideration of resection with vascular reconstruction if the tumor responds.

▶ Case 2

A 44-year-old woman with history of heavy alcohol intake (1 pint of vodka daily) presents with chronic abdominal pain. She reports that it radiates to the back, and is not relieved with oral pain medication. Additionally she has

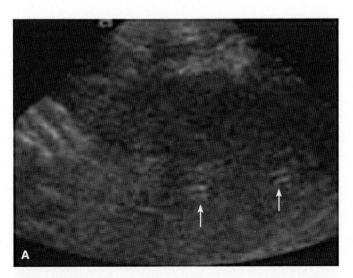

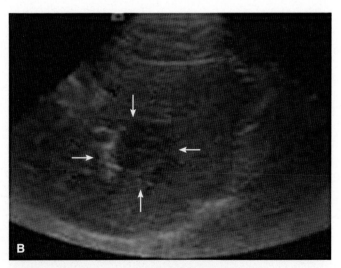

Figure 8-18. Ultrasonographic monitoring of irreversible electroporation. **(A)** Two hyperechoic probe tips of dual probe system (white arrow); **(B-F)** PIE ablated hypoechoic areas with relatively minimal hyperechoic microbubbles in the close proximity of the probes. A spherical hypoechoic area is well delineated and the ultrasound measurements of the ablated area were well correlated with pathological measurement. (Reprinted with permission from Lee EW, Loh CT, Kee ST. Imaging guided percutaneous irreversible electroporation: ultrasound and immunohistological correlation. *Technol Cancer Res Treat.* 2007 Aug;6(4):287–294.)

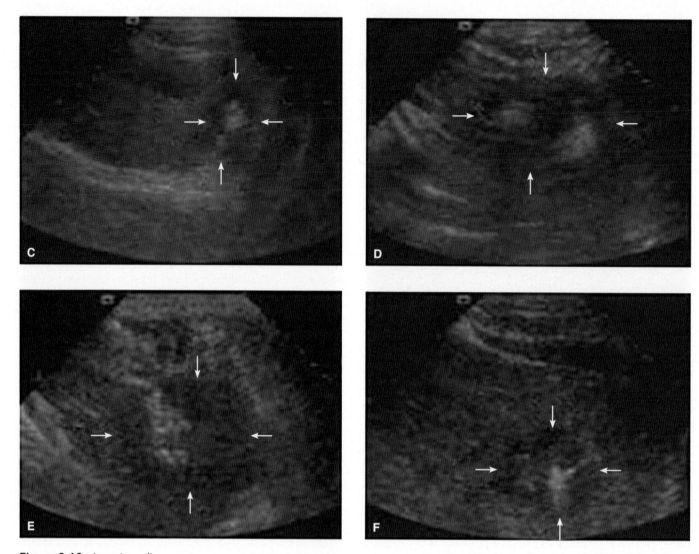

Figure 8-18. (continued)

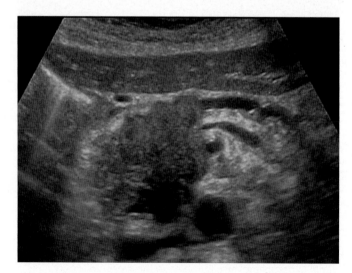

Figure 8-19. Transabdominal intrasound evaluation reveals a large mass in the head of the pancreas with a double duct sign. Note the blurring of the border between tumor and superior mesenteric vein. (Image courtesy of www.ultrsoundcases.info/)

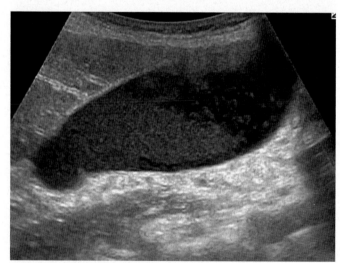

Figure 8-20. Transabdominal ultrasound of a distended gallbladder filled with sludge. (Image courtesy of www.ultrsoundcases.info/)

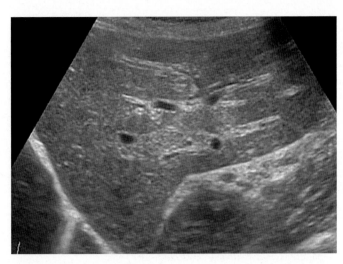

Figure 8-21. Transabdominal ultrasound of the liver revealing dilation of the intrahepatic bile ducts. (Image courtesy of www.ultrsoundcases.info/)

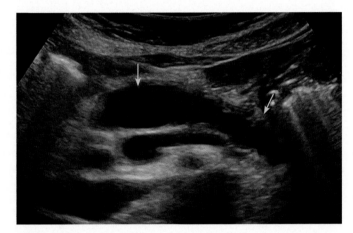

Figure 8-22. Transabdominal ultrasound of the pancreas, showing a dilated pancreatic duct. Note accompanying atrophy of the gland. (Image courtesy of www.ultrsoundcases.info/)

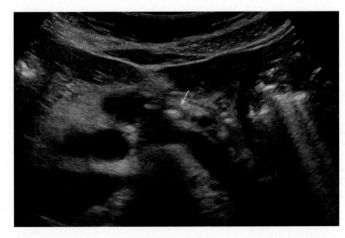

Figure 8-23. Calcification seen in the pancreatic parenchyma, outside of the dilated duct. (Image courtesy of www.ultrsoundcases.info/)

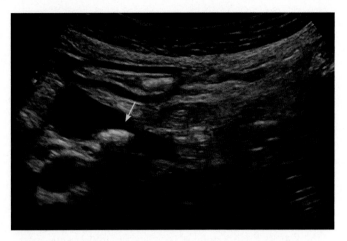

Figure 8-24. Calculus in pancreatic duct, with characteristic shadowing. (Image courtesy of www.ultrsoundcases.info/)

been experiencing malabsorptive type symptoms, including bloating and chronic diarrhea, as well as food intolerance and resulting weight loss. Ultrasound imaging revealed an extremely dilated pancreatic duct with accompanying pancreatic atrophy (Figure 8-22), with diffuse parenchymal calcification (Figure 8-23) and multiple pancreatic duct calculi (Figure 8-24), consistent with chronic pancreatitis. She was referred for a drainage procedure (longitudinal pancreaticojejunostomy) to palliate her symptoms.

SUGGESTED READINGS

Abu-Yousef MM, El-Zein Y. Improved US visualization of the pancreatic tail with simethicone, water and patient rotation. *Radiology*. 2000 Dec;217(3):780–785.

Amin Z. Pancreas. In: *Clinical Ultrasound*. 3rd ed. Edinburgh; 2011:285–323.

Bates J. *Abdominal Ultrasound, How, Why and When*. 3rd ed. Leeds, UK: Chuchill Livingstone; 2011.

Block B. *The Practice of Ultrasound, A Step-by-Step Guide to Abdominal Scanning*. Stutgart, Germany: Georg Thieme Verlag; 2004.

Brugge WR. EUS-guided pancreatic cyst ablation. *Techniques in Gastrointestinal Endoscopy*. 2007 Jan; 9(1):46–50. http://ultrasound-images.com/index.html

Brugge WR. The use of EUS to diagnose cystic neoplasms of the pancreas. *Gastrointest Endosc*. 2009 Feb;69(2 Suppl): S203–S209.

Chang KJ, Nguyen P, Erickson RA, Durbin TE, Katz KD. The clinical utility of endoscopic ultrasound-guided fine-needle aspiration in the diagnosis and staging of pancreatic carcinoma. *Gastrointest Endosc*. 1997 May;45(5):387–393.

Darren DB, Jonathan BK, Robert AK. Intraoperative ultrasound of the pancreas. *Ultrasound Clinics*. 2006 July;1(3):533–545.

Etienne D, John A, Menias CO, Ward R, Tubbs RS, Loukas M. Annular pancreas: a review of its molecular embryology, genetic basis and clinical considerations. *Ann Anat*. 2012 Sep;194(5):422–428.

Flay NW, Gorelick FS. Pancreas, anatomy. In: Leonard Johnson, Editor-in-Chief. *Encyclopedia of Gastroenterology*. New York; 2004:25–29.

Jang JY. Treatment guidelines for branch duct type intraductal papillary mucinous neoplasms of the pancreas: when can we operate or observe? *Ann Surg Oncol.* 2008 Jan;15(1):199–205.

Lee EW, Loh CT, Kee ST. Imaging guided percutaneous irreversible electroporation: ultrasound and immunohistological correlation. *Technol Cancer Res Treat.* 2007 Aug;6(4):287–294.

Long EE, Van Dam J, Weinstein S, Jeffrey B, Desser T, Norton JA. Computed tomography, endoscopic, laparoscopic, and intra-operative sonography for assessing resectability of pancreatic cancer. *Surg Oncol.* 2005 Aug;14(2):105–113.

Machi J, Oishi AJ, Furumoto NL, Oishi RH. Intraoperative ultrasound. *Surg Clin North Am.* 2004 Aug;84(4): 1085–1111.

Martinez-Noguera A, Montserrat E, Torrubia S, Monill JM, Estrada P. Ultrasound of the pancreas: update and controversies. *European Radiology.* 2011;11(9):1594–1606.

McAuley G, Delaney H, Colville J, Lyburn I, Worsley D, Govender P, Torreggiani WC. Multimodality preoperative imaging of pancreatic insulinomas. *Clin Radiol.* 2005 Oct;60(10):1039–1050.

Rodriguez JR, Salvia R, Crippa S, et al. Branch-duct intraductal papillary mucinous neoplasms: observations in 145 patients who underwent resection. *Gastroenterology.* 2007;133:72–79.

Schaberg FJ, Doyle MBM, Chapman WC, Vollmer CM, Zalieckas JM, Birkett DH, Miner TJ, Mazzaglia PJ. Incidental findings at surgery—part 1. *Current Problems in Surgery.* 2008 May; 45(5):325–374.

Schattner M, Belletrutti B, Gerdes H. Endoscopic ultrasound of the biliary tract and pancreas. In: Jarnagin WR, Blumgart LH, eds. *Blumgarts Surgery of the Liver, Pancreas and Biliary Tract.* 5th ed. 2012:232–240

Tanaka M, Chari S, Adsay V, Fernandez-del Castillo C, Falconi M, Shimizu M, Yamaguchi K, Yamao K, Matsuno S. International association of pancreatology. International consensus guidelines for management of intraductal papillary mucinous neoplasms and mucinous cystic neoplasms of the pancreas. *Pancreatology.* 2006;6(1-2):17–32.

9

TRAUMA ULTRASOUND

RONDI B. GELBARD

CLINICAL INDICATIONS FOR ULTRASOUND

Medical ultrasound was introduced in the 1950s but it wasn't until the early 1970s that the first case of visceral injury detected by ultrasound was described.[1] Throughout the next decade, technological advances made "real-time" images, and therefore the more practical application of ultrasound, possible. The utility of ultrasound in trauma began investigation in the late 1980s and in 1992 the first prospective study utilizing ultrasound for the detection of hemoperitoneum was published.[2]

We have come a long way in our understanding of ultrasound since then, and countless reports and studies of ultrasound for the rapid evaluation of intra-abdominal injury have emerged. Up to 40% of patients who have sustained traumatic injury to the abdomen may have no significant findings on physical examination. Furthermore, invasive or traditional radiographic methods of evaluation may be impractical in the unstable patient. Therefore, there is a role for a rapid, noninvasive test to detect the presence of free intraperitoneal, pericardial, and pleural fluid in the setting of acute blunt or penetrating chest and abdominal trauma. The Focused Assessment with Sonography for Trauma (FAST) examination has proven to be the most sensitive and specific test for this purpose, and is supported by the American College of Surgeons (ACS) in the advanced trauma life support (ATLS) course.

Trauma ultrasound has proven to be particularly useful in hemodynamically unstable patients, those with hypotension of unknown etiology, and in the setting of an equivocal physical examination.[3] Studies have shown the FAST examination to be 69–95% sensitive with a specificity of 95–100% for identifying intraperitoneal bleeding in hemodynamically unstable patients.[3] Emergency ultrasound is now used widely for multiple diagnostic purposes and to help guide various bedside procedures. In addition to accurately detecting free fluid in the abdomen, it has become an established tool in the evaluation of biliary disease, aortic aneurysms, ectopic pregnancy, cardiac pathology, pneumothorax, and hemothorax. In fact, it is nearly 100% sensitive for detecting a pericardial effusion or hemothorax and is equivalent to chest radiography in identifying a traumatic pneumothorax.[4] The FAST examination can accurately recognize cardiac injuries from penetrating trauma and has become the basis of the extended FAST (E-FAST), which includes thoracic views for the identification of pneumothorax, in some trauma centers.[5]

Ultrasound is both portable and noninvasive and can be used easily in the evaluation of trauma victims without interfering with definitive therapy. On average, the FAST examination can be performed within 2–4 minutes, usually simultaneously with other resuscitative measures, and can provide useful information without the delay imposed by other imaging modalities such as CT scan or diagnostic peritoneal lavage (DPL). In one recent randomized controlled trial, point-of-care limited ultrasonography was found to decrease the time to definitive surgical treatment by 64% in patients with torso trauma, reduce the number of CT scans obtained, decrease the length of hospital stay, and result in fewer complications.[6]

Studies have also shown that nonradiologist clinicians can accurately perform and interpret bedside ultrasound examinations after adequate didactic and practical experience. While there are no consensus guidelines regarding the number of ultrasound examinations required to achieve maximum proficiency, studies indicate that there is a steep learning curve during the first 30 to 50 examinations that plateaus after 200 examinations have been performed.[7] Given its ease of use, availability, and steep learning curve, ultrasound is an effective and efficient tool for guiding clinical decision making in the trauma patient. With adequate training and an understanding of its limitations, ultrasound can be an effective, safe, and accurate screening test for injury.

▶ Specific Indications

Chest and cardiac trauma

The majority of patients who sustain a penetrating cardiac injury do not survive to receive medical care due to exsanguinating hemorrhage. Hemodynamically unstable patients who survive transport to the hospital should proceed immediately to the operating room for exploration without any further imaging. For patients who remain hemodynamically stable after penetrating thoracic injuries, there is a definite role for rapid bedside ultrasound as part of their evaluation.

Of those that survive penetrating injury to the heart, approximately 2% of patients will develop pericardial tamponade. Often the signs and symptoms of pericardial tamponade can be delayed by hours or even days. Patients may be completely asymptomatic until rapid decompensation ensues with the development of shock and potentially cardiac arrest. It is crucial to detect a pericardial effusion as quickly as possible to prevent this from occurring. Ultrasound can provide evidence of tamponade, such as right ventricular diastolic or atrial collapse, well before clinical symptoms appear. A 10-year retrospective review by Plummer et al. in 1992 found that bedside ultrasound significantly decreased the time to diagnosis of penetrating cardiac injury and had a direct impact on the survival rate and neurologic outcome of survivors.[8]

One prospective cohort study of consecutive penetrating torso injury patients at a Level I trauma center found that ultrasound examination had a sensitivity of 48% and therefore lacked sufficient sensitivity to be used alone in determining the need for operative intervention after penetrating torso injury.[9] Nevertheless, the FAST examination can still be used to screen trauma victims with penetrating chest injury for a pericardial effusion or other cardiac defects and determine the need for pericardial window or more extensive operative intervention.

Blunt trauma to the heart is a relatively uncommon mechanism of injury but can be underestimated and often missed due to a wide range of clinical presentations and nonspecific symptoms. Injuries can include myocardial contusions with resulting wall motion abnormalities, aortic transection, valvular injuries, or ventricular wall rupture. Symptoms may range from palpitations to life-threatening arrhythmias to cardiogenic shock. To date there is no gold standard test for accurate diagnosis of blunt cardiac injury. Aortography is the preferred diagnostic test for suspected aortic transection but is costly, time-consuming, and not always readily available. Along with a high index of suspicion various studies have shown a beneficial role for ultrasound (in addition to cardiac enzymes and electrocardiography) in the diagnosis of blunt cardiac injury.[10] Two dimensional echocardiography can provide a direct view of wall motion abnormalities, intimal flaps, valve abnormalities, pericardial effusions, and severe global dysfunction, and should be performed on all patients that sustain blunt chest trauma.

While the FAST examination was initially meant to be a bedside tool for the detection of hemoperitoneum and hemopericardium, its use has recently expanded to include the identification of blood, fluid, or air in the pleural space as part of the E-FAST examination. In fact, ultrasound has a sensitivity equivalent to that of chest x-ray for detecting pneumothoraces[4] and is even more sensitive than x-ray for visualizing fluid in the pleural space.

A chest radiograph requires more than 150 mL of fluid to be present in the pleural cavity in order to detect an effusion.[11] With a sensitivity of 93% for pleural effusion, ultrasound can detect as little as 20 mL of fluid and can be carried out much more rapidly.[11] While a chest radiograph should still be done as part of the initial assessment of the trauma patient, ultrasound is more frequently being used to determine the need for an immediate tube thoracostomy.[11,12]

Abdominal trauma

The FAST examination has been most widely utilized and studied in the diagnosis and management of blunt abdominal trauma. Many algorithms have been developed to assess patients that have sustained blunt abdominal trauma (Figure 9-1), the majority of which suggest that a hemodynamically unstable patient with a positive FAST warrants a laparotomy. Although not yet well validated, several hemoperitoneum scoring systems have found that the amount of free fluid detected on ultrasound can accurately predict the need for therapeutic laparotomy.[13] According to such algorithms, patients with a negative ultrasound should undergo DPL followed by further evaluation for an extra-abdominal source of bleeding (ie, into the chest or extremity) if the DPL is negative. It is also important to note that patients suffering from spinal shock or head trauma can present with hemodynamic instability and a negative FAST examination. These patients may require further imaging after resuscitation and stabilization to further elucidate the extent of their injuries. While the role of ultrasound in the evaluation of unstable patients is well established, its reliability in the assessment of stable trauma patients is less clear. Several studies have questioned the routine use of ultrasound as a primary tool in assessing hemodynamically stable patients, especially multiply injured patients with a high Injury Severity Score (ISS), who are more likely to have ultrasound-occult injuries.[14,15] These studies have found that it may lead to the underdiagnosis of abdominal injury, in part due to its lower sensitivity for detecting parenchymal injury.[14] Therefore, a positive FAST in a hemodynamically stable patient should generally be followed by a CT scan to further evaluate the site of injury and minimize the rate of negative laparotomies, whereas a stable patient with a negative FAST can be observed with serial examinations and/or further imaging depending on clinical suspicion and mechanism of injury. While ultrasound is less sensitive than CT scan for

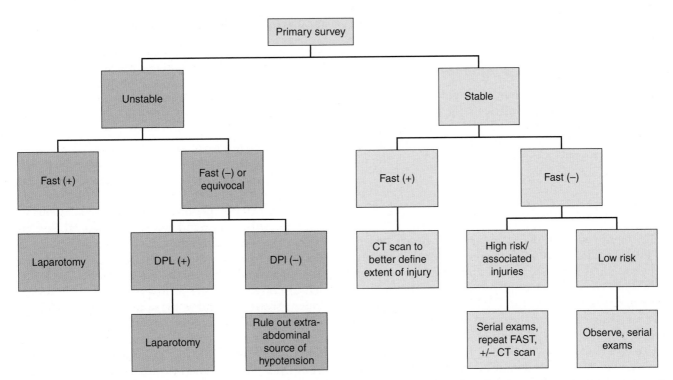

Figure 9-1. Algorithm for the management of patients with blunt abdominal injury based on their hemodynamic status and results of FAST examination.

detecting parenchymal injury and retroperitoneal bleeding, it has proven to be extremely useful in identifying intraperitoneal fluid that might otherwise be missed by other screening modalities.

The FAST examination has been proven to be highly specific, but less sensitive for detecting hemoperitoneum in patients with penetrating abdominal injuries. One study found the sensitivity of FAST alone for the evaluation of penetrating torso injury to be 67%, with a positive predictive value of 92%, and a negative predictive value of 89%.[16] The authors determined that the routine use of ultrasound in penetrating torso injury was useful for the detection of peritoneal fluid and it can be considered an important tool for guiding management in the setting of multiple penetrating injuries. However, it is important to note that a negative FAST examination does not rule out abdominal injury, such as a diaphragm or hollow viscus injury, and further evaluation is recommended.

Orthopedic injury

While it is not considered one of the primary goals of trauma resuscitation, the evaluation of skeletal injuries is an important adjunct to the secondary survey. Even non-life-threatening orthopedic injuries should be evaluated and managed without significant delay. Radiography has traditionally been the diagnostic test of choice for assessing bone fractures. However, there is growing interest in bedside ultrasound as a more rapid, noninvasive method for diagnosing orthopedic injuries. Ultrasound tends to be less reliable in the setting of compound fractures and injuries in close proximity to joints, but recent studies have demonstrated that it may be comparable to radiography for the diagnosis of long bone fractures with sensitivity and specificity of 89% and 100%, respectively.[17]

Ultrasound has also proven to be useful for guiding the manipulation and reduction (M&R) of distal radius fractures in adults and forearm fractures in children.[18,19] Ang et al. prospectively studied the use of ultrasound-guided M&R in 62 patients with distal forearm fractures and compared it to the blind manual palpation technique. They found that post-reduction radiographic findings were similar after both techniques, but there was slightly improved volar tilt in the ultrasound group ($P = .048$). The rate of operative intervention was also lower among those who underwent ultrasound-guided reduction (4.9% versus 16.7%; $P = .02$).[18] Ultrasound reduced the need for repeat M&R and therefore decreased the need for sedation and analgesia.

▶ Patient Populations Who Benefit from Trauma Ultrasound

The FAST examination is most useful in the rapid evaluation of hemodynamically unstable patients when the etiology of shock is unclear. Ultrasound is also useful in patients who have an unreliable examination (ie, in the setting of intoxication or head injury) and who require frequent re-assessments. In patients who require urgent transfer to a trauma center, it can also be a useful test during air or ground transport due to its portability and ease of use.

Fast examination and pregnancy

Pregnant women comprise another population of patients in whom ultrasound is particularly useful. DPL is relatively contraindicated in pregnancy and while CT scan should be performed if clinically indicated, there are potential teratogenic effects of radiation that can be avoided with the use of ultrasound.

Ultrasound and pediatric trauma

While the use of the FAST examination is clearly beneficial in the evaluation of adult trauma patients, the utility of trauma ultrasound has not been studied as extensively in children. The presence of physiologic free fluid in their pelvis makes interpreting the FAST examination slightly more challenging in pediatric patients. Limited studies have determined the sensitivity of FAST to range from 30% to 80%, and specificity 95% to 100% in children who have sustained blunt abdominal trauma.[20] When fluid is visualized outside of the pelvis in children, the sensitivity for solid organ injury increases to 90% and there is an 87% and 97% positive and negative predictive value, respectively.[21]

It is important to note that a positive FAST examination in a hemodynamically stable pediatric trauma patient should still be followed by a CT to further evaluate the source of hemoperitoneum. A negative FAST, however, does not always preclude the need for a CT scan but it may help to avoid unnecessary radiation exposure in patients who have a very low likelihood of intraperitoneal injury. In hemodynamically unstable pediatric trauma patients, the FAST examination can rapidly help guide decisions regarding the need for operative intervention. Further studies are clearly needed to evaluate the clinical utility of the FAST examination for pediatric trauma patients, especially given that most intra-abdominal injuries in children are managed nonoperatively.

More recent studies have demonstrated a role for bedside ultrasound in the evaluation and management of fractures in pediatric trauma patients. Not only is it highly sensitive for detecting certain types of orthopedic injuries, but it can be done rapidly and minimizes the risk of radiation exposure to pediatric patients. Clavicle fractures are one of the most common orthopedic injuries in children. A recent study by Cross et al. demonstrated that bedside ultrasound can accurately diagnose pediatric clavicle fractures with 95% sensitivity and 96% specificity, especially in patients with a high likelihood of fracture.[22] Another study prospectively evaluated the use of ultrasound for the reduction of forearm fractures in children and found it to have an initial success rate of 92% (95% CI, 75–99%).[19] It could be used to immediately assess for realignment of the bones and minimize the use of postreduction x-rays.

Disaster and mass casualty incidents

Mass Casualty Incidents (MCIs) are situations that require the rapid triage of large numbers of injured patients where the volume of injuries exceeds the resources and capabilities of medical responders and personnel in the field. A rapid, accurate screening and diagnostic tool is necessary to identify those who require immediate intervention, and thereby improve patient safety and outcomes.

Sarkisian et al was among the first to describe point-of-care ultrasound in a mass casualty setting, after an earthquake in northwestern Armenia in 1988 that injured more than 150,000 people.[23] Four hundred patients were evaluated with ultrasound in a 72-hour period, 96 examinations showed positive findings and 16 operations were performed based on these results with 1% false negative rate.[22] This and other more recent studies have shown that ultrasound is both sensitive and specific in resource-limited situations, and is becoming a more widely used tool by first responders in remote settings after natural disasters, terrorist attacks, and military mass casualties. It has been used both for initial assessment and surgical decision making, and prioritizing the need for further imaging. It can also be performed by adequately trained nonphysician and prehospital personnel in the setting of mass casualty incidents.

A recent paper by Stawicki et al. proposed the concept of a comprehensive ultrasound assessment of the chest, abdomen, vena cava, and extremities in acute triage (CAVEAT).[24] In addition to the standard FAST views, they proposed that evaluation of the inferior vena cava could yield important information about filling pressures and intravascular volume status, and help identify those who are likely to respond to volume expansion. Despite taking several minutes longer than the traditional FAST examination, the CAVEAT protocol could also be used to identify occult fractures when radiography is unavailable and thus lead to more timely management and utilization of resources.[24]

Data on its use in military deployment are sparse, but recent reports indicate that handheld ultrasound is becoming a more routinely used tool by forward medical units in combat environments.[24] Images can be transmitted by satellite from remote areas for expert interpretation and help influence treatment and evacuation strategies. Training courses currently exist to teach military surgeons the FAST technique.

▶ Contrast-Enhanced Ultrasound

The role of contrast-enhanced ultrasound (CEUS) in the assessment of trauma patients is also a recent subject of interest. CEUS uses contrast agents containing highly stable microbubbles filled with an inert gas that resonate at low acoustic pressure. Continuous real-time images are produced based on the microbubble signal that can provide important information on solid organ injury.[25] A growing body of evidence suggests that CEUS has increased

TABLE 9-1

Traumatic Lesions and Their Appearance on Contrast-Enhanced Ultrasound.

Lesion	Ultrasound
Laceration	Hypoechoic, linear filling defect often oriented perpendicularly to surface of organ
Infarction	Anechoic wedge-shaped mass with base at organ surface
Hematoma	Non-enhancing concave areas extending medially from organ surface
Active hemorrhage	Hyperechoic pool or jet
Scars	Anechoic, linear band at surface of organ

sensitivity for detecting subtle parenchymal injuries, as well as vascular lesions, active hemorrhage, and delayed pseudoaneurysms.[26,27] With sensitivities ranging from 63–99%, studies have shown CEUS to be more sensitive than ultrasound for detecting solid organ injury.[25,26] Solid organ lacerations and hematomas are nonenhancing due to lack of blood supply and appear as dark anechoic areas on contrast-enhanced ultrasound (Table 9-1 and Figure 9-2). Advantages of CEUS include its lack of ionizing radiation

and nephrotoxicity, which make it preferable for use in children and pregnant women, its ease of use, and ability to visualize arterial and venous phases.

Limitations to CEUS include its inability to adequately visualize retroperitoneal structures and skeletal injuries. It also requires intravenous access and may take slightly longer to obtain that traditional grayscale imaging. Therefore, its use should be restricted to hemodynamically stable trauma patients with a high likelihood of parenchymal injury in whom CT is unavailable or contraindicated due to iodinated contrast allergy.

NORMAL ANATOMY

Free intraperitoneal fluid collects in dependent areas formed by peritoneal reflections and mesenteric attachments, including the retrovesicular space (in men), the rectouterine pouch or the pouch of Douglas (in women), and right and left paracolic gutters. The right paracolic gutter connects Morison pouch with the pelvis. The left paracolic gutter courses to the splenorenal recess. The retrovesical pouch is the most dependent area of the male in supine position, while the pouch of Douglas is the most dependent area in the supine female.

Free fluid that accumulates on the right side of the intraperitoneal cavity will flow into the hapatorenal recess (Morison pouch) before traveling down the right paracolic gutter into the pelvis. Morison pouch is the most common

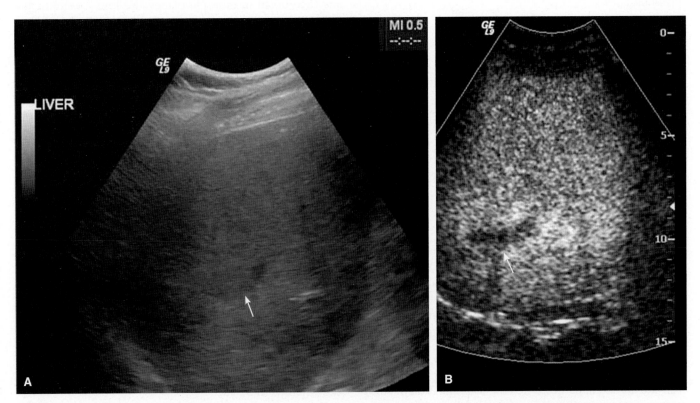

Figure 9-2. (**A**) Grayscale ultrasound showing subtle area of abnormal hepatic echostructure (white arrow); (**B**) CEUS with hypoechoic region consistent with parenchymal laceration (white arrow). (From Cokkinos D, et al. *Ultraschall Med.* 2012;33(1):60–67.)

location for free fluid to collect in the setting of parenchymal injury due to blunt trauma. Free fluid in the left upper quadrant will collect in the left subphrenic space and less commonly in the splenorenal space. With smaller collections, the phrenocolic ligament will often block the flow of fluid from the left paracolic gutter to the splenorenal recess, so fluid will usually spread across the midline to the right upper quadrant.

NORMAL APPEARANCE OF ULTRASOUND

▶ Simple Fluid

Intraperitoneal free fluid is anechoic on ultrasound. It is jet black and has a "pointy" appearance, forming around bowel and viscera in contrast to the "rounded" appearance of fluid within the lumen of a vessel or organ.

▶ Complex Fluid

Complex fluid on ultrasound is usually indicative of hemoperitoneum. Immediately after traumatic injury, blood appears sonolucent (hypoechoic) but becomes echogenic as clot begins to form over several hours. As it forms a hematoma, it may even appear hyperechoic. Blood becomes sonolucent again as fibrinolysis occurs approximately 12–24 hours from the time of injury.[28] It is important to recognize that echogenic blood is likely to be located at the site of injury and can therefore help guide intervention; however, it may be similar in echotexture to the surrounding parenchyma and can also be missed on ultrasound.

▶ Solid Organ Appearance

The spleen lies in a posterolateral position and has an echogenic capsule with a homogeneous cortex. Despite its gray echotexture similar in appearance to the liver, it is smaller in size and the intraparenchymal vessels are less visible. The kidneys lie inferior to the liver and spleen in a retroperitoneal location. The renal cortex has a similar echotexture but is slightly more hypoechoic than the liver or spleen and is outlined by the brightly echogenic Gerota's fascia.

▶ Hollow Organ Appearance

The bowel varies in appearance depending on whether it is filled with air, fluid, or solid matter. When the bowel lumen contains air, it may distort the appearance of surrounding structures. If it contains fluid or solid material, the bowel may have a cystic appearance but peristaltic waves are visible, distinguishing it from a stationary cystic structure.

▶ Parenchymal Findings

While the utility of ultrasound for detecting free fluid is well documented, its utility for the identification of solid organ injury is less clear. Moreover, both splenic and liver lacerations can occur with or without hemoperitoneum;

therefore, relying on the presence of free intraperitoneal fluid for the diagnosis of solid organ injury can be misleading.

If done accurately, the identification of parenchymal architectural abnormalities can help guide us to the site of injury and can be instrumental in planning surgical intervention if necessary. Lacerations often appear as an irregular contour or hyper- or hypoechoic areas within the visceral organ, whereas subcapsular hematomas may look like an echogenic rim.[28] Splenic parenchymal injuries can be diffusely heterogeneous or disorganized patterns with cystic or hypoechoic areas. This is in contrast to liver parenchymal injuries that usually appear as focal hyperechoic lesions.[28]

Injuries to the kidney can appear as a focal lesion or heterogeneity of the parenchyma that replaces normal kidney in the renal fossa, and adrenal injuries typically present as discreet mass above the kidney. A pseudoaneurysm may appear as a cyst-like anechoic mass within an organ, but can be differentiated from a cyst using Doppler to demonstrate flow within the pseudoaneurysm.[28] In situations where the presence of parenchymal injury is not clear, a higher frequency probe (7.5-MHz linear array probe) may more accurately detect tissue irregularities, especially in thin patients.[29]

SCANNING TECHNIQUES AND COMMON FINDINGS

Unlike a comprehensive ultrasound study that must visualize each organ in multiple planes, the FAST examination can be done with limited scanning planes with a patient lying supine in order to detect the presence or absence of free fluid. The FAST typically encompasses four views: the pericardial view, the perihepatic view, the perisplenic view, and the pelvic view. An anterior thoracic view is sometimes added to the standard views to assess for the presence of a pneumothorax. Each of these will be discussed in more detail below.

▶ Pericardial View

Technique

The pericardial view looks at the space between the right ventricle and the liver in order to rule out the presence of a pericardial effusion. With the patient lying supine, the probe (with the marker dot pointing toward the right) should be placed in the subxiphoid area and angled toward the patient's left shoulder (Figure 9-3). Ensure that the transducer is lying flush with the skin. Pressing firmly just below the xiphoid should reveal the right ventricle next to the left hepatic lobe. To improve the image, consider having the patient inhale deeply and hold their breath (if possible), with the transducer positioned further toward the patient's right side.

If the patient is uncooperative or the subxiphoid view cannot be obtained, a useful alternative is the parasternal

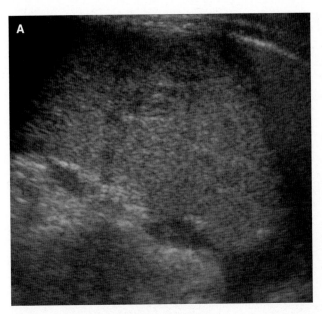

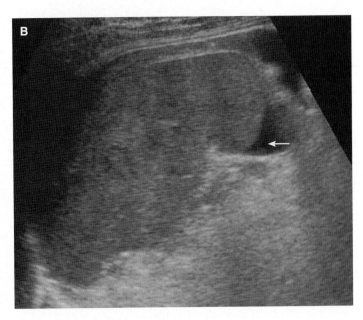

Figure 9-12. (**A**) Longitudinal view showing abnormal free fluid surrounding the spleen. (Used with permission from www.ultrasoundcases.info/Slide-View.aspx?cat=182&case=481) *ID: /2555.jpg;* (**B**) Inhomogeneous spleen with perisplenic free fluid (white arrow). (Used with permission from www.ultrasoundcases.info/*Slide-View.aspx?cat=182&case=480) ID: /2545.jpg*

▶ Pelvic View

Technique

The pelvic view is used to assess for free fluid around the bladder. The pelvis is the most dependent part of the abdomen overall and intraperitoneal fluid is therefore likely to collect there. In order to obtain this view, place the probe on the pubic bone in the midline, with the marker dot pointed toward the patient's head. To obtain a good longitudinal view of the pelvis, slowly slide the probe cephalad until it is approximately 2 cm from the pubic symphysis, at which point the bladder should come into view (Figure 9-13).

An empty bladder lies posterior to the pubic symphysis and has a thickened, irregular wall, whereas a full bladder appears triangular in shape and is anechoic with thin, smooth walls. The bladder should be distended prior to examination to provide an acoustic window. A full bladder also prevents reflection artifact from the sacrum and keeps the air-filled small intestine from dropping into the pelvis and obscuring the view (Figure 9-14). If a foley catheter

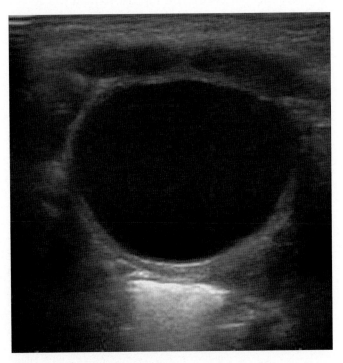

Figure 9-14. Ultrasound view of the normal bladder. (Used with permission from www.ultrasoundcases.info/Slide-View.aspx?cat=479&case=5496) *ID: /39678-Afbeelding8.jpg*

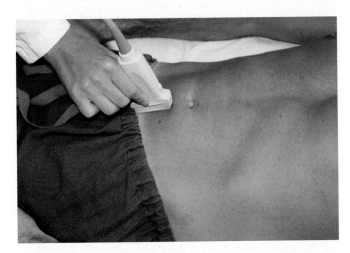

Figure 9-13. Probe position for longitudinal view of the pelvis.

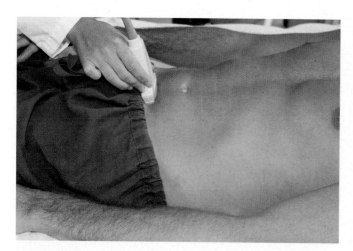

Figure 9-15. Probe position for transverse view of the pelvis.

has already been inserted, the bladder can be re-filled by instilling 200 cc of normal saline through the catheter and clamping it just prior to imaging. Avoid over-distending the bladder as it can also give a false-negative result by obscuring the retrovesical pouch.

To obtain a transverse view of the pelvis, rotate the probe 90 degrees so the marker dot is pointed toward the patient's right side (Figure 9-15).

Common findings and abnormalities

The inferior angle of the bladder will mark the interface between the intraperitoneal space (on the left) and the pelvic structures (on the right). In a man, free fluid will collect in the space posterior to the bladder wall. In a woman, the uterus lies posterior to the bladder, so fluid will collect around the uterus, or in the space posterior to the uterus, called the recto-uterine pouch or the pouch of Douglas

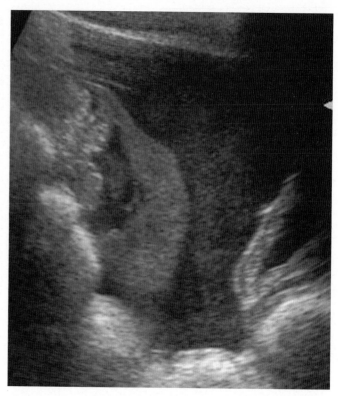

Figure 9-16. Large amount of free fluid (black) in the rectouterine pouch (pouch of Douglas). (Used with permission from www.ultrasoundcases.info/Slide-View.aspx?cat=182&case=483) *ID: /2567.jpg*

(Figure 9-16). Be aware that a small amount of free fluid in the pouch of Douglas may be physiologic in a premenopausal woman and is not necessarily a sign of injury.

The transverse view will usually show fluid posterior to the bladder or uterus (Figure 9-17). Be careful not to mistake

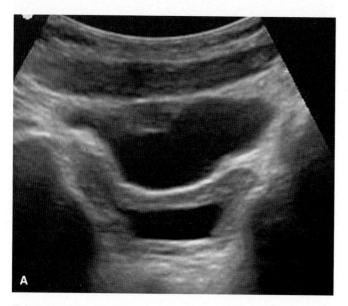

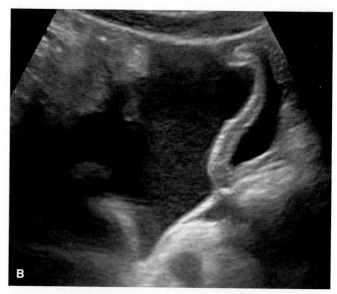

Figure 9-17. (**A**) Transverse view of hemoperitoneum posterior to the bladder. (Used with permission from www.ultrasoundcases. info/Slide-View.aspx?cat=182&case=4143) *ID: /23989.jpg*; (**B**) longitudinal view of fluid surrounding bladder. (Used with permission from www.ultrasoundcases.info/Slide-View.aspx?cat=182&case=4143) *ID: /23990.jpg*

the contents of an ovarian cyst or the iliopsoas muscle for free fluid, as they may be similar in appearance. Turning the gain down on the ultrasound machine may help minimize artifact and improve the image, and placing the patient in Trendelenburg position may also help if the pelvic view cannot be obtained easily. This will help empty the pelvis of any small intestine that might be obscuring the view.

▶ Anterior Thoracic View

Technique

In order to evaluate for the presence of a pneumothorax, place the probe on the anterior chest wall in a longitudinal position with the marker dot pointed cephalad. Start in the 3rd to 4th intercostal space at the midclavicular line and slowly slide the transducer inferiorly. Use the rib shadows to find the pleural plane. Adjust the probe until one rib lies on either side of the image and the pleural interface is visible at the posterior border of the ribs.

Common findings and abnormalities

The pleural surface should look like a bright line between the chest wall and the lung. In this position, it is possible to look for an echogenic line and a sliding motion of the visceral pleura against the parietal pleura. The absence of this "sliding sign" suggests the presence of a pneumothorax. Either a standard curvilinear abdominal probe or a high-frequency linear transducer may be used to obtain this view, and the depth should be decreased to a maximum of 4 cm.

COMMON PITFALLS

An accurate FAST examination can provide a great deal of information to help guide further use of resources and influence the management of secondary injuries. It can help limit the number of missed injuries and minimize the overuse of more expensive diagnostic tests. For these reasons, it is important to recognize certain limitations and pitfalls that could interfere with the benefits of this diagnostic modality.

▶ Factors Leading to False Negative Results

- The accuracy of ultrasound is limited in morbidly obese patients, as adipose tissue increases the distance between the probe and the region being evaluated, thereby decreasing acoustic penetration.

- The accuracy of ultrasound is also affected by intestinal gas or pneumoperitoneum, as well as subcutaneous emphysema that can obscure underlying structures and limit penetration of the sound waves.

- Hemoperitoneum can easily be missed in patients without a full bladder due to the lack of an acoustic window.

- Too much gain leads to the presence of noise artifact and can limit the detection of anechoic fluid.

- Ultrasound performance is operator dependent and requires adequate training in order to become proficient in the technique.

- Ultrasound provides a very limited view of the retroperitoneum, and can miss up to 1/3rd of isolated retroperitoneal injuries.[28]

- Ultrasound is less sensitive for detecting visceral injury, including pancreatic and renal pedicle injuries.

- Ultrasound may miss up to 14% of injuries involving the bowel or mesentery, and up to 58% of solid organ injuries that have no associated hemoperitoneum.[28]

- Small amounts of free fluid, especially less than 400 mL, can easily be missed on ultrasound.

- Ultrasound is not sensitive for detecting spinal or pelvic fractures, or diaphragmatic rupture.

▶ Ultrasound Findings Leading to False Positive Results

- Stomach and other fluid-filled bowel can be mistaken for free fluid on ultrasound.

- The diaphragm can appear hypoechoic and be mistaken for perisplenic or perihepatic fluid.

- Mirror image artifact can falsely indicate the presence of hyperechoic substance in the pleural cavity (where the liver is reflected back from the diaphragm), or fluid in the pelvis (where a full bladder is reflected back from the sacrum or rectum).

- Lack of pleural sliding is suggestive of a pneumothorax, but can also occur with poor ventilation or mainstem intubation.

- Ultrasound cannot distinguish between types of intraperitoneal fluid. A small amount of free pelvic fluid in a woman may be physiologic and not necessarily hemoperitoneum. Alternatively, pathologic free fluid can be due to ascites, a ruptured ovarian cyst, peritoneal dialysate, or even bladder injury.

- Hemangiomas and metastatic lesions can sometimes be misinterpreted as hematomas or parenchymal injuries in the liver or spleen.

- Adrenal adenomas, and perinephric and intra-abdominal fat can appear echogenic and be mistaken for hematoma despite their lack of an anechoic rim.

- A focal anterior hypoechoic region around the heart may be mistakenly identified as a pericardial effusion when it is actually normal pericardial fat.

CLINICAL PEARLS

- To differentiate stomach from free fluid, inject air or saline through a nasogastric tube under ultrasound guidance.

- Free fluid in Morison pouch can be distinguished from the gallbladder by its angular appearance and sharp corners compared to the rounded fundus of the gallbladder. Similarly, fluid-filled bowel has an echogenic border with perpendicular echogenic lines that represent the valvulae conniventes.

- Complete the pelvic view prior to placing a Foley catheter to ensure a full bladder. Alternatively, instill sterile normal saline into the bladder and clamp the catheter for the duration of the examination.

- Even in the case of inadvertent high-gain settings and noise artifact, simple fluid can be heralded by posterior enhancement.

- Place the patient in Trendelenburg position while obtaining the perihepatic and perisplenic views, and consider reverse Trendelenburg position during evaluation for hemothorax or free pelvic fluid.

- Have the patient take a slow, deep breath in and hold it to help bring the hepatorenal and splenorenal recesses into view.

- To minimize rib shadowing, rotate the probe 30 degrees to fit between the ribs or try using a phased array probe (with smaller footprint).

- To distinguish ascites from free fluid due to injury, assess for other signs of chronic liver disease such as nodular cirrhosis, gallbladder wall thickening, hepatosplenomegaly, and portal vein enlargement.

- To differentiate adrenal masses or abdominal fat from hematoma, compare them to the contralateral side.

- Perinephric fat can be distinguished from hematoma by its homogenous echodensity and lack of anechoic rim. It also remains stationary with respiratory variation.

- To distinguish pericardial fat from an effusion, assess whether or not it is circumferential and envelops the apex of the heart (this would be consistent with a pericardial effusion).

- Complete the FAST examination in every view and image any abnormal findings in more than one plane.

- In cases where it is difficult to distinguish normal structures from pathologic findings, a CT should be done to definitively exclude injury.

- Hemoperitoneum may not accumulate immediately. If the initial FAST is negative but the clinical suspicion for injury is high, wait for a short period of time and repeat the FAST. This is especially true if a patient's clinical status or examination changes. Serial examinations increase the sensitivity of FAST for detecting free intraperitoneal fluid due to blunt abdominal injury.

THERAPEUTIC MANEUVERS AND ULTRASOUND-GUIDED PROCEDURES

The use of ultrasound to guide therapeutic maneuvers and procedures has become increasingly popular over the past several years. Ultrasound is often favored over computerized tomography or fluoroscopy due to its ease of use, portability, and lack of radiation exposure to the patients and operator. Thoracostomy and pericardiocentesis are a few of the transthoracic procedures performed on trauma patients for which ultrasound has proven useful.

While ultrasound-guided tube thoracostomy is more likely to be performed in the nonacute setting for complicated effusions or empyema, it does have a role in the management of pneumo- or hemothorax. The transducer is used to visualize the guidewire entering the pleural cavity and ensure its proper location before advancing the catheter or various dilators (if a percutaneous thoracostomy tube is being used). To better visualize the wire, the transducer should be rotated along its long axis. The use of ultrasound in the setting of pneumothorax is slightly more challenging because intrapleural air obscures the interface between the visceral and parietal pleura; however, ultrasound can be used to ensure that you are above the diaphragm and that the intrapleural space at the site of insertion is clear of any other structures.

Ultrasound was first used for the drainage of a postoperative pericardial effusion in 1979.[30] Since then, ultrasound has been found to be superior to fluoroscopy (limited to a subcostal approach) with a lower mortality and complication rate in the hands of a trained physician. By providing direct visualization of the heart and surrounding structures, it has become the procedure of choice for the drainage of postprocedure and iatrogenic pericardial effusions, and its utility in the trauma setting has become evident as well. A 2.5- to 5-MHz transducer can be used and either a pericardiocentesis or central venous insertion kit. The optimal site for needle insertion is where the largest fluid collection is in closest proximity to the surface of the body, usually best seen with an apical or parasternal view. If the fluid accumulates in suboptimal locations for adequate visualization, placing the patient in a left lateral decubitus position may help to improve the apical view.

Care must be taken to avoid underestimating the distance from the skin to the pericardium. It is also important to visualize and avoid surrounding structures such as the lungs, the liver (during a subcostal approach), and the internal mammary artery (during the parasternal approach). Once the best site and trajectory have been determined, and ultrasound demonstrates a minimum of 1 cm of fluid between the heart and insertion site, the needle is inserted to the minimal depth required to withdraw fluid. If the needle is not within the pericardial space, it should be withdrawn and reinserted. Once correct positioning is confirmed, wire insertion followed by catheter insertion can be completed. The injection of agitated saline under direct ultrasound visualization can help confirm correct placement of the catheter.

Potential complications include laceration of the myocardium, pneumothorax, and vasovagal response, but the incidence of major complications is less than 2%.[31]

CONCLUSIONS AND THE FUTURE OF TRAUMA ULTRASOUND

Over the past 30 years, emergency ultrasound has become an integral part of trauma and emergency medical care. It is an accurate, sensitive diagnostic tool that allows for the rapid assessment and management of trauma victims with potentially life-threatening injuries. Emergency ultrasound is now considered the diagnostic test of choice for evaluating hemodynamically unstable patients and has helped to dramatically improve the outcome of blunt abdominal injuries.

Formal ultrasound training is a required component of all accredited emergency medicine residency programs and is already incorporated into the educational curriculum of surgery residents throughout Europe and the United States. Future research will help define standard criteria for achieving proficiency in the performance and interpretation of ultrasound for nonradiologist clinicians.

With rapid advances in technology, the role for trauma ultrasound will undoubtedly continue to evolve. The use of emergency ultrasound in pediatric and orthopedic trauma will become better defined, and will continue to replace more expensive and invasive conventional techniques for various procedures including fracture reduction, thoracostomy tube, and pericardiocentesis in adults and children. As smaller, more portable ultrasound units become readily available, it will have an increasing role in guiding prehospital care. Ultrasound may eventually become the gold standard for screening large numbers of patients in the setting of mass casualties.

CASE STUDIES

▶ Case 1

A 39-year-old man is brought in by EMS after a motor vehicle accident in which he was the unrestrained passenger. On arrival to the trauma bay, he is awake, alert, and responsive, and complaining of pain in his left lower extremity. His blood pressure is 120/68 with a heart rate of 102 beats per minute. Two large-bore intravenous lines are placed and 2 liters of crystalloid are infusing. On examination, he has multiple abrasions over his left chest, an open fracture of his left tibia, and tenderness in his left upper quadrant without guarding or rebound. A FAST examination is negative for free fluid, and radiographs of his chest and pelvis are normal.

Over the next several minutes, his oxygen saturation drops to 91% but improves to 95% on 2 liters of oxygen via nasal cannula. He is slightly diaphoretic, but his systolic blood pressure is 116/61 and his heart rate is 109. He continues to complain of abdominal pain and the decision is made to obtain a CT scan of the abdomen and pelvis on the way to the operating room for fixation of his lower extremity fracture.

On the way to the CT scanner, he becomes confused and progressively lethargic. His blood pressure is now 95/48 and his heart rate is 132. He is wheeled immediately back to the trauma bay where he is intubated emergently. A repeat FAST examination is performed simultaneously, revealing free fluid in Morison pouch and posterior to the bladder (Figure 9-18). He is taken immediately to the operating room where an exploratory laparotomy reveals

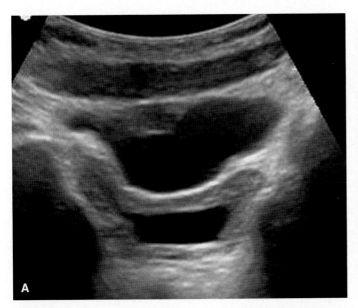
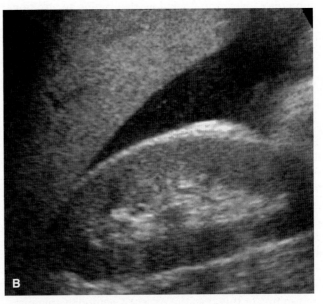

Figure 9-18. (**A**) Transverse view of hemoperitoneum posterior to the bladder. (Used with permission from www.ultrasoundcases.info/Slide-View.aspx?cat=182&case=4143) *ID: /23989.jpg;* (**B**) hemoperitoneum with blood in Morison pouch. (Used with permission from www.ultrasoundcases.info/Slide-View.aspx?cat=182&case=480); *ID: /2547.jpg*

a Grade 4 splenic laceration with significant hemoperitoneum. A splenectomy is performed and he recovers in the Trauma ICU over the next several days.

Discussion

This case illustrates the role of the FAST examination in the evaluation of a patient who becomes hemodynamically unstable and requires a more rapid test than CT scan to determine the need for immediate operative intervention. The FAST examination can be performed in less than three minutes and will not delay the time to definitive management. It also highlights the role for repeating the primary survey, including FAST examination, if a patient's clinical picture suddenly changes.

▶ Case 2

A 28-year-old woman presents to the emergency department complaining of worsening chest pain, dyspnea, and cough for two days. She reports being stabbed in the epigastric region with a small pocket knife during an altercation two days ago. There was minimal bleeding that stopped spontaneously and she did not seek further medical treatment. On arrival, she is awake but diaphoretic with a heart rate of 107, blood pressure of 95/68, a respiratory rate of 36, and an oxygen saturation of 89%. Further examination reveals mild jugular venous distention, decreased breath sounds over the left hemithorax, and a 1-cm laceration of her anterior chest wall, 3 cm to the left of the xiphoid. She is emergently intubated and FAST examination reveals a 2.3-cm pericardial effusion with right atrial diastolic collapse. A pericardiocentesis is performed in the emergency room that is positive for hemorrhagic fluid and 200 mL is removed with immediate improvement in her hemodynamic status. She is then taken to the operating room for a subxiphoid pericardial window that drains an additional 500 mL of serosanguinous fluid. A pericardial drain is left in place and an echocardiogram obtained on hospital day 3 shows complete resolution of the effusion.

Discussion

This patient presented with delayed cardiac tamponade from a penetrating chest injury. Cardiac tamponade occurs in up to 80% of patients who sustain penetrating injury to the heart. It may cause immediate cardiovascular collapse and death, or can accumulate slowly over time and offer a protective effect until clinical symptoms become apparent. Ultrasound, as part of the FAST examination, can accurately detect small amounts of fluid around the heart with a sensitivity and specificity of 100% and 99.3%, respectively. In addition to detecting hemopericardium, it can evaluate the hemodynamic effects of the pericardial effusion and should be performed in all cases of suspected penetrating chest injury. In this case, the patient's hemodynamic instability required emergent pericardiocentesis to temporize until more definitive treatment (pericardial window or thoracotomy and drain placement) could be obtained.

REFERENCES

1. Tso P, Rodrigues A, Cooper C, et al. Sonography in blunt abdominal trauma: a preliminary progress report. *J Trauma.* 1992;33:39–44.

2. Kristensen JK, Beumann B, Kuehl E. Ultrasonic scanning in the diagnosis of splenic haematomas. *Acta Chir Scand.* 1971;137:653–657

3. Rozycki GS, Ochsner MG, Jaffin JH, Champion HR. Prospective evaluation of surgeons' use of ultrasound in the evaluation of trauma patients. *J Trauma.* 1993;34(4):516–526; discussion 26-27.

4. Dulchavsky SA, Schwarz KL, Kirkpatrick AW, et al. Prospective evaluation of thoracic ultrasound in the detection of pneumothorax. *J Trauma.* 2001;50(2):201–205.

5. Kirkpatrick AW, Sirois M, Laupland KB, et al. Hand-held thoracic sonography for detecting post-traumatic pneumothoraces: the Extended Focused Assessment with Sonography for Trauma (EFAST). *J Trauma.* 2004;57:288–295.

6. Melniker LA, Leibner E, McKenney MG, Lopez P, Briggs WM, Mancuso CA. Randomized controlled clinical trial of point-of-care, limited ultrasonography for trauma in the emergency department: the first sonography outcomes assessment program trial. *Ann Emerg Med.* 2006;48(3):227–235.

7. Rose J, Ultrasound in abdominal trauma. *Emerg Med Clin N. Am.* 2004;22(3):581–599.

8. Plummer D, Brunette D, Asinger R, Ruiz E. Emergency department echocardiography improves outcome in penetrating cardiac injury. *Ann Emerg Med.* 1992;21: 709–712.

9. Soffer D, McKenney MG, Cohn S, et al. A prospective evaluation of ultrasonography for the diagnosis of penetrating torso injury. *J Trauma.* 2004;56:953–959.

10. Sybrandy KC, Cramer MJ, Burgersdijk C. Diagnosing cardiac contusion: old wisdom and new insights. *Heart.* 2003;89(5):485–489.

11. Ma OJ, Mateer JR. Trauma ultrasound examination versus chest radiography in the detection of hemothorax. *Ann Emerg Med.* 1997;29:312–316.

12. Moscati R, Reardon R. Clinical application of the FAST exam. In: Jehle D, Heller M, eds. *Ultrasonography in Trauma: The FAST.* 2003:39–60.

13. McKenney KL, McKenney MG, Cohn SM, et al. Hemoperitoneum score helps determine need for therapeutic laparotomy. *J Trauma.* 2001;50(4):650–654.

14. Becker A, Lin G, McKenney MG, Marttos A, Schulman CI. Is the FAST exam reliable in severely injured patients? *Injury.* 2010;41(5):479–483.

15. Miller T, Pasquale MD, Bromberg WJ, Wasser TE, Cox J. Not so fast. *J Trauma.* 2003;54:52–60.

16. Boulanger BR, Kearney PA, Tsuei B, Ochoa JB. The routine use of sonography in penetrating torso injury is beneficial. *J Trauma.* 2001;51(2):320–325.

17. Sinha TP, Bhoi S, Kumar S, et al. Diagnostic accuracy of bedside emergency ultrasound screening for fractures in pediatric trauma patients. *J Emerg Trauma Shock.* 2011;4(4):443–445.

18. Ang SH, Lee SW, Lam KY. Ultrasound-guided reduction of distal radius fractures. *Am J Emerg Med.* 2010;28(9): 1002–1008.

19. Chen L, Kim Y, Moore CL. Diagnosis and guided reduction of forearm fractures in children using bedside ultrasound. *Pediatr Emerg Care.* 2007;23(8):528–531.

20. Scaife ER, Fenton SJ, Hansen KW, Metzger RR. Use of focused abdominal sonography for trauma at pediatric and adult trauma centers: a survey. *J Pediatr Surg.* 2009;44(9):1746–1749.

21. Rathaus V, Zissin R, Werner M, et al. Minimal pelvic fluid in blunt abdominal trauma in children: the significance of this sonographic finding. *J Pediatr Surg.* 2001;36(9):1387–1389.

22. Cross KP, Warkentine FH, Kim IK, Gracely E, Paul RI. Bedside ultrasound diagnosis of clavicle fractures in the pediatric emergency department. *Acad Emerg Med.* 2010;17(7):687–693.

23. Sarkisian AE, Khondkarian RA, Amirbekian NM, Bagdasarian NB, Khojayan RL, Oganesian YT. Sonographic screening of mass casualties for abdominal and renal injuries following the 1988 Armenian earthquake. *J Trauma.* 1991;31:247.

24. Stawicki S, Howard J, Pryor J, Bahner D, Whitmill M, Dean A. Portable ultrasonography in mass casualty incidents: the CAVEAT examination. *World J Orthop.* 2010;1(1):10–19.

25. Cokkins D, Antypa E, Stefanidis K, et al. Contrast-enhanced ultrasound for imaging blunt abdominal trauma-indications, description of the technique and imaging review. *Ultraschall in Med.* 2012;33:60–67.

26. Catalano O, Aiani L, Barozzi L, et al. CEUS in abdominal trauma: multicenter study. *Abdon Imaging.* 2009;34(2): 225-234.

27. You JS, Chung YE, Lee HJ, et al. Liver trauma diagnosis with contrast-enhanced ultrasound: interobserver variability between radiologist and emergency physician in an animal study. *Am J Emerg Med.* 2012;30(7):1229-1234.

28. Brown MA, Sirlin CB, Hoyt DB, Casola G. Screening ultrasound in blunt abdominal trauma. *J Intensive Care Med.* 2003;18(5):253-260.

29. Stengel D, Bauwens K, Sehouli J, Nantke J, Ekkernkamp A. Discriminatory power of 3.5 MHz convex and 7.5 MHz linear ultrasound probes for the imaging of traumatic splenic lesions: a feasibility study. *J Trauma.* 2001;51(1):37–43.

30. Tsang TS, Freeman WK, Sinak LJ, Seward JB. Echocardiographically guided pericardiocentesis: evolution and state-of-the-art technique. *Mayo Clin Proc.* 1998;73:647–652.

31. Nguyen CT, Lee E, Luo H, Siegel RJ. Echocardiographic guidance for diagnostic and therapeutic percutaneous procedures. *Cardiovasc Diagn Ther.* 2011;10:2223–3652. 09.02

10

CRITICAL CARE ULTRASONOGRAPHY

OLIVER PANZER

INTRODUCTION AND CLINICAL INDICATIONS

The ultrasonographic examination by an intensive care physician differs significantly from other clinical disciplines such as cardiology, gastroenterology, or radiology. These specialties generally focus on one organ system in particular, and the examination is done systematically and in great detail. During the evaluation of an acutely and severely ill patient, however, ultrasonography is used to quickly narrow the differential diagnosis list, monitor the disease progress, and assist in difficult procedures. The intensivist uses this diagnostic tool at the bedside to answer specific questions (eg, why is this patient acutely short of breath?) as quickly as possible to tailor the therapy specifically to his patient. The intensivist performs ultrasonography as a part of the overall assessment of the patient, having a "quick look" at specific organs that may cause the acute illness or clinical change. To accomplish this task the intensivist needs an interdisciplinary approach to ultrasonography focusing on basic features/techniques of imaging the heart, lungs and thoracic wall, abdomen, and vascular structures. This chapter focuses on thoracic ultrasonography and echocardiography in the critical care setting.

▶ Thoracic Ultrasonography

Until recently ultrasonography of the lungs did not gain widespread acceptance, since its usefulness was questioned given the fact that ultrasound cannot transmit through air-filled spaces or penetrate bony structures. Dr. Lichtenstein and other authors, however, showed that simply evaluating pleural structures and ultrasound artifacts generated at the soft tissue-air interface of the chest wall and pleura may provide important diagnostic information to the clinician. A growing number of scientific papers describe the value of imaging the lung with ultrasonography instead of the conventional studies such as chest x-ray or the thoracic CT scan,[1,2] thus avoiding unnecessary exposure to ionizing radiation. Lung ultrasonography is easily performed at the bedside and given the lack of negative effects on the patient, it may be repeatedly used to monitor therapeutic progress in patients with lung pathology.[3]

Normal lung pattern on ultrasonography

Each intercostal space is visualized by first illustrating the upper and the lower ribs along a longitudinal plane. The proximal rib surface is identified as a bright white (hyperechoic) convex line followed by a clean, black acoustic shadow (Figure 10-1). In between the ribs, the pleura is identified as a hyperechoic line approximately 0.5 to 1 cm deep to the rib surface. During the respiratory cycle a to-and-fro movement of the visceral pleura against the parietal pleura on the chest wall can be seen in the real time or B-mode, and is referred to as the "lung sliding" sign. This finding can only be seen if both pleural sheaths are in direct contact, and thus effectively excludes a pneumothorax at that level.[4] If the examiner is unsure about the presence of lung sliding, the time motion mode (M-mode) can be used. With the cursor placed over the pleural line, the "Seashore sign" (Figure 10-2) should become apparent.[4] The resulting picture consists of continuous hyperechoic horizontal lines above the pleura representing the static chest wall, followed by a granulous pattern below the pleural line. This "sandy" pattern is created by the moving lung tissue during respiration. The significant difference in tissue densities between the pleura and the air-filled lung tissue creates a reverberation artifact, producing repetitive horizontal hyperechoic lines, called "A-lines," originating from the pleural line, depicted distal to the pleura at equally spaced intervals (Figure 10-3). A normal lung pattern on ultrasonography, therefore, appears as horizontal A-lines together with lung sliding, also referred to as the A-profile.[5]

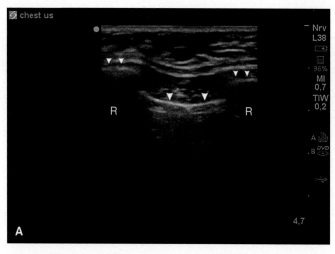

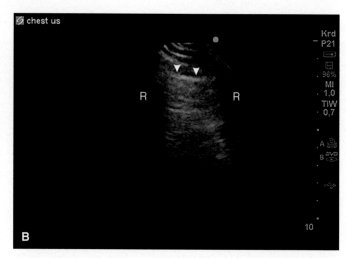

Figure 10-1. (**A**) Typical view of the intercostal space in the longitudinal plane using a linear array probe. The proximal rib surface (small arrows) is well seen with the following acoustic shadow (R). The pleural line (large arrows) is 0.5 to 1 cm deeper than the rib surface; (**B**) same view using a phased array probe. The rib surface is not well seen, but the pleural line is (large arrows).

Technique and equipment

Lung or thoracic ultrasonography can be performed with any modern medical ultrasound device supplied with a linear, phased array or curved linear array probe. Which probe should be used depends mainly on the patient's body habitus. A linear array probe is characterized by high resolution and poor penetration (max 9 cm) into tissue; thus, it is very useful for lean patients where superficial structures are of interest (eg, the pleura and chest wall). In contrast, a phased array probe has a poorer resolution but a better penetration into tissues (up to 25 cm) and is typically used for transthoracic echocardiography given its small footprint. This probe is useful if deeper structures need to be investigated such as consolidations and large pleural effusions. The curved linear array probe is a combination of both aforementioned probes, with a somewhat better resolution than the phased array

and a better penetration than the linear array probe. It is characterized by a large footprint and is mostly used for abdominal ultrasonography. Since lung ultrasonography is typically performed as part of a general ultrasound examination including echocardiography, we recommend to start with one probe that fits all—the phased array probe—and change the probe once the findings warrant a more detailed analysis.

Three different sonographic modes are used in lung ultrasonography: the real-time B-mode, the time motion mode (M-mode), and the color Doppler mode. For a more detailed description please refer to other chapters in this book.

In order to improve inter-interpreter variability and reproducibility of the ultrasound findings, each

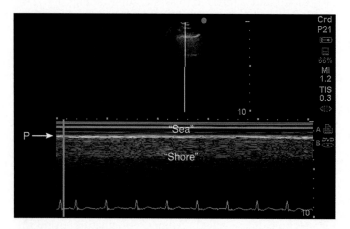

Figure 10-2. Sea-shore sign: To confirm lung sliding, the M-mode cursor is placed across the pleural line und the A-lines. The resulting image shows the so-called "sea shore sign", describing continuous horizontal lines above (sea) and a granulous pattern below (shore) the pleural line (P).

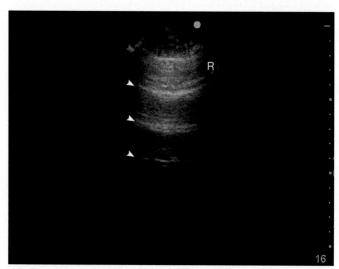

Figure 10-3. A-lines: A reverberation artifact originating from the strong reflection of ultrasound beams at the pleural-lung interface causes the depiction of multiple hyperechoic lines (arrows) at identical distance from each other underneath the pleural line (red arrow). R = rib.

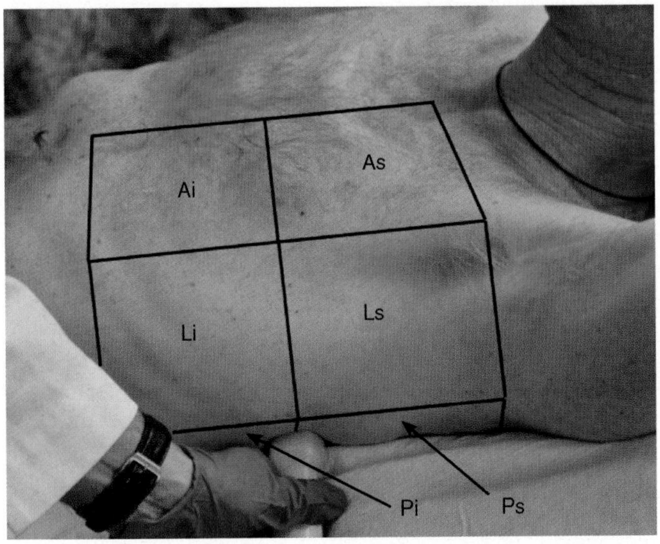

Alveolar-interstitial syndrome

Alveolar-interstitial syndrome (AIS) is a nonspecific finding on ultrasound associated with conditions such as acute lung injury (ALI) and acute respiratory distress syndrome (ARDS), interstitial pneumonia, pulmonary edema, as well as chronic diseases such as pulmonary fibrosis. In both instances the interlobular septi are thickened and cause a reverberation artifact leading to the formation of so-called B-lines. B-lines (also known as "comet tails" or "lung rockets") are ultrasound artifacts caused by the reflection of ultrasound beams within thickened interlobular septa just under the pleura and are seen as hyperechoic vertical lines arising from the pleural line.[6] These lines span the entirety of the ultrasound image without fading, are well defined, efface A-lines, and move with the visceral pleura. They may be part of a normal lung picture if they occur occasionally, mostly in the dependent lung zones. Their significance changes as they become more numerous; typically more than three in one window.

Their morphological correlate changes depending on the distance between the B-lines at the pleural line. B-lines ≥7 mm apart (B7 lines) represent thickened interlobular septi on CT scan[6] mostly caused by interstitial pulmonary edema of different etiologies. Comet tails, 3 mm or less apart (B3 lines), are typically caused by alveolar flooding or ground glass opacities on CT scan (Figure 10-5).

Assessing the presence and topographic distribution of the B-lines on the chest wall and taking into account clinical findings may help the clinician to narrow the differential diagnosis quickly in patients with respiratory distress. While AIS is present in both ALI/ARDS and cardiogenic pulmonary edema (findings such as "spared areas" with a normal lung pattern), a heterogenic mixture of B3 and B7 lines together with lung consolidations and focal absence of lung sliding points strongly toward lung injury, whereas a ubiquitous homogenous spread of B7 lines without any of the aforementioned ultrasound findings makes a cardiac pulmonary edema more likely.[7] A normal ultrasound pattern (no B-lines) in a patient with acute respiratory distress, on the other hand, would make a COPD exacerbation or a pulmonary embolus more likely than pulmonary edema of any cause.[8,9]

Lung ultrasonography may also assist in optimizing mechanical ventilator settings and monitoring treatment success. In patients with ALI/ARDS it may differentiate focal from disseminated disease and, therefore, help titrate positive end-expiratory pressure (PEEP) to avoid hyperinflation of the normal lung parenchyma ("baby lung").[10] The changes in lung aeration scores based on ultrasound findings correlate with changes found on chest CT scans after interventions such as pleural drainage or antimicrobial therapy for ventilator-associated pneumonia.[11]

Atelectasis and lung consolidation

Atelectasis (ATX) and lung consolidations are frequent findings in ventilated critically ill or postoperative patients and

Figure 10-4. Lung zones: Each hemithorax is divided into three zones: anterior (A), lateral (L), and posterior (P). Each zone is divided into a superior (s) and an inferior (i) area.

hemithorax is divided into three zones: the anterior zone, reaching from the sternal line to the anterior axillary line; the lateral zone, reaching from the anterior axillary line to the posterior axillary line; and the posterior zone, reaching from the posterior axillary line to the spine. Each zone is divided into a superior and an inferior area (Figure 10-4).

An ultrasonic examination is performed with the patient in supine or semirecumbent position. Depending on the clinical scenario the patient may need to be turned into a lateral decubitus position to access the posterior chest wall. However, the scapula limits the accessibility significantly in most cases. Each examination begins with the identification of the diaphragm on the corresponding side to differentiate the intrathoracic from the intra-abdominal space. Subsequently each intercostal space is thoroughly examined. The ultrasound examination is performed along close longitudinal (caudal to cranial direction) and transverse lines starting at the posterolateral aspect of the thorax and moving toward the sternum. A comprehensive examination of both lungs typically takes approximately 15 minutes, although in skilled hands, it may be performed more quickly.

Common pathological findings on chest ultrasonography

As described above, normal lung tissue may not be seen on ultrasound, since air-filled spaces are poorly penetrated by ultrasound waves. Only if the lung injury or pathological changes extend to the periphery (pleura) can they be seen on ultrasound. Processes such as interstitial pulmonary edema, alveolar flooding and resulting lung consolidation, pneumothoraces, and pleural effusions are characterized by specific ultrasound findings or a combination of them.

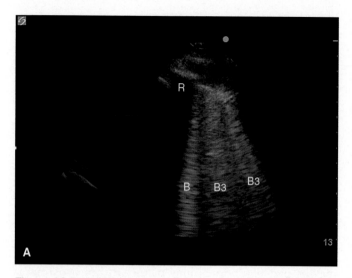
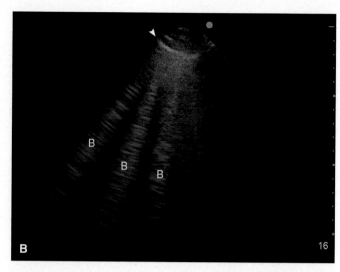

Figure 10-5. (**A**) B3 lines in a patient with alveolar interstitial syndrome. The B-lines are 3 or less mm apart at the pleural line and correlate to alveolar flooding or ground glass opacities on CT; (**B**) B-lines about 7 mm apart at the pleural line correlate to interstitial edema with thickened interlobular septi.

may be associated with significant morbidities such as induction of atelect-trauma and lung injury, if left untreated. Two forms of atelectasis are recognized: (a) passive ATX, produced by external compression, mostly due to a large pleural effusion or empyema; and (b) active or obstructive ATX, secondary to the resorption of oxygen. The ensuing lung collapse through loss of aeration leads to the consolidation of the lung tissue and thus allows ultrasound to travel through it and create a picture. A lung consolidation caused by compressive ATX is shown as hypoechoic (shades of dark gray) tissue floating in a large pleural effusion ("waving hand").[12] In obstructive ATX, additional interspersed hyperechoic spots, representing air bronchograms, are present (Figure 10-6) and the accompanying effusion tends to be smaller. Pneumonia also presents as a lung consolidation of different size and location, but is associated with dynamic air bronchograms

describing a reinforcement of the hyperechoic spots during inspiration.[3] In contrast, this reinforcement of the air bronchograms does not take place in complete ATX, since there is no air flow per se.[13] In complete obstruction of a lung segment, eg, after mainstem intubation, the so-called "lung pulse" is seen early on. In this case lung sliding is abolished and a pulsating movement of the pleura is detected, generated by the transmission of cardiac pulsations through the lung tissue.[14] This sign is best assessed using the time motion mode. The lung pulse is seen as intermittent vertical lines of granular pattern interrupting the straight horizontal lines underneath the pleural line in synchrony with cardiac contractions on the EKG tracing on the monitor. The clinical value lies in its ability to detect nonventilated lung areas early on, long before the collapse and consolidation of the lung segment occurs. This may be of particular interest in patients with marginal respiratory function, since already consolidated lung areas are much less likely to be re-recruited.[10]

Pleural effusion

To assess a pleural effusion sonographically, it is useful to identify the diaphragm first, since the fluid accumulates in the dependent areas, and to differentiate intra-abdominal from intrathoracic fluid (Figure 10-7). Fluid is typically anechoic and thus a pleural effusion will present itself as a black (anechoic) band surrounded by the visceral pleura, the diaphragm, and the parietal pleura during in- and expiration. Since fluid facilitates the propagation of ultrasound, deeper thoracic structures may well be seen. If the lung is still aerated, the visceral pleura is seen as a hyperechoic line followed by the previously described artifacts. If the pleural effusion is large and compressive, floating lung consolidations are seen. Vascular structures such as the descending thoracic aorta may be identified on the left side. Distinction of well-perfused and thus almost

Figure 10-6. Consolidated left lung within a large pleural effusion. The lung segment is hypoechoic, resembling the liver on ultrasound ("hepatization of the lung"). The hyperechoic spots within the atelectatic lung (white arrows) correspond to "air bronchograms," caused by microbubbles of air trapped in mucous inside the airways. PE = pleural effusion; S = spine.

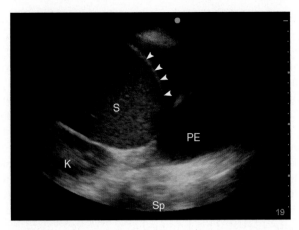

Figure 10-7. Identification of the diaphragm: Before assessing the pleural effusion, the diaphragm needs to be identified. In this picture, the diaphragm (arrows) clearly separates the intra-abdominal space with the spleen (S) to form the intrathoracic space with a pleural effusion (PE). Sp = Spine; K = Kidney.

anechoic organs or structures may be difficult. Applying color Doppler may help by identifying vessels within the organs such as the spleen or liver. To differentiate a small loculated effusion from edematous and thickened pleura, the "color fluid" sign may help. A positive sign elicits color Doppler signals within the space in question, caused by phasic respiratory movements within the pleural fluid. In addition, the sinusoid sign on M-mode shows the movement of the lung tissue toward the periphery during inspiration (Figure 10-8), confirming the presence of fluid. Although the sonographic characteristics cannot differentiate between transudate and exudate, they may guide

further diagnostic workup. Depending on the echogenicity of the pleural fluid, a pleural effusion may be described as anechoic, complex nonseptated, complex septated, and homogenously echogenic. The fluid is anechoic if no echogenic materials are found within the effusion, complex nonseptated if some echogenic material is floating within the effusion, complex septated if fibrin strands connect to the visceral and parietal pleura, and homogenously echogenic if echogenic particles are equally distributed within the pleural space.[15] In a study evaluating 320 patients with pleural effusions, findings of complex nonseptated, complex septated, and homogenously echogenic pleural fluid always defined an exudate, whereas anechoic fluid could be an exudate or a transudate.[15] Homogenously echogenic pleural effusions are typically caused by an hemorrhagic effusion or an empyema (Figure 10-9).

Ultrasound may also be used for the quantification of the pleural fluid. Two methods have been described achieving good estimates of the actually drained pleural effusion volume and/or estimated volume on CT scan. In 58 postcardiac surgery patients with signs of pleural effusion on chest x-ray (CXR), the prepuncture pleural volume was estimated using the formula $V_{pre} = (15.06 \times D[mm]) + 21.45$, where D is the distance measured via ultrasound between the midheight of the diaphragm and the visceral pleura at end-expiration in a sitting patient. Only patients with >30 mm distance were tapped and evaluated; a strong correlation between tapped and estimated volume was observed with a correlation coefficient $r = 0.89$, $P < 0.001$.[16] However, most of the methods using the maximal effusion depth have a poor correlation with smaller effusions. Using the cross-sectional area (cm²) of the pleural effusion (PE) instead, a significantly better

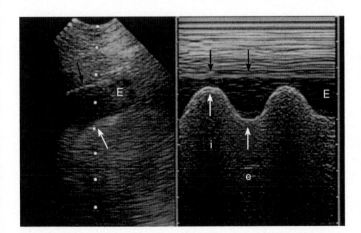

Figure 10-8. Sinusoid sign: the picture on the left shows an anechoic band (E) representing a pleural effusion with the visceral pleura underneath (white arrow) and the parietal pleura above (black arrow). The picture on the right shows the "sinusoid sign," a sign specific for a liquid-filled pleural space, caused by an inspiratory narrowing of the pleural effusion (i) and expiratory widening (e). (With permission: Lichtenstein DA. Ultrasound in the management of thoracic disease. *Crit Care Med.* 2007 May;35(Suppl):S250–S261.)

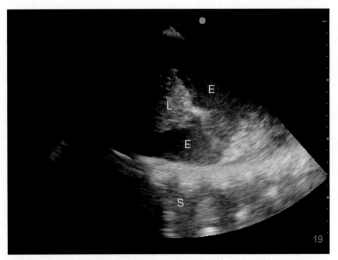

Figure 10-9. Empyema: In this longitudinal view of the right hemithorax, pleural fluid is surrounding the collapsed lung areas (L); however, the fluid is not anechoic but homogenously hypoechoic with floating particles (E). This picture was taken of a 55-year-old gentleman with persistent fevers despite adequate antibiotic treatment.

correlation was reached between the measured PE volume (PEV) on CT and the measured volume on ultrasound. The measurements were taken in supine patients along the posterior axillary line in a transverse plane. The PEV on ultrasound was measured using the formula: $PEV = A_{us} \times L_{us}$, A_{us} referring to the cross-sectional area of the PE at the midlevel between the apical and caudal limits of the PE spread, and L_{us} standing for the maximal length of the PE in craniocaudal direction. With this method, small, moderate, and large PEs could be accurately predicted compared to CT, with a correlation coefficient of 0.96 and $P < 0.001$.[17]

CXRs as well as physical examination have a poor accuracy in predicting the extent of the effusion and determining a safe puncture site for thoracocentesis. Lung ultrasound, on the other hand, has several advantages, and since it may be rapidly performed at the bedside, it allows accurate estimates of the extent and finding of a safe puncture site, avoiding procedure-related complications such as a pneumothorax. Even though thoracocentesis is considered safe, accidental pneumothoraces occur in up to 30% of clinically guided attempts.[18] Using ultrasound guidance for thoracocentesis led to a 10% reduction in accidental organ puncture and avoided puncture at an inappropriate site in 15% of patients.[19] Moreover, in 58% of clinically attempted "dry taps," subsequent ultrasound examination showed the puncture site to be below the diaphragm.[20]

There are two ways of using ultrasound for thoracocentesis. Most intensivists do not use real-time ultrasonography for the tapping of a pleural effusion, but rather mark the best puncture site on the patient's skin and then insert the needle afterward. Since the patient may change his/her position or the mark may fade, the puncture should follow immediately after the site has been marked. In fact, significant delay eliminates the benefit of using ultrasound to avoid a pneumothorax compared to the conventional approach. The other option is to perform the tap under real-time ultrasonography, allowing for control of the needle tip throughout the procedure. The skill set required for this approach is somewhat more advanced, but easily achieved even without formal training.[21] The patient may be brought into the sitting position or the supine position with a slight head elevation to tap the effusions.

Pneumothorax

A pneumothorax (PTX) may be caused by trauma, ARDS, mechanical ventilation, severe pneumonia, and procedures such as placing a central line or performing a thoracentesis.[22] The sensitivity of AP CXRs to detect a PTX varies from 25% to 60% and is often associated with a significant delay until the diagnosis is established. The gold standard for diagnosing PTX is the CT scan, yet increased transportation risk and exposure to ionizing radiation are limiting factors, especially if repetitive evaluation is necessary. Detecting a pneumothorax on transthoracic ultrasound is much quicker and more sensitive than using a CXR, especially in the emergency setting.[23,24] By definition a PTX causes the visceral pleura to separate

from the parietal pleura, thereby effectively abolishing the lung sliding seen on ultrasonography. On M-mode the granular pattern below the pleural line is replaced by straight horizontal lines, creating the so-called "barcode sign" (Figure 10-10Ab). In addition, A-lines should be seen without any occasional B-lines or other pleural artifacts ("A-line" sign in PTX). However, absent lung sliding may also be caused by large bullae, severe COPD and overdistention, mainstem intubation, pleural adherences, or a chest tube. A sign of partial pneumothorax is the so-called "lung point" where the normal lung pattern (lung sliding and A-lines) intermittently changes into a pattern of a pneumothorax (absent lung sliding with A-lines) (Figure 10-10). This finding has a 79% sensitivity and a 100% specificity.[25] Tracking the lung points in the different intercostal spaces may help delineate the size of the partial PTX. For this purpose the patient should be supine during the examination. The major advantage in the diagnosis of PTX by ultrasonography lies in its high negative predictive value. The presence of lung sliding, B-lines, or the lung pulse effectively excludes a PTX. To improve the positive predictive value of the absence of lung sliding during procedures with a high risk of PTX, it is crucial to perform the examination before and after the intervention. If lung sliding is present before the procedure and is absent afterward, the likelihood of PTX is very high.

Pulmonary embolism

Recent evidence suggests that thoracic ultrasound may be useful to evaluate the possibility of pulmonary embolism (PE) in the critically ill. Even though ultrasound can only evaluate the lung periphery and certainly not the central pulmonary vessels, about 80% of the patients with a central embolus also have evidence of smaller peripheral emboli,[26] resulting in small pulmonary hemorrhages. In fact up to 66% of the peripheral lesions occur in the lower lobes of the lung,[27] potentially allowing their detection on thoracic ultrasound. To optimize access to the lower thorax the patient should be sitting at the bedside with both hands behind his/her head to open up the intercostal spaces. The sonomorphology of a PE lesion has characteristic features: hypoechoic, pleural based, wedge-shaped (85%), or round-shaped (11%) lesions with the majority located in an area of pleuritic chest pain.[28] These lesions have to be differentiated from lesions associated with bronchial cancer, lung metastases, and pneumonic infiltrate. A pneumonic lesion typically has an irregular border, is inhomogeneous, and is well perfused on color-Doppler imaging. Thus, it is easily differentiated from a PE-related lesion. Occasionally an air bronchogram may be found inside the lesion. In case of neoplastic disease, the lesion may either have an irregular or polycyclic shape with diffuse borders in case of bronchogenic carcinoma or have a sharp border and a round/oval shape in case of lung metastases (which may therefore be confused with PE lesions). Invasive growth into adjacent tissues such as the parietal pleura or chest wall may give further clues to a neoplastic mass. Accepting either

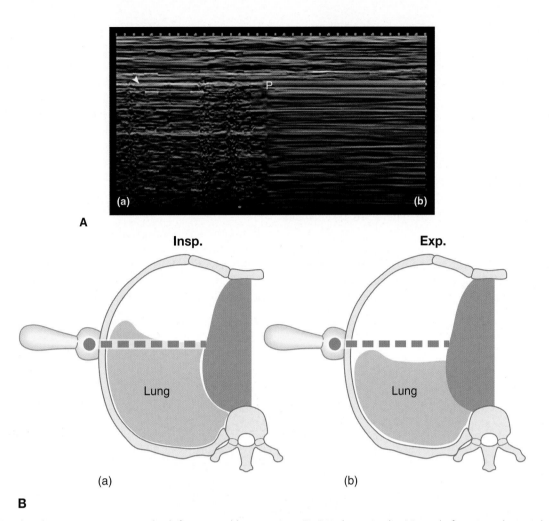

Insp.   **Exp.**

(a)   (b)

B

Figure 10-10. The "lung point" sign: on the left a normal lung pattern (Aa) is shown in the M-mode function, the seashore sign as described above. In case of a partial pneumothorax the seashore sign intermittently changes with the "barcode" sign (Ab) in the area where the pneumothorax borders with the still expanded lung. The "barcode sign" develops as the lung drops below the scanning plane (Bb) during expiration and describes continuous horizontal lines above and below the pleura. (Ultrasound picture with permission from Bouhemad B, Zhang M, Lu Q, Rouby J-J. Clinical review: bedside lung ultrasound in critical care practice. *Crit Care*. 2007;11(1):205.)

two or more typical wedge-shaped or rounded subpleural lesions or one typical lesion with a corresponding small pleural effusion as sonographic criteria for PE in patients with confirmed PE on CT pulmonary angiography resulted in a 74% sensitivity and 95% specificity of transthoracic ultrasound for diagnosing PE.[27] Since only roughly two-thirds of the thorax can be evaluated by ultrasound (due to the ribs and scapula preventing the depiction of the lung), and the fact that peripheral pulmonary hemorrhages may be reabsorbed within a few hours or days, a negative finding on ultrasound does not rule out a PE.[27,28] In acutely dyspneic patients, however, the finding of a normal lung profile (A-lines and lung sliding) over both hemithoraces and a deep vein thrombosis on duplex sonography of the femoral veins yielded a positive predictive value of 94%, a sensitivity of 81%, and a specificity of 99% for the diagnosis of PE.[5] This implies that lung ultrasound should be performed together with the duplex sonography of the lower extremity veins if a PE is suspected. This approach should

be used in patients with respiratory distress but hemodynamic stability. If the patient is in shock, though, an echocardiography should be done first, looking for signs of acute right ventricular failure and, if present, thrombolysis or embolectomy may be initiated on these findings alone (see focused echocardiography section).

▶ Focused Transthoracic Echocardiography

Indications

Every critically ill patient who is hemodynamically unstable may benefit from a focused transthoracic echocardiography (FTTE) by the intensivist, especially after the first measures of resuscitation prove to be ineffective. FTTE may be used to obtain a momentary status of the cardiovascular performance or may be used to monitor treatment efficacy. Hüttemann et al showed in a meta-analysis of medical and surgical critical care patients that in case of acute hypotension, echocardiography resulted in a management change in 36% of patients, and led to a surgical intervention in 14% of cases.[29] Used as a monitoring tool, TEE detected severe previously unknown heart dysfunction in 8% of newly admitted intensive care patients.

Technique and normal anatomy

The heart is visualized through acoustic windows in the anterior chest wall that allow for a clear view of the heart with minimal interference from lung tissue or bony structures. The sites on the thorax and the related pictures from the heart have been standardized. There are three main access sites (Figure 10-11).

(1) Left parasternal window (left 2nd to 4th intercostal space in proximity to the sternum). (2) Apical window (placing the US probe on the point of maximal impact of the cardiac apex, typically 4th to 6th left intercostal space

between the midclavicular and the anterior axillary line). (3) Subcostal window (placing the US probe just underneath the xiphoid process in the epigastric area).

To scan the heart from the parasternal and apical window the patient should be brought into the left lateral decubitus position, since this maneuver pushes the heart toward the left anterior chest wall and thus minimizes interference with aerated lung tissue. For the subcostal window the patient should be in the supine position, with the legs bent to relax the abdominal wall.

Left parasternal window

Using the left parasternal window, two basic views (imaging planes) have been described: parasternal long-axis (PLAX) and short-axis (PSAX) views. The parasternal long axis is a cut (of the ultrasound beam) through the longitudinal axis of the heart, meaning from the base

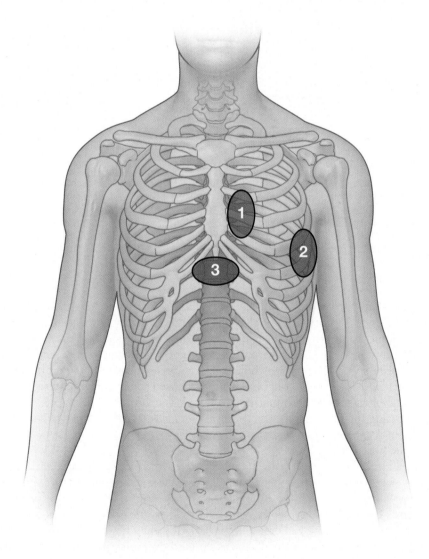

Figure 10-11. Transducer positions on the chest wall: 1. Parasternal area: two views may be taken from here: the parasternal long-axis view and the parasternal short-axis view; 2. apical area: the apical four-chamber view is taken here; 3. subcostal area: subcostal four-chamber view.

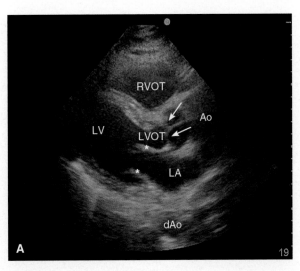 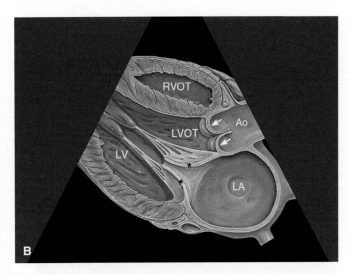

Figure 10-12. Parasternal long-axis view (PLAX). (**A**) real ultrasonographic picture; (**B**) corresponding animated picture. RVOT = Right ventricular outflow tract; Ao = ascending aorta; LVOT = left ventricular outflow tract; LV = left ventricle; LA = left atrium; stars = mitral valve; arrows = aortic valve. ((B) Reproduced with permission from Patrick Lynch, Medical Illustrator/Wikimedia Commons.)

(valvular plane) to the apex of the heart. In this view, according to the American Society of Echocardiography, the index marker on the US probe should point toward the right shoulder of the patient, with the screen marker on the US screen located on the right side. This view is defined by the visualization of the right ventricular outflow tract (RVOT), the interventricular septum (IVS) and the aortic valve (AV) and root, the left ventricle (LV), the mitral valve (MV), and the left atrium (LA) with the adjacent descending aorta (descAo), going from anterior to posterior or from top to bottom on the ultrasound screen (Figure 10-12).

To visualize the heart in the short-axis plane, the US probe is rotated clockwise toward the left shoulder by 90 degrees at the same position on the chest wall. In this

imaging plane, a total of five different short-axis levels have been described. For the purpose of the focused echocardiography examination, the midventricular or papillary muscle level and the aortic valve level, however provide enough information. In the papillary muscle level, the LV is depicted in a circular fashion ("doughnut sign"), the landmark for this cross-sectional cut being the two round-shaped papillary muscles in the lower half of the LV lumen (Mickey Mouse sign) (Figure 10-13).

If the LV lumen is ellipsoid in shape, the imaging plane is not exactly perpendicular to the long axis of the heart and can be adjusted by slightly rotating the US probe. The RV has a crescent shape in this view, and many times, the free right ventricular wall is not well seen. This view is particularly useful for the analysis of the contractile

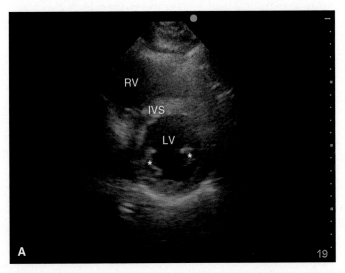 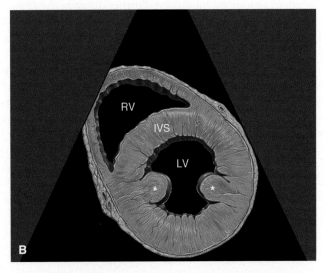

Figure 10-13. Parasternal short-axis view (PSAX): midpapillary level. RV = right ventricle; IVS = interventricular septum; LV = left ventricle; star = papillary muscles. ((B) Reproduced with permission from Patrick Lynch, Medical Illustrator/Wikimedia Commons.)

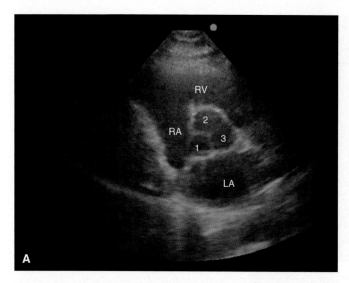
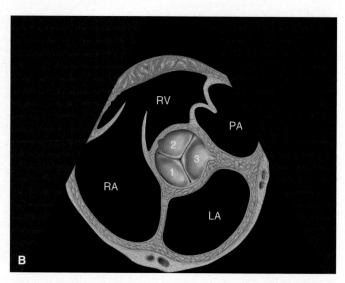

Figure 10-14. Parasternal short-axis view—aortic valve level: by tilting the ultrasound beam slightly toward the right shoulder of the patient, the picture changes from the papillary muscle level to the aortic valve level. Using the clock analogy, the RV inflow and outflow tract wrap around the central aortic valve starting at approximately 7 o'clock to approximately 2 o'clock. RA = right atrium; RV = right ventricle; PA = pulmonary artery; LA = left atrium; 1 = noncoronary cusp; 2 = right coronary cusp; 3 = left coronary cusp.

function. The LV contraction is complex, consisting of a longitudinal, torsional, and radial component. About 90% of the contractile force is generated by the circumferentially aligned myocardial fibers; hence, the PSAX view at the midpapillary level is particularly useful to evaluate the LV contractility. However, Doppler measurements are typically of limited value, since most of the time the blood flow is perpendicular or in a steep angle to the ultrasound beam.

The PSAX aortic valve level view is sometimes difficult to obtain given that the heart base is often positioned behind the sternum. At this level, all three cusps of the AV are seen. During systole the valve opens to an almost circular orifice and the cross-sectional area of the AV opening may be measured. During diastole the closed cusps form an inverse Y sign ("Mercedes-Benz Sign"). The AV and pulmonary valves lie perpendicular to each other; hence, the PV is seen in a longitudinal cut at the left coronary cusp. The RV inflow and outflow tract wrap around the AV valve clockwise. The inflow tract starts with the RA and TV adjacent to the noncoronary cusp and followed by the RV chamber and the outflow tract with the PV and the beginning of the pulmonary artery close to the left coronary cusp. Posterior to the AV is the LA. This view is particularly useful to assess the blood flow through the TV and PV, since the ultrasound beam is almost parallel to the direction of the blood flow (Figure 10-14).

Apical window

From this window the apical four-chamber (A4C) and five-chamber (A5C) view may be visualized. All four chambers are seen in the axial plane of the heart, plus the LVOT in the A5C view. Whenever possible the patient should be brought into the left lateral decubitus position with the left arm abducted. The US probe should ideally be placed over the point of maximal impulse of the heart apex. Generally it should be in the fifth intercostal space or more caudal between the left midclavicular line and the medial axillary line. The probe should be angled toward the right shoulder, whereas the index marker should be pointing toward the left lateral chest wall. The US probe may have to be rotated slightly to visualize all four chambers. The following structures should be seen going from the top to the bottom of the picture on the ultrasound screen: cardiac apex, RV, and RA on the left side and the LV and LA on the right side of the screen, and the descending aorta posterior to the LA, TV, and MV leaflets and the IVS (Figure 10-15).

To obtain the five-chamber view the probe is slightly angled cranially and the LVOT with the AV and the aortic root will appear at the base of the heart between the MV and TV (Figure 10-16). The apical views are particularly useful for the evaluation of the right heart function and to assess valvular pathologies in the Doppler mode, since the blood flow runs in parallel to the ultrasound beam (color Doppler, continuous wave Doppler mode).

Subcostal window

Similar to the parasternal views, long-axis and short-axis views of the heart may be obtained. The subcostal or subxiphoid long-axis view shows all four chambers in the same axial plane as the A4C view. However, instead of originating at the apex of the heart, the ultrasound beam

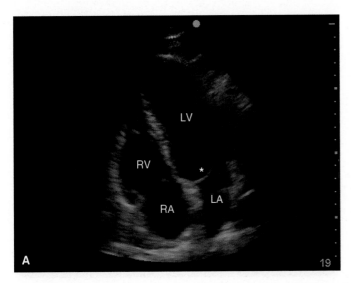

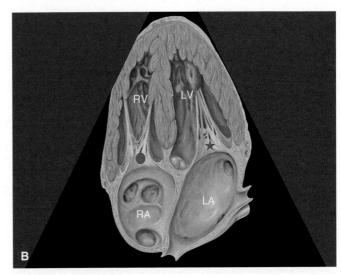

Figure 10-15. Apical four-chamber (A4C) view: RV = right ventricle; LV = left ventricle; RA = right atrium; LA = left atrium.

is coming from the right side of the heart and moves through the heart toward the left lateral wall of the LV (Figure 10-17).

Contrary to the prior views, the patient should stay supine, with the knees bent to relax the abdominal wall. The probe is placed in the epigastric area just underneath the xiphoid process and angled cranially pointing toward the left shoulder. Before orienting the probe cephalad, enough pressure must be exerted to push the probe somewhat into the abdomen to scan posterior to the rib cage, thus avoiding interference with the bony structures. This view is particularly helpful in patients with COPD or pneumothoraxes, since intrathoracic air cannot interfere significantly in this approach (posterior pericardium is attached to the diaphragm). However, other aspects such as a recent meal and subsequent air in the stomach, recent

laparotomy, or mediastinal chest tubes may limit the value of this approach.

Common findings

An increasing number of practicing intensivists rely on focused echocardiography to assess a hemodynamically unstable patient. An ultrasound examination performed by the intensivist himself has the advantage that it permits immediate and 24-hour availability of an effective, noninvasive, and repeatable hemodynamic bedside tool. Apart from the visualization of the heart, the combination of the two-dimensional depiction of the cardiac structures and their function plus the dynamic assessment of blood flow via Doppler echocardiography allows for a detailed insight into the cardiac function in real time.

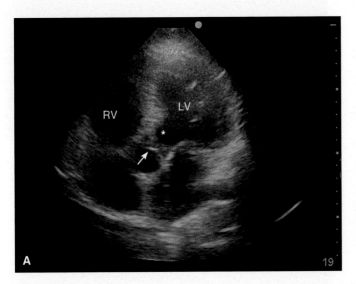

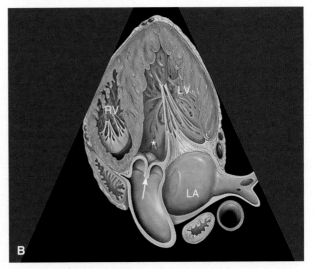

Figure 10-16. Apical five-chamber (A5C) view: By tilting the US probe slightly cranially the A5C view is obtained. RV = right ventricle; LV = left ventricle; star = left ventricular outflow tract; arrow = aortic valve. (Reproduced with permission from Patrick Lynch, Medical Illustrator/Wikimedia Commons.)

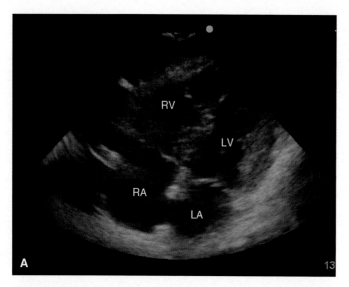

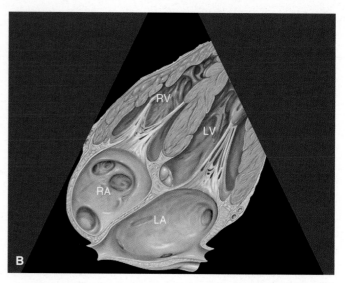

Figure 10-17. Subcostal four-chamber view: RV = right ventricle; LV = left ventricle; RA = right atrium; LA = left atrium.

During interpretation of the acquired images, the examiner should always proceed systematically to avoid mistakes. For the use in the ICU the following seems the most effective:

- Assessment of LV size and function
- Assessment of RV size and function
- Assessment of the pericardial space
- Assessment of the valvular function

LV size and function

LV function depends on many factors including preload and afterload, contractile function during systole and diastole, etc. Ultrasonography may give clues about global function by assessing ejection fraction (LVEF), cardiac output (CO) and stroke volume (SV), left ventricular filling pressures, and regional myocardial dysfunction in the setting of ischemic disease.

Visual estimation of global function/contractility (hypo-, hyperdynamic)

Visual estimation of left ventricular function can be done using the "eyeballing" method. This visual estimation of left ventricular ejection fraction using the PLAX, PSAX view, and the A4C view shows a good correlation with formal assessment methods of systolic left ventricular function (Simpson method, fractional shortening method).[30] Left ventricular function is graded as hyperdynamic, normal, and mildly, moderately, or severely hypokinetic. Formal assessment methods are based on the calculated ejection faction (LVEF), for example, by dividing the stroke volume (SV) through the left ventricular end-diastolic volume (Simpson). The exact determination of the systolic and diastolic LV volumes, however, is time-consuming and subject to significant interobserver variability. Simpler methods such as the calculation of the fractional area change (FAC) or the

fractional shorting (FS) (Figure 10-18) correlate well with radionuclide ejection fraction (gold standard). Since it is readily and quickly performed, eyeballing ejection fraction seems more appropriate in emergency situations and could be used for routine echocardiography instead of formal methods.

The calculation of the patients CO (SV × heart rate) may give further clues to the hemodynamic instability (high output failure in sepsis or severe cirrhosis, low output

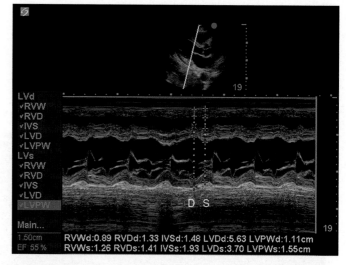

Figure 10-18. Calculation of LVEF: using the M-mode function, the LV EF may be estimated by calculating the fractional shortening (FS): LVDd – LVDs/LVDd = LVEF (%). Ideally this should be done in the PLAX and PSAX – midpapillary muscle level view (picture). Normal values are between 30% and 45%. Similarly, the fractional area change (FAC) method may be used, FAC: LVEF (%) = LVA^{2}d – LVA^{2}s/LVA^{2}d. The endocardial borders have to be traced on the PSAX view using the area mode on the ultrasound machine. Normal values are between 55% and 65%. LVDd = diastolic left ventricular diameter; LVDs = systolic left ventricular diameter; LVA^{2}d = diastolic left ventricular area; LVA^{2}s = systolic LVA; D = diastolic measurements; S = systolic measurements.

failure in cardiogenic shock). Using echocardiography, the SV is calculated by multiplying the cross-sectional area of the LVOT (CSA_{LVOT}) with the velocity time integral in the LVOT (VTI_{LVOT})

$$SV \ (cm^3 = mL) = VTI_{LVOT} \ (cm) \times CSA_{LVOT} \ (cm^2)$$

The diameter of the LVOT ($LVOT_D$) is measured in the PLAX view directly under the aortic valve ring. The LVOT is round during systole so that the area can be calculated using the formula for a circle:

$$CSA_{LVOT} \ (cm^2) = \pi r^2 = \pi \ (D_{LVOT}/2)^2$$

Visual estimation of size

Impaired left ventricular function can be associated with increased left ventricular size. End-stage impairment of left ventricular function can result in an increased size of the left atrium and left ventricle. This increase in size is typical of dilated cardiomyopathy and long-lasting aortic or mitral valve regurgitation. The failing left ventricle may also present with severe hypertrophy of the myocardium associated with the underlying disease, with only mild increase in size but reduced contractility.

Left ventricular filling pressures

Impaired ventricular function is associated with impaired systolic and diastolic performance, resulting in an increase in left ventricular filling pressures. Up to 50% of the patients with heart failure present with isolated diastolic dysfunction. Elevated filling pressures of the LV are the main consequence of diastolic dysfunction. The ratio of early velocity of transmitral left ventricular filling (E wave on continuous wave Doppler through MV) and the early velocity of the mitral annulus (E' wave on Doppler tissue imaging) (E/E' ratio) can be used to estimate the left ventricular end-diastolic pressure and estimate LV relaxation/

stiffness independent of pre- and afterload conditions. Normal values are smaller than or equal to 8; values above 15 represent severe diastolic dysfunction and are accompanied by increased LV end-diastolic filling pressures. Furthermore, the pulmonary capillary wedge pressure (PCWP) may be calculated based on the E/E' ratio

$$PCWP = 1.24 \times (E/E') + 1.9 \ mm \ Hg$$

These measurements are taken in the A4C view as shown in Figure 10-19.

Regional myocardial dysfunction

Ischemic heart disease is still the most common reason for acute heart failure and cardiogenic shock in critically ill patients. Early diagnosis and treatment is essential, since the time window for successful percutaneous angiography and stenting is limited and the resulting hemodynamic disturbances have a significant impact on patient outcome. Once the blood flow though a coronary artery is reduced or even absent, the dependent myocardium loses its ability to contract. On echocardiography this may be seen as a regional loss of systolic inward movement during contraction and systolic wall thickening. In an emergency situation it is sufficient to assess the heart in the PSAX at the mid-papillary level. The three main coronary arteries and their respective segments are represented in this view; hence, 50–70% of all new onset ischemic changes are detected.

Right ventricular size and function

In 20–30% of hemodynamically unstable ICU patients, right heart failure is the sole cause and is often overlooked. It may be caused by an acute increase in afterload or an ischemic event. The right ventricle has a limited contractile reserve and quickly goes into pump failure when faced with acute increases in pulmonary vascular resistance.

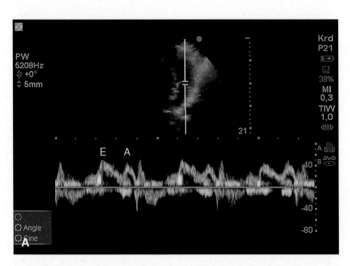

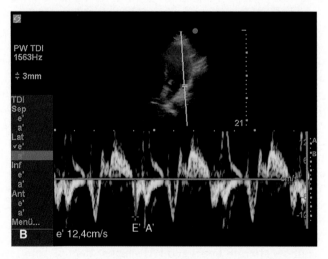

Figure 10-19. (**A**) Showing the transmitral flow profile on pulsed wave (PW) Doppler. The E wave is produced during early diastolic filling, whereas the A wave represents the atrial kick at end-diastole. The sample window is placed at the tip of the mitral valve leaflets; (**B**) Showing a tracing of the mitral valve annulus on PW tissue Doppler. It represents the velocity at which the myocardium relaxes during diastolic filling. The stiffer the LV wall, the slower the velocity. As a result the E/E' ratio would increase as a sign of worsening diastolic dysfunction. In this case the E/E' ratio is 4.5 (a value above eight is considered abnormal).

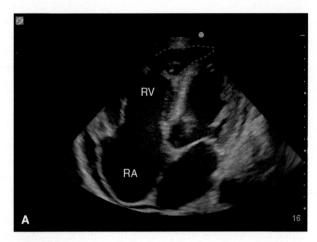
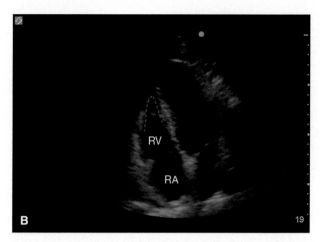

Figure 10-20. (A) A4C view with severe RV dilation: the RV has surpassed the LV in size and the heart apex is completely occupied by the RV; **(B)** in contrast, a normal RV in the A4C view. The RV is less than 60% of the LV size and the heart apex is completely occupied by the LV.

Common processes involved are pulmonary emboli, acute respiratory distress syndrome, sepsis, or high airway pressures during mechanical ventilation. Since treatment differs from LV failure, early diagnosis and the differentiation between acute and chronic processes are important.

Echocardiography can help establish the diagnosis through visual analysis on two-dimensional ultrasound and via alterations on color and continuous wave Doppler of the TV.

Visual estimation of right ventricular function

Secondary to its limited contractile reserve, the failing right ventricle quickly dilates. Comparison of RV to LV size on the A4C view may be used and is graded as mild, moderate, and severe dilatation. The compensated RV should be less than 60% in size compared to the LV. If RV failure is severe, the dilated RV may compress the LV and push the IVS into the LV lumen, giving the LV a D-shape on PSAX views.

This, however, may be inaccurate if a dilated cardiomyopathy is present; also, the apical morphology of the heart is altered with worsening RV failure. While the apex is solely occupied by the LV apex with normal RV function, the opposite is true in severe right heart failure (Figure 10-20).

The RV has the capability to adapt to slow progressive increases in afterload, such as in primary pulmonary hypertension or secondary pulmonary hypertension caused by chronic pulmonary diseases or severe mitral valve disease. The RV dilation is then accompanied by a progressive free wall hypertrophy (>6 mm thickness). In this setting the RV may be able to maintain high mean pulmonary pressures (>60 mm Hg). In acute RV failure hypertrophy only manifests after 48 hours and PAPs higher than 60 mm Hg are rare. Decompensation invariably leads to dilation of the tricuspid valve annulus and tricuspid valve insufficiency. Two-dimensional analysis of the RV is best done in the A4C view or the subcostal four-chamber view.

Estimation of pulmonary pressures and severity of Tricuspid valve regurgitation

Estimation of systolic pulmonary artery pressures (PAPs) plays an important role in the assessment of the right ventricular function. High PAPs may trigger further workup of the underlying pulmonary hypertension as a reason for the poor RV function. On the other hand, high PAPs require adequate blood flow (pressure = flow × resistance) and thus may also stand for a preserved RV pump function. PAPs may be calculated by measuring the peak velocity of the tricuspid regurgitant jet (v_{max}) in m/s using continuous wave Doppler imaging. Following the calculation of the pressure gradient over the TV using the simplified Bernoulli equation, the central venous pressure (CVP) is added:

$$PAPs = \Delta P + CVP = (4 \times v_{max}^2) + CVP$$

To accurately determine PAPs, parallel alignment of the ultrasound beam to the regurgitant jet has to be accomplished, which may be technically challenging. In patients lacking a central line, direct measurement of the RAP/CVP is not possible, but may be estimated by measuring IVC diameter and collapsibility during respirations. For this purpose the IVC is visualized in a longitudinal or cross-sectional view as it passes through the liver. The ultrasound probe is placed in the epigastric area, slightly to the right of the midline in a sagittal plane just underneath the xiphoid process. The size and the inspiratory collapsibility of the IVC correlate to a certain central venous pressure in spontaneously breathing patients as shown in Table 10-1 and may be used instead of the directly measured CVP.

The severity of the tricuspid regurgitation (TR) as an indicator for the degree of RV failure is best determined using color Doppler imaging. In emergent situations the semiquantitative method using color flow mapping within the RA area may be most useful. Mild TR is characterized by a small systolic jet area just around the TV (<5 cm^2),

TABLE 10-1

Correlation of RAP with IVC Diameter and Collapsibility

RAP (mm Hg)	IVC Diameter	Collapsibility Index (%)
<5	Small-normal	High
<10	Big	High
	Small-normal	Normal
10–15	Big	Normal
10–20	Big	low

Correlation of RAP with IVC diameter (IVCD) and collapsibility index (IVC-CI) measured in spontaneously breathing patients. The IVC diameter was measured using the M-mode at end-expiration and end-inspiration. The collapsibility index was calculated as : IVCDexp – IVCDinsp/IVCDexp = IVC-CI. The IVC diameter was categorized as small (<1.7 cm), normal (1.7–2.1 cm), and big (>2.1cm). The IVC-CI was categorized as high (>55%), normal (35–55%), and low (<35%).[31]

moderate TR by a jet area filling less than 40% of the RA (5–10 cm^2), and severe TR filling out more than 40% of the RA (>10 cm^2). In fact severe TR may cause systolic flow reversal in the IVC and hepatic vein. Before coming to a conclusion, TR should be examined in multiple views. Of note, the peak velocity of the tricuspid regurgitant jet does not quantify the severity of the TR, but solely describes the pressure gradient across the TV and is thus a measure of RV afterload. Severe TR may very well be associated with low PAPs, for example in the case of an endocarditis. The A4C view is best suited to perform these measurements.

Pericardial space

The pericardial space (PS) is a potential space between the two pericardial layers (visceral and parietal). The pericardial sac surrounds the entire heart from the apex to the base and invests around the aortic root, the main pulmonary artery, and the superior and inferior vena cava inflow into the RA. The parietal pericardium consists mainly of stiff connective tissue such as collagen and is attached to the diaphragm, the anterior mediastinum, and sternum, and anchors the heart in the central thorax. Under normal conditions the PS is filled with roughly 50 mL of serous fluid, which accumulates mostly in the interatrial or atrioventricular groove.

Pericardial effusion

Pericardial effusions are one of the most common pericardial pathologies with which an intensivist is confronted. Under normal conditions the pericardial sac is relatively stiff and thus only tolerates minimal accumulation of excess fluid before the effusion compresses the heart and leads to circulatory collapse secondary to cardiac tamponade. If the fluid increases slowly, however, relatively large amounts of fluid can accumulate. The nature of the fluid may be serous fluid (anechoic), blood, or rarely pus (hypoechoic, inhomogeneous). Echocardiography may be particularly useful in roughly estimating the size of the effusion and give hints toward its nature. The size of the pericardial effusion is graded as small, moderate, or large. A small effusion is less than 100 mL of fluid and is typically localized. In a supine patient (most critically ill patients), a small effusion would accumulate in the posterior aspect of the PS and may be viewed best on a PLAX or PSAX view. A moderate effusion contains 100–500 mL of fluid, spreads circumferentially around the heart, and measures less than 2 cm in width between the epicardial border and the pericardium (Figure 10-21).

A large effusion is also circumferential but the maximum width is more than 2 cm. The so-called "swinging heart" may be seen on the A4C view or the subcostal

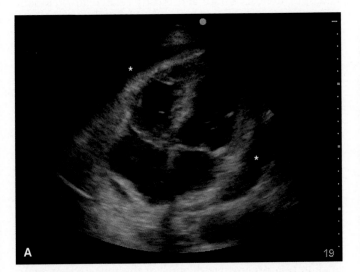
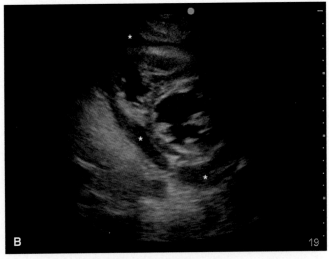

Figure 10-21. Pericardial effusion: (**A**) a pericardial effusion (asterix) shown on the A4C view. The effusion spreads circumferentially; (**B**) Pericardial effusion (asterix) on the PSAX view at the midpapillary level. As on the A4C view the effusion spreads circumferentially as marked by the asterix. The fluid appears anechoic and thus represents serous fluid most likely. Since the effusion appears circumferential in multiple views and measures less than 2 cm in width, this represents a moderate pericardial effusion of approximately 100–500 mL of fluid. Depending on the clinical presentation, this effusion may need to be drained.

four-chamber view. Importantly echocardiography may help differentiate between a pericardial and a pleural effusion. Both the pleura and the pericardium are hyperechoic. On both the PLAX and the A4C view, fluid in the pericardium extends between the LA and the descending aorta. A pleural effusion only extends posterior (as seen on the PLAX) or lateral (as seen on the A4C) to the descending aorta.

Tamponade

As mentioned above cardiac tamponade occurs once the accumulated pericardial fluid leads to impaired cardiac filling and a progressive reduction in cardiac output. The development of tamponade depends on the rate of accumulation as well as on the total amount of fluid; 25–30% of patients with a large pericardial effusion develop tamponade physiology, enhancing the effects of the pulsus paradoxus and interdependence of the cardiac chambers. As the pericardial pressure increases, the total intracardiac volume is fixed. This means that as one chamber increases in size the other is being compressed and underfilled. Early signs on echocardiography are seen by examining the TV and MV using continuous wave Doppler on A4C view. While during spontaneous inspiration venous return increases and leads to better filling and enlargement of the RV, the LV is subsequently compressed and LV stroke volume and cardiac output decrease. Therefore, the diastolic TV flow velocity increases, whereas MV flow velocity decreases. The opposite is true during spontaneous expiration, where intrathoracic pressure increases. Late signs of tamponade are the visual diastolic compression of the right heart chambers followed by the compression of the left-sided chambers with worsening tamponade. Compression of the chambers typically occurs in the following order: late diastolic collapse of the RA, early diastolic collapse of the RV, followed by LA and LV compression. Most patients with tamponade have a large pericardial effusion with the heart swinging within the pericardial sac. This may not be true in post cardiac surgery patients, where an isolated hemopericardium behind RA leads to its compression and cardiogenic shock secondary to impaired RV inflow. Although echocardiography provides important information about the pericardial space, cardiac tamponade remains largely a clinical diagnosis. When a pericardial effusion is detected in a hemodynamically unstable patient, with low urine output and high filling pressures, cardiac tamponade is likely and warrants a pericardial tap, even if the echocardiographic signs are not conclusive.

Evaluation of valve function

The intensivist should be able to determine the presence or absence of severe valvulopathy. In other words, if no signs of mitral regurgitation (MR) are present on echocardiography, the diagnosis can be ruled out. If there are signs of MR, however, the intensivist should include the diagnosis in his differential until a more detailed examination

by an experienced echocardiographer has determined the severity. Only the most common valvular pathologies are discussed here and the focus is on identification and semiquantitative assessment of severe valve dysfunction at the bedside. To screen for valvular regurgitation color flow imaging is used. Regurgitation is graded as mild, moderate, or severe, depending on the size of the color jet area relative to the size of the receiving chamber, for example, the LA in case of MR. Detection of abnormal flow patterns on color flow imaging may be limited by misinterpretation of the timing or origin of the flow signal. Therefore, abnormal flow pattern should be confirmed on at least two different views. Regurgitation may be missed because of low signal strength, especially if the structures are deep or the acoustic window is small. Additionally, several parameters such as the frame rate, the Nyquist limit, and the color gain need to be optimally set, and should be standardized for all users on one ICU to avoid mistakes. For more accurate determination of severity, quantitative parameters such as the vena contracta width, regurgitant volume, regurgitant fraction, and regurgitant orifice should be evaluated by an experienced echocardiographer and should not be part of the "emergent" assessment.

To detect valvular stenosis continuous wave (CW) Doppler imaging or two-dimensional echocardiography is used. The velocity time integral is recorded and the stenotic valve area is calculated using the continuity equation. Alternatively, the stenotic orifice may be traced on the two-dimensional image in the parasternal short-axis plane. Evaluation of pressure gradients has been described to assess valvular stenosis; however, this parameter is dependent on ventricular pump function and may be less accurate.

Tricuspid valve

The intensivist should be aware how to evaluate TR, since tricuspid stenosis is rare and mostly related to rheumatic heart disease. TR is mostly caused by RV failure secondary to ischemia, cor pulmonale or pulmonary hypertension, infective endocarditis, volume overload secondary to atrial septal or ventricular septal defects, or connective tissue diseases. Evaluation of the TV starts with two-dimensional imaging. Findings such as flail or mal-coapting leaflets, vegetations or masses, heavy calcifications of the TV ring, or presence of pacing wires may all lead to some degree of TR and should be confirmed in multiple views. The severity of TR is best assessed with color Doppler and has been discussed previously (evaluation of right ventricular function).

Mitral valve

Mitral valve regurgitation (MR) is a common finding in the ICU patient. In most patients this is a chronic process, leading to a progressive dilation of the mitral valve annulus, preventing the coaptation of the two leaflets during systole. Chronic MR is a chronic process mostly and may be caused by ischemic heart disease, nonischemic dilated cardiomyopathy, or annular calcifications, with rheumatic heart disease and endocarditis being the most common etiologies. Structural changes such as the dilation of the LA and LV secondary to volume overload, regional wall motion abnormalities secondary to ischemia, thickened and calcified or flail leaflets, vegetations, ruptured chordae tendinae, or papillary muscles may be found on 2D imaging and indicate MR. Only Doppler imaging may detect severe MR. According to the ASE guidelines a jet area of less than 4 m² or filling less than 20% of the LA area is considered mild, whereas a jet area of more than 8 m² or filling more than 40% of the LA area is most likely severe. This method is most accurate in determining mild regurgitation, but there is significant overlap between moderate and severe MR regarding the jet area. The mitral valve is best examined in the PLAX and A4C view. Acute MR secondary to papillary muscle (ischemic) or chordae tendinae rupture (endocarditis/rheumatic heart disease) is a life-threatening complication, and warrants immediate diagnosis and surgical intervention. Certain signs described above, such as LA and LV dilation, are slow to develop and may not be present.

Aortic valve

Aortic valve regurgitation and stenosis are common in critically ill patients. While the PSAX and PLAX views are best suited to evaluate the AV on two-dimensional echo, the PLAX and A5C views should be used for the Doppler evaluation. AV regurgitation (AR) is considered mild if the color jet width (measured immediately below the AV) to LVOT diameter ratio is less than 25% (PLAX and PSAX), and severe if the ratio is greater than 60%. AR may be acute or chronic. Several indices on echo may help make the differentiation: chronic AR typically goes along with a dilated LV, near-normal LV end-diastolic pressures (see above), wide pulse pressure, and a rather flat CW Doppler slope. In acute AR the LV size is normal, but the LVEDP is

elevated with a narrow pulse pressure and a steep continuous wave Doppler slope.

Aortic stenosis is a chronic process that may go unrecognized until it is unmasked by an additional insult such as myocardial ischemia or sepsis. Most cases of AS are related to a valvular process, like progressive calcification of the AV secondary to aging (degenerative), rheumatic heart disease, or bicuspid AV. In some instances AS originates from a subvalvular stenosis caused by a membrane or hypertrophied septal myocardium bulging into the LVOT. Supravalvular AS is typically of congenital origin and is rare. Once the cross-sectional area of the AV (CSA_{Ao}) is less than 0.7 cm², the AS is considered severe. The CSA_{Ao} can be measured on the PSAX view aortic valve level by tracing the valve opening during systole. Alternatively, the CSA_{Ao} can be calculated using the continuity equation:

$$CSA_{Ao} = CSA_{LVOT} \times VTI_{LVOT}/VTI_{Ao}$$
$$CSA_{LVOT} = (D_{LVOT}/2)^2 \times \pi$$

To calculate the LVOT cross-sectional area the LVOT diameter is measured in the PLAX view. The velocity time integral at the aortic valve level (VTI_{Ao}) and the LVOT (VTI_{LVOT}) are measured in the A5C view using PW Doppler (Figure 10-22).

In addition to the calculated valve area, a ratio VTI_{LVOT} to the VTI_{Ao} of less than 25% is also considered severe. Furthermore, severe AS is accompanied by LV dilation and hypertrophy, thickened and calcified cups with restricted motion, and a poststenotic dilation of the aortic root on two-dimensional echo.

Common pitfalls

Chest ultrasound in general has several limitations. (1) Ultrasound poorly penetrates air; thus, central lesions that do not extend to the periphery may not be seen on

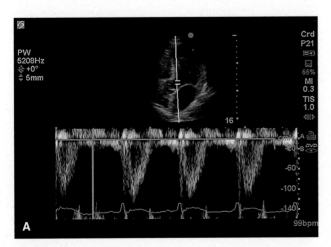
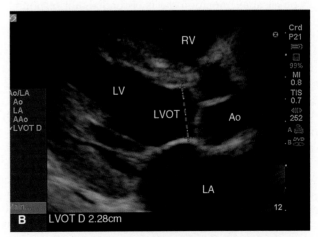

Figure 10-22. Measurements for the calculation of the aortic cross-sectional area (CSA_{Ao}) by the continuity equation. (**A**) VTI measurement in the LVOT. As seen on this picture the sample volume is placed proximal to the aortic valve in the LVOT. Many times, the ultrasound beam is not perfectly parallel to the blood flow. This may lead to smaller VTI values and underestimation of the CSA_{Ao}; (**B**) Measurement of the LVOT diameter directly under the insertion of the aortic valve leaflets.

ultrasound. A subcutaneous emphysema may limit the utility of chest ultrasonography for the same reason. (2) It is important not to mistake a hyperechoic fascia in the soft tissue of the chest wall for the pleura and draw wrong conclusions. Identification of the ribs with the typical acoustic shadow will help find the true pleural line. (3) Bony or calcified structures are impermeable to ultrasound. The ribs, in general, and the scapula, in particular, will limit the access to the lung. Maneuvers such as abduction of both arms help overcome this limitation. (4) Other conditions such as large thoracic dressings, chest tubes, pleurodesis, or obesity will make the evaluation of the chest more difficult. (5) Doppler imaging is dependent on many factors such as gain settings, the Nyquist limit, intercept angle between blood flow and ultrasound beam, etc; therefore, conclusions based on Doppler measurements should be confirmed in at least two views or more. (6) The IVC may be confused with the abdominal aorta, since both run in close proximity to each other. The aorta, however, has a thick wall and is separated by a connective tissue layer from the liver. In addition, the hepatic veins drain into the IVC immediately below the diaphragm, whereas the aorta does not receive any vessels at this level. The view through the subcostal window may be obscured by an air-filled stomach. The insertion of a gastric tube may help resolve this problem.

▶ Clinical Cases

Case 1

A 70-year-old woman with a history of heavy smoking, nonischemic CHF with an EF of 50%, NIDDM is brought to the ICU with acute shortness of breath. She was admitted two weeks ago for a hip fracture, and is now status post total hip replacement. During the last 12 hours she has been getting progressively more short of breath. She was started on CPAP via facemask an hour before the nurse found her to be increasingly obtunded.

On physical examination she is obtunded, not responding to voice or pain, with rapid shallow breathing; her extremities are warm and well perfused, and pulses palpable; and on auscultation, there are no breathing sounds on both sides. Her vitals are: HR 110 bpm, BP 160/75, SpO_2: 82% on 100% Facemask, no fever. A blood gas and labs are drawn as the team prepares the intubation. In the meanwhile a quick thoracic ultrasound examination is performed. Each hemithorax shows a typical normal lung pattern, with A-lines and occasional B-lines mainly at the bases, and weak but detectable lung sliding in all lung zones. The diaphragms appear to be pushed downward into the abdominal space. No pleural effusion or lung consolidations were seen. A quick subcostal echocardiogram reveals a normal-sized LV with mild reduction in contractility, a normal-sized RV with normal function, trace TR, and trace MR; no pericardial effusion is seen.

Before more information is available through further diagnostic workup, the clinician already is guided by the results of the ultrasound examination. Given the clinical picture and the findings on ultrasound a COPD exacerbation is most likely. COPD presents with marked hyperinflation of the lung, resulting in a normal lung profile despite the acute shortness of breath. If marked COPD is present, lung sliding may be absent completely and may be confused with a PTX. However, a PTX can safely be ruled out in this patient, given the presence of lung sliding and occasional B-lines. A cardiogenic pulmonary edema or inflammatory pulmonary process is unlikely, since both processes are associated with a focal or global alveolar interstitial syndrome. However, in this patient all lung zones were free of B3 or B7 lines. According to Lichtenstein and coworkers, pulmonary emboli and COPD could present with identical findings on ultrasound. In the absence of deep vein thrombosis in the lower extremities on vascular ultrasound, COPD or asthma could be diagnosed with 89% sensitivity and 97% specificity.[5] In addition, no peripheral lesions associated with a PE could be found. Assuming that an ultrasound device is readily available, a sonographic examination can be quickly performed at the bedside, revealing real-time diagnostic clues that facilitate important management decisions. In this case, rather than giving diuretics or placing a chest tube, the therapy was tailored to the treatment of COPD with intravenous steroids and inhaled bronchiolytics before the chest x-ray and most of the laboratory test were available.

Case 2

An 85-year-old woman is brought to the PACU after she underwent a total hip replacement under general anesthesia for a traumatic hip fracture. Her intraoperative course was uneventful, estimated blood loss was approximately 1 liter. The patient is extubated, awake and alert, and comfortable when she arrives in the PACU. Shortly thereafter the patients becomes obtunded and hypotensive with a BP of 45/20 and an HR of 55. She responds to ephedrine 10 mg and 1 liter of crystalloid fluid boluses. However, 30 minutes later, the same episode repeats itself, this time with no significant response to fluids or vasoactive agents.

No past medical history is available. A preoperative chest x-ray was notable for a hyperinflated lung. On physical examination she is awake, responds to voice, and is not oriented. She is tachypneic at a rate of 25 breaths per minute; her extremities are cold, pulses are weakly palpable, and on auscultation, breathing sounds are diminished on both sides. Her vitals are: sinus rhythm of 70–90 bpm, BP 50/30, SpO_2: 92% on 100% facemask, no fever. A blood gas and labs are drawn. Given the acuity an inotropic agent is started after a central line has been placed and a focused sonographic examination is performed.

The focused echocardiogram reveals RV failure with a markedly dilated and thickened RV with reduced contractile function, a dilated RA, severe TR, and pulmonary hypertension (PHT) with calculated PAPs of 55 mm Hg. The LV is hypertrophied, small in size with a normal function and absent regional wall motion abnormalities. No valvular dysfunction was seen on Doppler imaging. On chest ultrasonography there are mostly normal patterns in all anterior segments; the left lung base reveals a small compressive ATX and pleural effusion, and few scattered B-lines in the right lung base.

In this case it seems that the hemodynamic compromise is caused by RV failure in the setting of PHT. PHT may have pulmonary or cardiac causes. COPD and pulmonary fibrosis or ARDS are common pulmonary causes, whereas pulmonary embolism (PE), left to right shunt (ASD/VSD), LV dysfunction, and MV or AV disease are cardiac etiologies leading to PHT. A chronic condition is most likely given the signs of adaptation such as the thickened RV wall, and enlarged RA. COPD is a possibility given the findings on chest ultrasound, whereas pulmonary fibrosis as well as ARDS would present with ubiquitous B-lines in all chest wall areas. In fact RV failure due to ARDS typically occurs in the setting of high ventilator pressures and subsequent pulmonary capillary compression, which is not the case here. Furthermore, there are no obvious signs of LV or valvular dysfunction. However, the decreased preload to the LV can mask an underlying cardiomyopathy and may become evident once the RV function improves and blood flow to the left heard increases.

Also, an acute event like RV ischemia/infarction or an acute PE may be superimposed on a chronic condition. Since the RCA supplies the inferior wall of the LV and the septum, ischemia is unlikely given the absence of regional wall motion abnormalities. In addition, elevated pulmonary artery pressures are unlikely during a RV infarction, since a poor contractile function would be the reason for RV failure. A PE secondary to fat or thrombotic material needs to be considered, and depending to the clinical scenario, treatment has to be started and further diagnostic workup has to be initiated such as a pulmonary angiography.

In this case, a PE was assumed, and while the patient awaited transport to the CT scan for pulmonary angiography, a heparin drip and an inhaled pulmonary vasodilator were started in addition to the inotropes and vasopressors. In addition, inhaled bronchodilators and stress dose steroids were administered for a possible COPD exacerbation.

REFERENCES

1. Kurian J, Levin TL, Han BK, Taragin BH, Weinstein S. Comparison of ultrasound and CT in the evaluation of pneumonia complicated by parapneumonic effusion in children. *AJR Am J Roentgenol.* 2009 Dec 1;193(6): 1648–1654.

2. Galbois A, Ait-Oufella H, Baudel J-L, Kofman T, Bottero J, Viennot S, et al. Pleural ultrasound compared with chest radiographic detection of pneumothorax resolution after drainage. *Chest.* 2010 Sep 1;138(3):648–655.

3. Bouhemad B, Zhang M, Lu Q, Rouby J-J. Clinical review: bedside lung ultrasound in critical care practice. *Crit Care.* 2007;11(1):205.

4. Lichtenstein DA, Menu Y. A bedside ultrasound sign ruling out pneumothorax in the critically iii: lung sliding. *Chest.* 1995 Nov 1;108(5):1345–1348.

5. Lichtenstein DA, Mezière GA. Relevance of lung ultrasound in the diagnosis of acute respiratory failure: the BLUE protocol. *Chest.* 2008 July 1;134(1): 117–125.

6. Lichtenstein D, Mézière G, Biderman P, Gepner A, Barré O. The comet-tail artifact. An ultrasound sign of alveolar-interstitial syndrome. *Am J Respir Crit Care Med.* 1997 Nov 1;156(5):1640–1646.

7. Copetti R, Soldati G, Copetti P. Chest sonography: a useful tool to differentiate acute cardiogenic pulmonary edema from acute respiratory distress syndrome. *Cardiovasc Ultrasound.* 2008;6(1):16.

8. Lichtenstein D, Mezière G. A lung ultrasound sign allowing bedside distinction between pulmonary edema and COPD: the comet-tail artifact. *Intens Care Med.* 1998 Dec 1; 24(12):1331–1334.

9. Lichtenstein DA, Mezière GA, Lagoueyte J-F, Biderman P, Goldstein I, Gepner A. A-lines and B-lines: lung ultrasound as a bedside tool for predicting pulmonary artery occlusion pressure in the critically ill. *Chest.* 2009 Oct;136(4): 1014–1020.

10. Bouhemad B, Brisson H, Le-Guen M, Arbelot C, Lu Q, Rouby J-J. Bedside ultrasound assessment of positive end-expiratory pressure-induced lung recruitment. *Am J Respir Crit Care Med.* 2011 Feb 1;183(3):341–347.

11. Bouhemad B, Liu Z-H, Arbelot C, Zhang M, Ferarri F, Le-Guen M, et al. Ultrasound assessment of antibiotic-induced pulmonary reaeration in ventilator-associated pneumonia. *Crit Care Med.* 2010 Jan;38(1):84–92.

12. Reissig A, Copetti R, Kroegel C. Current role of emergency ultrasound of the chest. *Crit Care Med.* 2011 April;39(4):839–845.

13. Lichtenstein D, Mezière G, Seitz J. The dynamic air bronchogram. A lung ultrasound sign of alveolar consolidation ruling out atelectasis. *Chest.* 2009 June 1;135(6):1421–1425.

14. Lichtenstein DA, Lascols N, Prin S, Mezière G. The "lung pulse": an early ultrasound sign of complete atelectasis. *Intens Care Med.* 2003 Dec 1;29(12):2187–2192.

15. Yang PC, Luh KT, Chang DB, Wu HD, Yu CJ, Kuo SH. Value of sonography in determining the nature of pleural effusion: analysis of 320 cases. *AJR Am J Roentgenol.* 1992 July;159(1):29–33.

16. Usta E, Mustafi M, Ziemer G. Ultrasound estimation of volume of postoperative pleural effusion in cardiac surgery patients. *Interact Cardiovasc Thorac Surg.* 2010 Feb 1;10(2):204–207.

17. Rémérand F, Dellamonica J, Mao Z, Ferrari F, Bouhemad B, Jianxin Y, et al. Multiplane ultrasound approach to quantify pleural effusion at the bedside. *Intens Care Med.* 2010 April;36(4):656–664.

18. Grogan DR, Irwin RS, Channick R, Raptopoulos V, Curley FJ, Bartter T, et al. Complications associated with thoracentesis. A prospective, randomized study comparing three different methods. *Arch. Intern. Med.* 1990 April;150(4):873–877.

19. Diacon AH, Brutsche MH, Solèr M. Accuracy of pleural puncture sites: a prospective comparison of clinical examination with ultrasound. *Chest.* 2003 Feb;123(2): 436–441.

20. Weingardt JP, Guico RR, Nemcek AA, Li YP, Chiu ST. Ultrasound findings following failed, clinically directed thoracenteses. *J Clin Ultrasound: JCU.* 1994 Sep;22(7):419–426.

21. Mayo PH, Goltz HR, Tafreshi M, Doelken P. Safety of ultrasound-guided thoracentesis in patients receiving mechanical ventilation. *Chest.* 2004 March;125(3): 1059–1062.

22. Stefanidis K, Dimopoulos S, Nanas S. Basic principles and current applications of lung ultrasonography in the intensive care unit. *Respirology.* 2011 Jan 27;16(2):249–256.

23. Kirkpatrick AW, Simons RK, Brown R, Nicolaou S, Dulchavsky S. The hand-held FAST: experience with hand-held trauma sonography in a level-I urban trauma center. *Injury.* 2002 May 1;33(4):303–308.

24. Agricola E, Arbelot C, Blaivas M, Bouhemad B, Copetti R, Dean A, et al. Ultrasound performs better than radiographs. *Thorax.* 2011 Sep;66(9):828–9; author reply 829.

25. Lichtenstein DA, Mezi Re G, Lascols N, Biderman P, Courret J-P, Gepner AS, et al. Ultrasound diagnosis of occult pneumothorax*. *Crit Care Med.* 2005 June 1;33(6): 1231–1238.

26. Reissig A, Heyne JP, Kroegel C. Sonography of lung and pleura in pulmonary embolism: sonomorphologic characterization and comparison with spiral CT scanning. *Chest.* 2001 Dec;120(6):1977–1983.

27. Mathis G, Blank W, Reissig A, Lechleitner P, Reuss J, Schuler A, et al. Thoracic ultrasound for diagnosing pulmonary embolism: a prospective multicenter study of 352 patients. *Chest.* 2005 Sep 1;128(3):1531–1538.

28. Reissig A, Kroegel C. Transthoracic ultrasound of lung and pleura in the diagnosis of pulmonary embolism: a novel non-invasive bedside approach. *Respiration.* 2003 Aug;70(5):441–452.

29. Hüttemann E, Schelenz C, Kara F, Chatzinikolaou K, Reinhart K. The use and safety of transoesophageal echocardiography in the general ICU—a minireview. *Acta anaesthesiologica Scandinavica.* 2004 Aug;48(7): 827–836.

30. Gudmundsson P, Rydberg E, Winter R, Willenheimer R. Visually estimated left ventricular ejection fraction by echocardiography is closely correlated with formal quantitative methods. *Int J Cardiol.* 2005 May;101(2): 209–212.

31. Brennan JM, Blair JE, Goonewardena S, et al. Reappraisal of the use of inferior vena cava for estimating right atrial pressure. *J Am Soc Echocardiogr.* 2007 Jul 1;20(7): 857–861.

11

ENDOSCOPIC ULTRASOUND: FOREGUT INCLUDING ESOPHAGUS, STOMACH, SMALL INTESTINE, AND PANCREATICOBILIARY

AMRITA SETHI

In order to access the accompanying videos for this chapter, please see the attached DVD.

CLINICAL INDICATIONS FOR EUS

Endoscopic ultrasound (EUS) has a wide array of indications for diseases of the foregut. It can be used for staging, diagnosing, and even treating aspects of both benign and malignant processes of the esophagus, mediastinum, stomach, duodenum, pancreas, and additional extraintestinal organs. This chapter will focus on some of the most common indications for the use of EUS and particularly in ways in which management might be effected.

▶ EUS in the Esophagus

Esophageal cancer

The TNM classification (Table 11-1) is currently used for the staging of esophageal cancer[1,2] and accurate staging is critical for directing patients to appropriate treatment protocols. For instance, 5-year survival is >95% for stage 0 disease, 50–80% for stage I disease, and 10–40% for stage II disease.[1-3] EUS has been demonstrated to be most reliable for locoregional staging, staging T3 and T4 lesions with accuracies of 89–94% and 88–100%, respectively.[4,5] T1 and T2 lesions can be differentiated from T3 and T4 lesions with an accuracy of 87%.[6] EUS is the most accurate modality for staging of regional lymph nodes compared to CT scan and PET.[7] The overall accuracy of N staging is 75–80% compared to CT (51–74%).[5] FNA improves the diagnostic performance of EUS by at least 13%.[8] Unfortunately, EUS's role for metastases (M) staging has been disappointing. PET scan and CT remain the most accurate methods for M staging. Small liver metastasis may be better detected by EUS.[9]

Mediastinal masses, nodes, and cysts

EUS is an excellent method of evaluating the posterior mediastinum. The role of EUS in the staging of lung cancer will not be discussed here but it has been used to sample not only primary lung masses but, most importantly, mediastinal lymph nodes in order to determine if there is metastatic involvement.[10,11] Lymph node sampling by EUS-FNA can also play a critical role in diagnosis of benign disease such as tuberculosis, lymphoma, sarcoidosis, and histoplasmosis.[12,13] Overall, the diagnostic accuracy of EUS-FNA for posterior mediastinal lymph nodes is approximately 93%.[14] In addition to primary metastatic lung cancer, posterior mediastinal masses can represent other metastatic disease or primary posterior mediastinal neoplasms, 75% of which are neurogenic tumors.[15] Foregut cysts, either bronchogenic, neuroenteric, or esophageal duplication cysts, make up 15% of posterior mediastinal masses and can be differentiated by EUS based on appearance, location, and fluid contents. Sampling by FNA is not highly recommended for simple cysts given an increased risk of infection.[16-18] If FNA is performed, then antibiotics are often given prophylactically.[19] Ten to 15% of benign mediastinal masses are congenital foregut cysts. Oftentimes mistaken for mediastinal masses, mediastinal cysts can be differentiated from mass lesions by EUS.

Other common esophageal lesions included leiomyomas and granular cell tumors. Esophageal leiomyoma is a benign tumor. It typically originates from the muscularis mucosae, which can be determined by EUS. Granular cell tumors are small neoplasms typically found incidentally on upper endoscopy. The malignancy rate was initially thought

TABLE 11-1

TNM Staging of Esophageal Cancer

Tumor (T) Stage of TNM Staging of Esophageal Adenocarcinoma

T0	No evidence of primary tumor
Tis	High-grade dysplasia
T1a	Tumor invades lamina propria or muscularis mucosae
T1b	Tumor invades submucosa
T2	Tumor invades muscularis propria
T3	Tumor invades adventitia
T4a	Resectable tumor that invades pleura, pericardium, or diaphragm
T4b	Unresectable tumor that invades other adjacent structures, ex aorta, trachea, vertebrae, etc

Stage	T	N	M
0	Tis	N0	M0
IA	T1	N0	M0
IB	T1	N0	M0
	T2	N0	M0
IIA*	T2	N0	M0
IIB	T3	N0	M0
	T1-2	N1[+]	M0
IIIA	T1-2	N2[++]	M0
	T3	N1	M0
	T4a	N0	M0
IIIB	T3	N2	M0
IIIC	T4a	N1-2	M0
	T4b	Any	M0
	Any	N3[+++]	M0
IV	Any	Any	M1

*Grade 3 vs Grade 1,2 for Stage IB; [+]N1: Metastases in 1-2 regional nodes; [++]N2: Metastases in 3-6 regional nodes; [+++]N3: Metastases in >7 regional nodes.
Based on American Joint Committee on Cancer (AJCC) Cancer Staging Atlas. A Companion to the 7th Edition of the AJCC Cancer Staging Manual and Handbook

to be small;[20,21] however, recent reports have suggested their propensity to be infiltrative.[22] Endoscopic ultrasound can provide information on the layer of origin and tumor extension. These lesions are usually confined to the mucosal and submucosal layers.

▶ EUS in the Stomach

Gastric adenocarcinoma

Gastric adenocarcinoma accounts for more than 90% of all gastric cancers.[23] In the United States there has been an increase in the incidence of gastric adenocarcinoma. As with other upper GI cancers, prognosis correlates with resectability. EUS is currently the most accurate method of staging localized gastric cancer,[24] therefore permitting the selection of lesions most amenable to endoscopic resection by either endoscopic musocal resection (EMR) or

endoscopic submucosal dissection (ESD). High-frequency transducers help characterize the degree of mucosal and submucosal involvement, allowing the differentiation of T1 and T2 lesions in which the tumor infiltrates into the muscularis propria. T2 lesions are no longer considered safe for endoscopic resection and require surgical management.[25] N staging of gastric cancer requires careful examination of nodes in the areas of greater and lesser curvatures, the celiac axis, the gastrohepatic ligament, and the splenic hilum. FNA of any suspicious lymph nodes is crucial in confirming malignant involvement. However, EUS remains less accurate for N staging than T staging.[24] Cross-sectional imaging remains the favored method to evaluate metastatic disease in gastric adenocarcinoma. If performed, EUS with FNA can help detect distal metastasis in the posterior mediastinum, left adrenal gland, and pancreas, and allow for sampling of ascites.[26,27]

Gastric lymphoma

Gastric lymphoma comprises <10% of GI malignancies, but is the most common site of gastrointestinal lymphoma.[28] Most gastric lymphomas are mucosal-associated lymphoid tumors (MALT) and are usually associated with chronic infection with *Helicobacter pylori* or with an autoimmune process.[28,29] EUS with FNA has a reported accuracy of 89% in the diagnosis of gastric non-Hodgkin lymphoma.[30] EUS-FNA, with flow cytometery, can be used to distinguish MALT from other gastric B-cell lymphomas.[29]

Subepithelial lesions

These lesions, oftentimes referred to as submucosal nodules, are bulges or masses that are visible on endoscopy from the GI lumen but that have overlying normal mucosa. The lesion can arise from within any of the intrinsic gastric wall layers or can be extrinsic to the GI wall causing an impression. Subepithelial lesions are most commonly determined to be mesenchymal tumors (54%) and include gastrointestinal stromal tumors (GISTs), leiomyomas, leiomyosarcomas, or schwannomas.[31] While EUS alone cannot differentiate between these tumors, immunohistochemical staining performed on FNA samples can be diagnostic with a sensitivity and accuracy of 95% and 87%, respectively.[32] Most GISTs stain positive for CD117 (*c-kit*) and CD 34, while leiomyomas express smooth muscle actin and desmin, and schwannomas are positive for S-100.[33] While GISTs are the most common type of mesenchymal tumor and malignant in 20–25%,[34] all GISTs are considered to have malignant potential. Endosonographic features can be used to help predict this potential risk for malignancy with sensitivities of 80–100%.[35-37] For example, regularity of border, a homogenous pattern, and size <30 mm have been shown to be associated with benign GISTs, whereas necrotic centers and hyperechoic foci that suggest calcifications have been associated with malignant lesions (Figure 11-1A, 11-1B, and 11-1C).[36,37] Additional subepithelial lesions include lipomas (5%), pancreatic rests

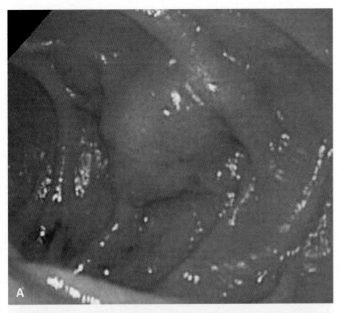

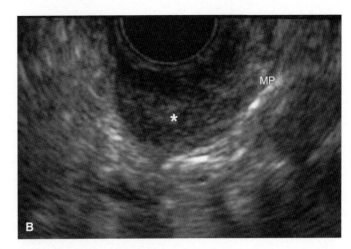

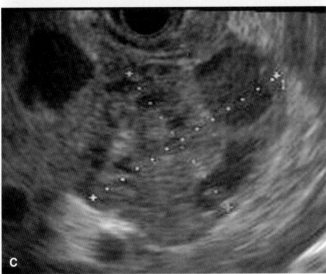

Figure 11-1. Endoscopic and EUS images of gastrointestinal stromal tumors (GIST). (**A**) Endoscopic view of submucosal nodule in duodenum; (**B**) EUS image of GIST (*) arising from muscularis propria (MP). The small size, Homogenous pattern and regular borders are consistent with benign histopathology; (**C**) EUS image of GIST of stomach wall with irregular borders, cystic component, large size, consistent with malignant histopathologic findings.

(incidence 0.6–13.7%), carcinoid lesions, and cysts such as duplication cysts, granular cell tumors, inflammatory polyps, and varices. Gastric carcinoid is the most common type of neuroendocrine tumors (Figure 11-2). EUS provides the depth of invasion and vascularity of carcinoid tumors and can lead to an informed decision as to whether to attempt endoscopic resection.[38] Extrinsic causes of subepithelial lesions include indentation by essentially any of the surrounding organs including spleen, splenic vessels, left liver lobe, gallbladder, and others. Extralumenal causes can easily be visualized by EUS.

▶ **EUS of the Ampulla and Duodenum**

Benign ampullary lesions include adenomas, GISTs, lipomas, and neuroendocrine tumors, with an overall incidence of 0.04–0.21% of patients on autopsy studies.[39] Ampullary adenomas are the most frequent of these and tend to follow

an adenoma-carcinoma sequence, with 35–90% of adenocarcinomas arising from preexisting adenomas.[40] Five-year survival ranges from 30–70% and is dependent on size and stage. Staging by EUS, based on the TNM classification system, has been demonstrated in a number of studies to have the greatest accuracy in T staging (78%) compared to CT (24%) and MRI (46%).[41] Nodal staging has been shown to be equivalent, however, between EUS and CT.[42,43]

▶ **EUS of the Pancreas**

Pancreatic malignancies

Pancreatic adenocarcinoma is the second leading cause of death among all GI cancers.[44] Adenocarcinoma accounts for 90% of all pancreatic cancers.[45] Additional malignancies include neuroendocrine tumors (NETs), exocrine tumors, lymphomas, and metastatic lesions.[46] Early diagnosis of

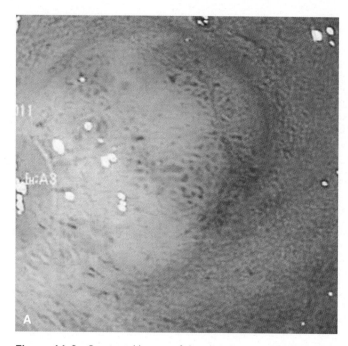

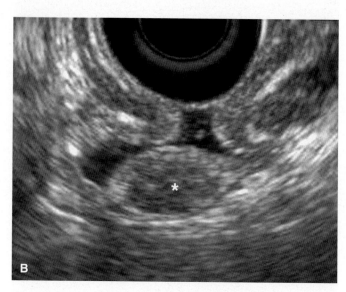

Figure 11-2. Carcinoid lesion of the duodenum. (**A**) Endoscopic view of submucosal lesion in duodenal bulb; (**B**) EUS image of the lesion characterized by defined margins, hypoechoic echogenicity, and arising from submucosal layer of duodenal wall.

resectable lesions and the avoidance of unnecessary debilitating surgery are the key roles of the EUS for pancreatic cancer. Pancreatic tumors can often appear as a hypoechoic mass with irregular borders. If located in the head of the pancreas, it is can be associated with either pancreatic or biliary dilation or both (Figure 11-3). EUS allows for both accurate tumor staging, as well as real-time tissue sampling. EUS allows for thorough evaluation of vessel involvement such as portal vein, splenic vein, and arterial involvement, as well as the detection of ascites and possible metastases to the liver. Its superiority, compared to CT, has been

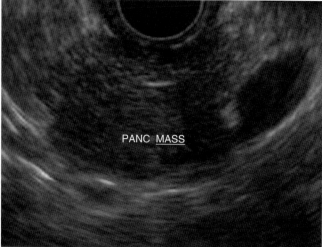

Figure 11-3. EUS image of pancreas mass. This lesion is described as hypoechoic with irregular borders arising within the body of the pancreas.

demonstrated in pancreatic lesions <25 mm.[47] The sensitivity and specificity of EUS and FNA is 85% and 98%, respectively, and has completely replaced pancreatic duct sampling during ERCP.[47] In cases in which the diagnosis is indeterminate between inflammation and malignancy, fine needle biopsy (FNB) can be used. Fine needle biopsy has been shown to have up to 100% sensitivity in diagnosing autoimmune pancreatitis (AIP) in the setting of a pancreatic mass, as it provides greater amount of tissue to demonstrated specific histologic features needed to diagnosis this form of chronic pancreatitis.[48,49]

Pancreatic cysts

The incidence of pancreatic cyst detection is increasing with more frequent use of cross-sectional imaging studies such as CT and MRI. The most common cystic lesions are pseudocysts (80–90%), while cystic neoplasms, including serous cystadenomas (SCA), mucinous cystadenomas (MCN), mucinous cystadenocarcinomas (MCAC), and intraductal papillary mucinous neoplasm (IPMN), occur in 10% of cases.[50,51] EUS not only can be used to help differentiate these lesions by morphological features, but can also provide fluid analysis via FNA to help determine malignant potential. Diagnosis based on morphology alone has an accuracy of 51–73%.[52] The addition of FNA increases this accuracy to 79–94 %.[52,53] Fluid analysis includes measurement of tumor markers such a CEA and amylase. In one prospective study, the optimal cutoff value of CEA level of 192 ng/mL, provided an accuracy of 79% to differentiate mucinous from nonmucinous cystic lesions.[52] Elevated amylase levels provide additional confirmation that the cystic lesion is likely a pseudocyst or IPMN.[54]

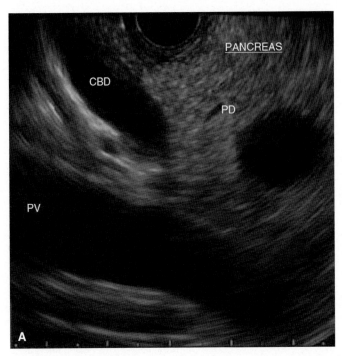
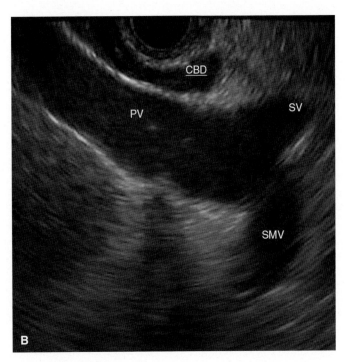

Figure 11-9. EUS imaging of head of pancreas. (**A**) Common bile duct (CBD) medial to portal vein (PV), with cross section of pancreatic duct (PD); (**B**) splenoportal confluence. Splenic vein, SV; superior mesenteric vein, SMV.

as hypoechoic, anechoic, hyperechoic, or isoechoic. Vasculature, ducts, and cysts are typically anechoic and appear black. If they are fluid-filled, posterior enhancement can usually be appreciated. Solid tumor masses are typically hypoechoic compared to the surrounding organ tissue. Fat-containing structures such as lipomas are typically hyperechoic (bright) (Figure 11-10A and 11-10B). By grouping together various descriptive features, an EUS-based diagnosis can be rendered.

Esophageal malignancies are typically seen as hypoechoic masses with irregular borders that disrupt normal wall architecture. Malignant lymph nodes can be defined by regular borders, round or oval shaped, size >1 cm, and homogenous hypoechoic echogenicity (Figure 11-11).[86] EUS-based diagnosis of submucosal nodules similarly can be made based on echogenicity and wall-layer origin

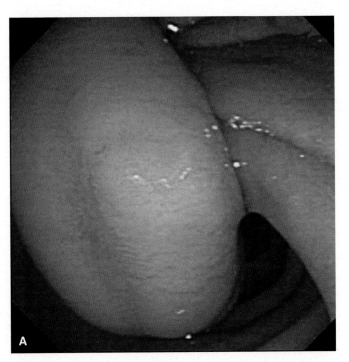
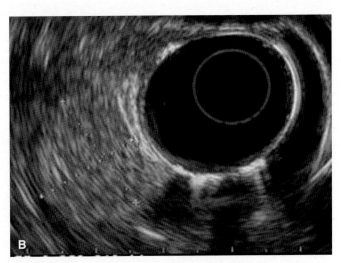

Figure 11-10. Lipoma. (**A**) Endoscopic view of large polypoid lesion in duodenum, with normal overlying mucosa; (**B**) EUS demonstrates lesion to be hyperechoic, arising from submucosa, consistent with lipomatous lesion.

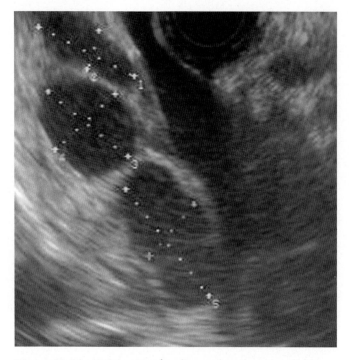

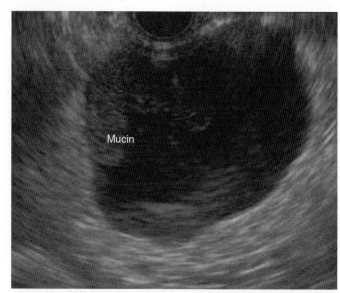

Figure 11-12. EUS image of pancreatic cyst with anechoic (black) center representing fluid. Debris or nodules can often be seen along the wall of the cyst. FNA of the fluid in this cyst confirmed it to be a mucinous lesion. The debris likely represents collections of mucin.

Figure 11-11. EUS image of malignant lymph nodes. Notes regular borders, homogenous and hypoechoic pattern, and large size (>1 cm) consistent with malignant appearance.

(Table 11-2).[87] Neoplastic lesions of the pancreas are also typically hypoechoic and have irregular borders. Neuroendocrine tumors, however, can variably have discrete borders with a homogenous pattern, and with increased vascularity.[88] EUS of cystic lesions of the pancreas demonstrates an anechoic center and can often have debris or nodules seen along the wall (Figure 11-12 and Video 11-3). Common EUS features of chronic pancreatitis are described above. Calcifications of the bile duct, pancreatic duct, and gallbladder appear as hyperechoic foci with acoustic shadow-

ing. Similarly debris within pseudocysts and sludge within the biliary system can appear hyperechoic; however, they typically do not cause shadowing.[89]

PITFALLS AND CLINICAL PEARLS

Pitfalls in endosonography vary widely and can be encountered from issues including, but not limited to, sedation of the patient, imaging details, orientation, scope selection,

TABLE 11-2			
Characteristic Layers of Origin and EUS Patterns of Submucosal Tumors			
Tumor Type	**Layer**	**Echogenicity**	**Pattern**
Lipoma	**Submucosa (third)**	Hyperechoic	Homogenous
Pancreatic rest	**Submucosa (third)**	Hypoechoic, isoechoic, and mixed	Heterogeneous with indistinct border
	Deep mucosa (second)		
	Muscularis propria (fourth)		
Carcinoid	**Submucosa (third)**	Hypoechoic	Homogenous
	Any		
Cysts	**Submucosa (third)**	Anechoic, hypoechoic	Homogenous
	Any		
Granular cell tumors	**Submucosa (third)**	Hypoechoic, isoechoic	Heterogeneous
Stromal tumors (GISTs)	**Muscularis propria (fourth)**	Hypoechoic, anechoic spaces	Homogenous, heterogeneous
	Deep mucosa (second)		
Vascular	Any	Anechoic	Doppler flow

The most common layer is in bold.
EUS indicates endoscopic ultrasound; GISTs, gastrointestinal stromal tumors.

and maneuvers. EUS tends to be a longer procedure with a slightly wider diameter scope. Thus, deeper sedation is often required than for a regular endoscopy. In order to prevent aspiration in the case of anticipated water instillation for gastric wall evaluation, or in the case of therapeutic maneuvers such as pseudocyst drainage, the endoscopist may consider general anesthesia with intubation. Insertion of the echoendoscope can often times be difficult, given the oblique endoscopic angle as well as the stiff bending portion of the echoendoscope. Intubation with the scope can sometimes employ a more blind approach than a forward-viewing endoscope and may require manipulation of the head and neck, or jaw thrust in order to facilitate passage of the scope into the esophagus. Gaining rapid orientation once inside the esophagus or stomach can also be frustrating for novice endosonographers. Early identification of anatomical landmarks, as discussed above, is the best way to orient oneself. Additionally, following a systematic approach with each examination until proficiency is obtained assists in orientation and also prevents accidental omission of elements of the examination.

Some consideration should be given to the choice of echoendoscope used for the examination, radial versus linear. Radial examinations are especially helpful with staging, particularly of the mediastinum, as the 360-degree views allow for a more global assessment of lymphadenopathy at each level. Use of the linear scope in this setting requires careful rotation of the scope to the right and the left, which may result in inadvertent duplication of imaging of a node that was already seen, or may result in missing critical angles. Use of the radial scope, however, does not allow for sampling of the lesion with FNA and would require withdrawal of the scope, and repeat localization of the lesion with the linear scope. All interventional maneuvers also require not only use of the linear scope, but specific use of the therapeutic linear array echoendoscope, which has a larger channel that can accommodate devices such as dilating catheters and 10-French stents.

Air artifact can often present a problem during EUS examination. Careful inspection of the balloon and ensuring the clearance of any bubbles, with the scope outside of the patient, can reduce this problem significantly. Additionally, inflation of the balloon in areas such as the duodenum can help maximize contact between the balloon and mucosa and assist in reducing luminal air. Lastly, water can be infused to replace the air and assist in visualization, particularly of mucosal or submucosal lesions.

Pitfalls can also be encountered when attempting FNA. Advancing the needle through a strongly angulated scope, such as when visualizing the head of pancreas or uncinate process from the duodenum, can oftentimes be difficult. The scope may have to be slightly withdrawn or advanced distally and the scope tip partially straightened with just slight advancement of the needle past the elevator, followed by repositioning the scope to the area of interest. Alternatively, a smaller needle, such as a 25-gauge (G) needle, should be chosen, as it is more flexible and traverses

the angulations of the scope more easily. When performing FNA of lymph nodes or highly vascular lesions, samples can often be excessively bloody. To prevent this, a 25-G needle can be selected, and the syringe can be set to either no suction or half suction.

THERAPEUTIC MANEUVERS

All of the diagnostic or therapeutic maneuvers that are performed using EUS are centered around the use of the EUS needles. These needles have a hollow bore, are long enough to fit through the channel of the echoendoscope, have handles to allow the endoscopist to perform "passes" and move the needle back and forth, and have echogenic tips to allow for visualization of the needle on EUS. These needles come in 19 G, 22 G, and 25 G sizes and can be blunt or bevel-tipped. They all contain a stylet that is usually maintained in the needle until the tip has been inserted into the area of interest. It can then be used to help clear the needle of unwanted tissue or to help retrieve aspirated tissue. Larger core biopsy needles are available that are used to provide more solid samples of tissue that can be sent for histology.

Fine needle aspiration (FNA)

Fine needle aspiration is performed by removing the cap of the scope channel, inserting the needle through the channel of the echoendoscope, and then locking it in place on the threads of the channel. The needle is then advanced so that the tip is visible on ultrasound view. Manipulation of the scope tip and elevator is then done to adjust the needle so that it follows a straight path into the target of interest when advanced forward. Typically, the lesion or target is placed in the 6 to 7-o'clock position in order to allow for the easiest and most direct passage of the needle (Video 11-4). Power flow should be used to confirm that the anticipated needle track is clear of blood vessels. The needle plunger is then unlocked and the needle sheath lock can be moved to a length of choice based on the location of the target. The needle is then advanced using the handle with some force in order to penetrate through the gastrointestinal lumen into the area of interest. Once it is correctly positioned, the stylet is first advanced to clear the needle and then is removed entirely. For FNA, a syringe prepared with negative pressure is attached to the top of the needle. The suction is opened and the needle is thrust in a "to-and-fro" manner within the target of interest. Each insertion of the needle into the target through the lumen wall is referred to as a "pass." When the needle is removed, the suction is turned off and the needle is quickly withdrawn and locked back into place, and finally removed from the channel of the echoendoscope.

Interventional EUS

Interventional EUS also utilizes the same puncture method with the needle as described above. Typically, the larger channel therapeutic EUS scope is used to accommodate for the necessary accessories such as dilating catheters, balloons, cautery devices, and stents. In addition, a 19-G needle is typically used to allow for insertion of a .035 guide wire in the area of interest, thereby allowing for wire-guided maneuvers to be performed. Examples of interventions that use this method include transduodenal choledocho-duodenostomy, transgastric or transgastric cystgastrostomy. These procedures are best performed with fluoroscopy, as EUS visualization of the lesion is often suboptimal after needle access is obtained and the wire is passed into the area of interest.

Pseudocyst drainage is performed by first visualizing the cyst on ultrasound. The needle is then inserted into the fluid collection and fluid is aspirated for confirmation of the location as well as analysis such as culture. A long .035 guide wire is then inserted into the collection through the needle and looped several times under fluoroscopic guidance. Once the wire is secure, the needle is removed from the collection and entirely from the channel of the echoendoscope while forward pressure is applied to the wire in an "exchange" fashion. The tract created by the wire is then opened by either cautery using a needle knife, cystotome, or by bougie dilation. These devices are similarly exchanged in and out of the scope over the wire. The fistula is then dilated with a balloon. There are a number of variations as to how these types of procedures are performed and the exact devices used. The goal at the end of the procedure is to place a number of stents across the newly created tract in order to maintain patency and allow for continued drainage (Video 11-5).

Celiac plexus block/neurolysis

Just as fluid and tissue can be aspirated, the access provided by EUS penetration of the needle can be used for injection as well (fine needle injection, FNI). The most common application of this is in performing celiac plexus neurolysis. The celiac axis and corresponding ganglion are identified endosonographically. The needle is then inserted and advanced adjacent to the takeoff of the celiac artery or directly into the ganglion. Aspiration is performed to ensure that a vessel has not been penetrated. Various agents can then be injected, but most typically include aliquots of bupivicaine followed by denatured alcohol (neurolysis) or triamcinalone (block), followed by a saline flush (Video 11-6).

CASE STUDIES

1. A 59-year-old man with a history of hypertension-experienced symptoms of hypoglycemia (mental status changes, blood glucose of 34) with elevated insulin levels during a hospital stay for knee surgery. Suspecting an insulinoma, an MRI and subsequently octreotide scan were performed that failed to demonstrate a potential lesion. He developed symptoms of hypoglycemia again

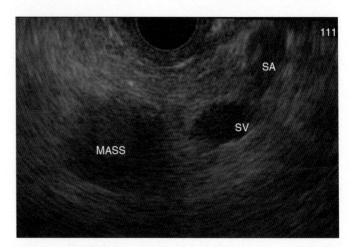

Figure 11-13. EUS image of pancreas mass in inferior body of pancreas. No vascular involvement was seen.

during a supervised 72-hour fast. EUS was performed to attempt to identify a lesion.

A 15 mm × 19 mm hypochoic lesion with well-defined borders was demonstrated in the body/tail junction of the pancreas (Figure 11-13). No vascular involvement was seen. FNA was performed and an on-site cytologist confirmed the presence of cells suspicious for a neuroendocine tumor. Immunohistochemical staining confirmed an insulinoma (Figure 11-14). EUS helped in identification of the location of a tumor and final diagnosis, thereby providing a therapeutic plan of surgical resection for this patient.

2. A 43-year-old woman with acute recurrent pancreatitis secondary to presumed sphincter of Oddi dysfunction returned with persistent abdominal pain requiring debilitating doses of narcotics. She was not amenable to endoscopic treatment of the pancreatitis. She elected to undergo EUS-guided celiac nerve block.

The region of the celiac axis was identified on EUS and a ganglion was visualized. The FNA needle was inserted directly into the ganglion. 10 mL of 0.25% bupivicaine was injected into the ganglion, followed by 25 mg of triamcinalone. A blush was seen with the two injections. The patient experienced no complications from the procedure. At 3-week follow-up she was pain-free and had been able to cut her oral pain medications by half as well as a transcutaneous patch.

CONCLUSION

This chapter discussed indications for EUS in the upper GI tract. EUS and FNA are important in the diagnosis, staging, and sampling of upper GI tract pathology. EUS imaging and sampling can help to direct further management of potential surgical lesions. In addition, interventional EUS allows access to lesions otherwise unreachable and facilitates alternative therapeutic methods.

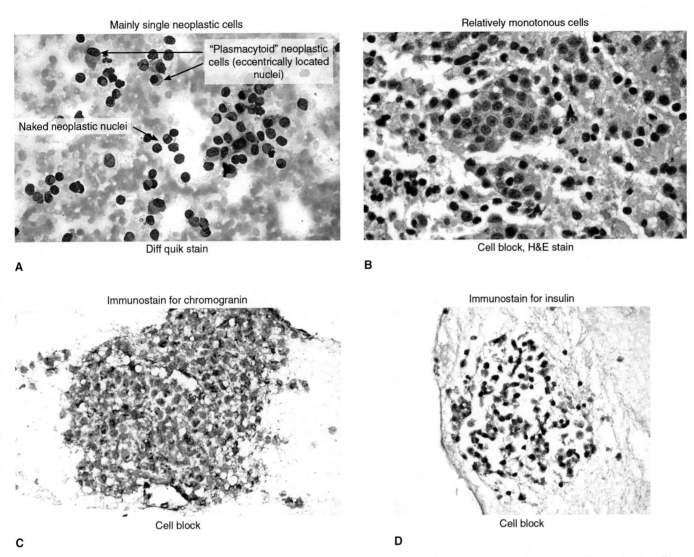

Figure 11-14. Cytology of pancreas mass confirms tumor of neuroendocrine origin. (**A**) multiple "plasmacytoid" neoplastic cells seen on Diff quick stain; (**B**) sheets of small cells with "salt and pepper" chromatin on cell block; (**C**) staining for chromagranin; and (**D**) insulin to confirm neuroendocrine origin. (With permission from Diane Hamele-Bena.)

SUGGESTED READINGS

Hawes RH, Van Dam J, Varadarajulu S, eds. *Diagnostic and Interventional Endoscopic Ultrasound. Supplement to Gastrointestinal Endoscopy.* 2009;69(2).

Hawes RH and Fockens P, eds. *Endosonography.* Philadelphia: Elselvier Saunders; 2011.

Shami VM and Kahaleh M, eds. *Endoscopic Ultrasound.* New York: Humana Press; 2011.

REFERENCES

1. Edge SB, Compton CC. The American Joint Committee on Cancer: the 7th edition of the AJCC cancer staging manual and the future of TNM. *Ann Surg Oncol.* 17(6):1471–1474.

2. Wittekind C, Compton CC, Greene FL, Sobin LH. TNM residual tumor classification revisited. *Cancer.* 2002;94(9): 2511–2516.

3. Shumaker DA, de Garmo P, Faigel DO. Potential impact of preoperative EUS on esophageal cancer management and cost. *Gastrointest Endosc.* 2002;56(3): 391–396.

4. Rosch T. Endosonographic staging of esophageal cancer: a review of literature results. *Gastrointest Endosc Clin N Am.* 1995;5(3):537–547.

5. Heidemann J, Schilling MK, Schmassmann A, Maurer CA, Buchler MW. Accuracy of endoscopic ultrasonography in preoperative staging of esophageal carcinoma. *Dig Surg.* 2000;17(3):219–224.

6. Rice TW, Blackstone EH, Adelstein DJ, Zuccaro G, Jr., Vargo JJ, Goldblum JR, Murthy SC, DeCamp MM, Rybicki LA. Role of clinically determined depth of tumor invasion in the treatment of esophageal carcinoma. *J Thorac Cardiovasc Surg.* 2003;125(5):1091–1102.

7. Lowe VJ, Booya F, Fletcher JG, Nathan M, Jensen E, Mullan B, Rohren E, Wiersema MJ, Vazquez-Sequeiros E, Murray JA, Allen MS, Levy MJ, Clain JE. Comparison of positron emission tomography, computed tomography, and endoscopic ultrasound in the initial staging of patients with esophageal cancer. *Mol Imaging Biol.* 2005;7(6):422–430.

8. Vazquez-Sequeiros E, Wiersema MJ, Clain JE, Norton ID, Levy MJ, Romero Y, Salomao D, Dierkhising R, Zinsmeister AR. Impact of lymph node staging on therapy of esophageal carcinoma. *Gastroenterology*. 2003;125(6):1626–1635.

9. Prasad P, Schmulewitz N, Patel A, Varadarajulu S, Wildi SM, Roberts S, Tutuian R, King P, Hawes RH, Hoffman BJ, Wallace MB. Detection of occult liver metastases during EUS for staging of malignancies. *Gastrointest Endosc*. 2004;59(1):49–53.

10. Hernandez A, Kahaleh M, Olazagasti J, Jones DR, Daniel T, Stelow E, White GE, Shami VM. EUS-FNA as the initial diagnostic modality in centrally located primary lung cancers. *J Clin Gastroenterol*. 2007;41(7):657–660.

11. Eloubeidi MA, Desmond R, Desai S, Mehra M, Bryant A, Cerfolio RJ. Impact of staging transesophageal EUS on treatment and survival in patients with non-small-cell lung cancer. *Gastrointest Endosc*. 2008;67(2):193–198.

12. Puri R, Vilmann P, Sud R, Kumar M, Taneja S, Verma K, Kaushik N. Endoscopic ultrasound-guided fine-needle aspiration cytology in the evaluation of suspected tuberculosis in patients with isolated mediastinal lymphadenopathy. *Endoscopy*. 42(6):462–467.

13. Fritscher-Ravens A, Sriram PV, Topalidis T, Hauber HP, Meyer A, Soehendra N, Pforte A. Diagnosing sarcoidosis using endosonography-guided fine-needle aspiration. *Chest*. 2000;118(4):928–935.

14. Wallace MB, Fritscher-Ravens A, Savides TJ. Endoscopic ultrasound for the staging of non-small-cell lung cancer. *Endoscopy*. 2003;35(7):606–610.

15. Macchiarini P, Ostertag H. Uncommon primary mediastinal tumours. *Lancet Oncol*. 2004;5(2):107–118.

16. Fazel A, Moezardalan K, Varadarajulu S, Draganov P, Eloubeidi MA. The utility and the safety of EUS-guided FNA in the evaluation of duplication cysts. *Gastrointest Endosc*. 2005;62(4):575–580.

17. Annema JT, Versteegh MI, Veselic M, Welker L, Mauad T, Sont JK, Willems LN, Rabe KF. Endoscopic ultrasound added to mediastinoscopy for preoperative staging of patients with lung cancer. *JAMA*. 2005;294(8):931–936.

18. Wildi SM, Hoda RS, Fickling W, Schmulewitz N, Varadarajulu S, Roberts SS, Ferguson B, Hoffman BJ, Hawes RH, Wallace MB. Diagnosis of benign cysts of the mediastinum: the role and risks of EUS and FNA. *Gastrointest Endosc*. 2003;58(3):362–368.

19. Banerjee S, Shen B, Baron TH, Nelson DB, Anderson MA, Cash BD, Dominitz JA, Gan SI, Harrison ME, Ikenberry SO, Jagannath SB, Lichtenstein D, Fanelli RD, Lee K, van Guilder T, Stewart LE. Antibiotic prophylaxis for GI endoscopy. *Gastrointest Endosc*. 2008;67(6):791–798.

20. Xu GQ, Zhang BL, Li YM, Chen LH, Ji F, Chen WX, Cai SP. Diagnostic value of endoscopic ultrasonography for gastrointestinal leiomyoma. *World J Gastroenterol*. 2003;9(9):2088–2091.

21. Ordonez NG, Mackay B. Granular cell tumor: a review of the pathology and histogenesis. *Ultrastruct Pathol*. 1999;23(4):207–222.

22. John BK, Dang NC, Hussain SA, Yang GC, Cham MD, Yantiss R, Joseph AS, Giashuddin SM, Lee PC, Fleming R, Somnay K. Multifocal granular cell tumor presenting as an esophageal stricture. *J Gastrointest Cancer*. 2008;39(1-4):107–113.

23. Crew KD, Neugut AI. Epidemiology of gastric cancer. *World J Gastroenterol*. 2006;12(3):354–362.

24. Aibe T FH, Noguchi T, et al. Endosonographic detection and staging of earl gastric cancer. In: Dancygier HCM, ed. *Fifth International Symposium on EUS*. Munich, 1989.

25. Tsendsuren T, Jun SM, Mian XH. Usefulness of endoscopic ultrasonography in preoperative TNM staging of gastric cancer. *World J Gastroenterol*. 2006;12(1):43–47.

26. Chen CH, Yang CC, Yeh YH. Preoperative staging of gastric cancer by endoscopic ultrasound: the prognostic usefulness of ascites detected by endoscopic ultrasound. *J Clin Gastroenterol*. 2002;35(4):321–327.

27. Chu KM, Kwok KF, Law S, Wong KH. A prospective evaluation of catheter probe EUS for the detection of ascites in patients with gastric carcinoma. *Gastrointest Endosc*. 2004;59(4):471–474.

28. Kita H. EUS to predict cure of gastric mucosa-associated lymphoma after Helicobacter pylori eradication. *Gastrointest Endosc*. 2007;65(1):97–98.

29. Caletti G, Fusaroli P, Togliani T. EUS in MALT lymphoma. *Gastrointest Endosc*. 2002;56(4 Suppl):S21–S26.

30. Wiersema MJ, Vilmann P, Giovannini M, Chang KJ, Wiersema LM. Endosonography-guided fine-needle aspiration biopsy: diagnostic accuracy and complication assessment. *Gastroenterology*. 1997;112(4):1087–1095.

31. Kim JH, Lim JS, Lee YC, Hyung WJ, Lee JH, Kim MJ, Chung JB. Endosonographic features of gastric ectopic pancreases distinguishable from mesenchymal tumors. *J Gastroenterol Hepatol*. 2008;23(8 Pt 2):e301–e307.

32. Brand B, Oesterhelweg L, Binmoeller KF, Sriram PV, Bohnacker S, Seewald S, De Weerth A, Soehendra N. Impact of endoscopic ultrasound for evaluation of submucosal lesions in gastrointestinal tract. *Dig Liver Dis*. 2002;34(4):290–297.

33. Miettinen M, Sarlomo-Rikala M, Lasota J. Gastrointestinal stromal tumors: recent advances in understanding of their biology. *Hum Pathol*. 1999;30(10):1213–1220.

34. Sepe PS, Moparty B, Pitman MB, Saltzman JR, Brugge WR. EUS-guided FNA for the diagnosis of GI stromal cell tumors: sensitivity and cytologic yield. *Gastrointest Endosc*. 2009;70(2):254–261.

35. Chak A, Canto MI, Rosch T, Dittler HJ, Hawes RH, Tio TL, Lightdale CJ, Boyce HW, Scheiman J, Carpenter SL, Van Dam J, Kochman ML, Sivak MV, Jr. Endosonographic differentiation of benign and malignant stromal cell tumors. *Gastrointest Endosc*. 1997;45(6):468–473.

36. Palazzo L, Landi B, Cellier C, Cuillerier E, Roseau G, Barbier JP. Endosonographic features predictive of benign and malignant gastrointestinal stromal cell tumours. *Gut*. 2000;46(1):88–92.

37. Yasuda K, Nakajima M, Yoshida S, Kiyota K, Kawai K. The diagnosis of submucosal tumors of the stomach by endoscopic ultrasonography. *Gastrointest Endosc*. 1989;35(1):10–15.

38. Varas MJ, Gornals JB, Pons C, Espinos JC, Abad R, Lorente FJ, Bargallo D. Usefulness of endoscopic ultrasonography (EUS) for selecting carcinoid tumors as candidates to endoscopic resection. *Rev Esp Enferm Dig*. 102(10):577–582.

39. Grobmyer SR, Stasik CN, Draganov P, Hemming AW, Dixon LR, Vogel SB, Hochwald SN. Contemporary results with ampullectomy for 29 "benign" neoplasms of the ampulla. *J Am Coll Surg*. 2008;206(3):466–471.

40. Defrain C, Chang CY, Srikureja W, Nguyen PT, Gu M. Cytologic features and diagnostic pitfalls of primary ampullary tumors by endoscopic ultrasound-guided fine-needle aspiration biopsy. *Cancer*. 2005;105(5):289–297.

41. Cannon ME, Carpenter SL, Elta GH, Nostrant TT, Kochman ML, Ginsberg GG, Stotland B, Rosato EF, Morris JB, Eckhauser F, Scheiman JM. EUS compared with CT, magnetic resonance imaging, and angiography and the influence of biliary stenting on staging accuracy of ampullary neoplasms. *Gastrointest Endosc*. 1999;50(1):27–33.

42. Rosch T, Braig C, Gain T, Feuerbach S, Siewert JR, Schusdziarra V, Classen M. Staging of pancreatic and ampullary carcinoma by endoscopic ultrasonography. Comparison with conventional sonography, computed tomography, and angiography. *Gastroenterology*. 1992;102(1):188–199.

43. Tio TL, Sie LH, Kallimanis G, Luiken GJ, Kimmings AN, Huibregtse K, Tytgat GN. Staging of ampullary and pancreatic carcinoma: comparison between endosonography and surgery. *Gastrointest Endosc*. 1996;44(6):706–713.

44. Jemal A, Siegel R, Ward E, Hao Y, Xu J, Murray T, Thun MJ. Cancer statistics, 2008. *CA Cancer J Clin*. 2008;58(2):71–96.

45. Kloppel G, Clemens A. The biological relevance of gastric neuroendocrine tumors. *Yale J Biol Med*. 1996;69(1):69–74.

46. Baylor SM, Berg JW. Cross-classification and survival characteristics of 5,000 cases of cancer of the pancreas. *J Surg Oncol*. 1973;5(4):335–358.

47. Dewitt J, Devereaux BM, Lehman GA, Sherman S, Imperiale TF. Comparison of endoscopic ultrasound and computed tomography for the preoperative evaluation of pancreatic cancer: a systematic review. *Clin Gastroenterol Hepatol*. 2006;4(6):717–725; quiz 664.

48. Detlefsen S, Mohr Drewes A, Vyberg M, Kloppel G. Diagnosis of autoimmune pancreatitis by core needle biopsy: application of six microscopic criteria. *Virchows Arch*. 2009;454(5):531–539.

49. Mizuno N, Bhatia V, Hosoda W, Sawaki A, Hoki N, Hara K, Takagi T, Ko SB, Yatabe Y, Goto H, Yamao K. Histological diagnosis of autoimmune pancreatitis using EUS-guided trucut biopsy: a comparison study with EUS-FNA. *J Gastroenterol*. 2009;44(7):742–750.

50. Balthazar EJ, Chako AC. Computed tomography of pancreatic masses. *Am J Gastroenterol*. 1990;85(4):343–349.

51. Brugge WR, Lauwers GY, Sahani D, Fernandez-del Castillo C, Warshaw AL. Cystic neoplasms of the pancreas. *N Engl J Med*. 2004;351(12):1218–1226.

52. Brugge WR. The role of EUS in the diagnosis of cystic lesions of the pancreas. *Gastrointest Endosc*. 2000; 52(6 Suppl):S18–S22.

53. Frossard JL, Amouyal P, Amouyal G, Palazzo L, Amaris J, Soldan M, Giostra E, Spahr L, Hadengue A, Fabre M. Performance of endosonography-guided fine needle aspiration and biopsy in the diagnosis of pancreatic cystic lesions. *Am J Gastroenterol*. 2003;98(7):1516–1524.

54. van der Waaij LA, van Dullemen HM, Porte RJ. Cyst fluid analysis in the differential diagnosis of pancreatic cystic lesions: a pooled analysis. *Gastrointest Endosc*. 2005;62(3):383–389.

55. Allen PJ, D'Angelica M, Gonen M, Jaques DP, Coit DG, Jarnagin WR, DeMatteo R, Fong Y, Blumgart LH, Brennan MF. A selective approach to the resection of cystic lesions of the pancreas: results from 539 consecutive patients. *Ann Surg*. 2006;244(4):572–582.

56. Varadarajulu S, Lopes TL, Wilcox CM, Drelichman ER, Kilgore ML, Christein JD. EUS versus surgical cyst-gastrostomy for management of pancreatic pseudocysts. *Gastrointest Endosc*. 2008;68(4):649–655.

57. Stevens T, Lopez R, Adler DG, Al-Haddad MA, Conway J, Dewitt JM, Forsmark CE, Kahaleh M, Lee LS, Levy MJ, Mishra G, Piraka CR, Papachristou GI, Shah RJ, Topazian MD, Vargo JJ, Vela SA. Multicenter comparison of the interobserver agreement of standard EUS scoring and Rosemont classification scoring for diagnosis of chronic pancreatitis. *Gastrointest Endosc*.71(3):519–526.

58. Wallace MB, Hawes RH, Durkalski V, Chak A, Mallery S, Catalano MF, Wiersema MJ, Bhutani MS, Ciaccia D, Kochman ML, Gress FG, Van Velse A, Hoffman BJ. The reliability of EUS for the diagnosis of chronic pancreatitis: interobserver agreement among experienced endosonographers. *Gastrointest Endosc*. 2001;53(3):294–299.

59. Garrow D, Miller S, Sinha D, Conway J, Hoffman BJ, Hawes RH, Romagnuolo J. Endoscopic ultrasound: a meta-analysis of test performance in suspected biliary obstruction. *Clin Gastroenterol Hepatol*. 2007;5(5):616–623.

60. Gleeson FC, Rajan E, Levy MJ, Clain JE, Topazian MD, Harewood GC, Papachristou GI, Takahashi N, Rosen CB, Gores GJ. EUS-guided FNA of regional lymph nodes in patients with unresectable hilar cholangiocarcinoma. *Gastrointest Endosc*. 2008;67(3):438–443.

61. Menzel J, Poremba C, Dietl KH, Domschke W. Preoperative diagnosis of bile duct strictures—comparison of intraductal ultrasonography with conventional endosonography. *Scand J Gastroenterol*. 2000;35(1):77–82.

62. Levy AD, Murakata LA, Rohrmann CA, Jr. Gallbladder carcinoma: radiologic-pathologic correlation. *Radiographics*. 2001;21(2):295–314; questionnaire, 549–555.

63. Shirai Y, Yoshida K, Tsukada K, Ohtani T, Muto T. Identification of the regional lymphatic system of the gallbladder by vital staining. *Br J Surg*. 1992;79(7): 659–662.

64. Bartlett DL. Gallbladder cancer. *Semin Surg Oncol*. 2000; 19(2):145–155.

65. Dixon E, Vollmer CM, Jr., Sahajpal A, Cattral M, Grant D, Doig C, Hemming A, Taylor B, Langer B, Greig P, Gallinger S. An aggressive surgical approach leads to improved survival in patients with gallbladder cancer: a 12-year study at a North American Center. *Ann Surg*. 2005;241(3):385–394.

66. Weber SM, DeMatteo RP, Fong Y, Blumgart LH, Jarnagin WR. Staging laparoscopy in patients with extrahepatic biliary carcinoma. Analysis of 100 patients. *Ann Surg*. 2002;235(3):392–399.

67. Soltan HM, Kow L, Toouli J. A simple scoring system for predicting bile duct stones in patients with cholelithiasis. *J Gastrointest Surg*. 2001;5(4):434–437.

68. Freeman ML, DiSario JA, Nelson DB, Fennerty MB, Lee JG, Bjorkman DJ, Overby CS, Aas J, Ryan ME, Bochna GS, Shaw MJ, Snady HW, Erickson RV, Moore JP, Roel JP. Risk factors for post-ERCP pancreatitis: a prospective, multicenter study. *Gastrointest Endosc*. 2001;54(4): 425–434.

69. Mazen Jamal M, Yoon EJ, Saadi A, Sy TY, Hashemzadeh M. Trends in the utilization of endoscopic retrograde cholangiopancreatography (ERCP) in the United States. *Am J Gastroenterol*. 2007;102(5):966–975.

70. Buscarini E, Tansini P, Vallisa D, Zambelli A, Buscarini L. EUS for suspected choledocholithiasis: do benefits outweigh costs? A prospective, controlled study. *Gastrointest Endosc.* 2003;57(4):510–518.

71. de Ledinghen V, Lecesne R, Raymond JM, Gense V, Amouretti M, Drouillard J, Couzigou P, Silvain C. Diagnosis of choledocholithiasis: EUS or magnetic resonance cholangiography? A prospective controlled study. *Gastrointest Endosc.* 1999;49(1):26–31.

72. Schmidt S, Chevallier P, Novellas S, Gelsi E, Vanbiervliet G, Tran A, Schnyder P, Bruneton JN. Choledocholithiasis: repetitive thick-slab single-shot projection magnetic resonance cholangiopancreaticography versus endoscopic ultrasonography. *Eur Radiol.* 2007; 17(1):241–250.

73. McMahon CJ. The relative roles of magnetic resonance cholangiopancreatography (MRCP) and endoscopic ultrasound in diagnosis of common bile duct calculi: a critically appraised topic. *Abdom Imaging.* 2008;33(1): 6–9.

74. Lopes CV, Pesenti C, Bories E, Caillol F, Giovannini M. Endoscopic-ultrasound-guided endoscopic transmural drainage of pancreatic pseudocysts and abscesses. *Scand J Gastroenterol.* 2007;42(4):524–529.

75. Maranki J, Hernandez AJ, Arslan B, Jaffan AA, Angle JF, Shami VM, Kahaleh M. Interventional endoscopic ultrasound-guided cholangiography: long-term experience of an emerging alternative to percutaneous transhepatic cholangiography. *Endoscopy.* 2009;41(6):532–538.

76. Kahaleh M, Hernandez AJ, Tokar J, Adams RB, Shami VM, Yeaton P. Interventional EUS-guided cholangiography: evaluation of a technique in evolution. *Gastrointest Endosc.* 2006;64(1):52–59.

77. Park do H, Koo JE, Oh J, Lee YH, Moon SH, Lee SS, Seo DW, Lee SK, Kim MH. EUS-guided biliary drainage with one-step placement of a fully covered metal stent for malignant biliary obstruction: a prospective feasibility study. *Am J Gastroenterol.* 2009;104(9):2168–2174.

78. Bories E, Pesenti C, Caillol F, Lopes C, Giovannini M. Transgastric endoscopic ultrasonography-guided biliary drainage: results of a pilot study. *Endoscopy.* 2007;39(4):287–291.

79. Kahaleh M, Shami VM, Conaway MR, Tokar J, Rockoff T, De La Rue SA, de Lange E, Bassignani M, Gay S, Adams RB, Yeaton P. Endoscopic ultrasound drainage of pancreatic pseudocyst: a prospective comparison with conventional endoscopic drainage. *Endoscopy.* 2006;38(4):355–359.

80. Kahaleh M, Hernandez AJ, Tokar J, Adams RB, Shami VM, Yeaton P. EUS-guided pancreaticogastrostomy: analysis of its efficacy to drain inaccessible pancreatic ducts. *Gastrointest Endosc.* 2007;65(2):224–230.

81. Tessier G, Bories E, Arvanitakis M, Hittelet A, Pesenti C, Le Moine O, Giovannini M, Deviere J. EUS-guided pancreatogastrostomy and pancreatobulbostomy for the treatment of pain in patients with pancreatic ductal dilatation inaccessible for transpapillary endoscopic therapy. *Gastrointest Endosc.* 2007;65(2):233–241.

82. Talreja JP KM. Endoscopic ultrasound-guided drainage of pancreatic fluid collections. In: Shami VM KM, ed. *Endoscopic Ultrasound.* New York: Humana Press; 2011.

83. Fritscher-Ravens A. EUS—experimental and evolving techniques. *Endoscopy.* 2006;38(1):S95–S99.

84. Tio TL, Tytgat GN. Endoscopic ultrasonography of normal and pathologic upper gastrointestinal wall structure. Comparison of studies in vivo and in vitro with histology. *Scand J Gastroenterol Suppl.* 1986;123:27–33.

85. Wiersema MJ, Wiersema LM. High-resolution 25-megahertz ultrasonography of the gastrointestinal wall: histologic correlates. *Gastrointest Endosc.* 1993; 39(4):499–504.

86. Stelow EB, Lai R, Bardales RH, Mallery S, Linzie BM, Crary G, Stanley MW. Endoscopic ultrasound-guided fine-needle aspiration of lymph nodes: the Hennepin County Medical Center experience. *Diagn Cytopathol.* 2004;30(5):301–306.

87. Hwang JH, Kimmey MB. The incidental upper gastrointestinal subepithelial mass. *Gastroenterology.* 2004;126(1):301–307.

88. Pais SA, Al-Haddad M, Mohamadnejad M, Leblanc JK, Sherman S, McHenry L, DeWitt JM. EUS for pancreatic neuroendocrine tumors: a single-center, 11-year experience. *Gastrointest Endosc.* 71(7):1185–1193.

89. Liu CL, Lo CM, Chan JK, Poon RT, Fan ST. EUS for detection of occult cholelithiasis in patients with idiopathic pancreatitis. *Gastrointest Endosc.* 2000;51(1):28–32.

12

ANORECTAL ULTRASOUND

CHRISTINA J. SEO

In a day and age where medicine and surgery have an increasing drive for less invasive measures, there is a rising need to find the greatest possible amount of information prior to definitive intervention. The use of ultrasound for the evaluation of anal and rectal disorders has become a mainstay in the workup of anorectal disease for many years and has seen numerous improvements in technology as well as in the understanding of normal and abnormal anatomy. As with many other innovations, this technology was initially borrowed from urologists, who had been using it as a means of examining the prostate. Since that time, adjustments have been made to optimize it for the evaluation of the rectum and anus.

CLINICAL INDICATIONS FOR ULTRASOUND

Endoluminal ultrasound, specifically of the rectum and anus, can be an extremely useful adjunct in the diagnosis of various conditions. As with any other ultrasound modality, this technique is very user-dependent, so specialized training is quite important for reproducible results. A practice that provides a consistent need for this test is also valuable.

Endoanal ultrasound is used most commonly in the evaluation of the anal sphincters in the workup of fecal incontinence. In women who have a history of vaginal delivery or any patient with a history of anal trauma, symptoms of incontinence may indicate scarring of the internal sphincters. Ultrasound, in conjunction with anal manometry, pudendal nerve testing, and defecography, can help determine the cause of the loss of fecal control and guide optimal surgical options.

Endorectal ultrasound is key to staging and evaluation of rectal cancers. In the hands of an experienced ultrasonographer, depth of invasion as well as nodal status can be measured with a fair degree of certainty. Advanced techniques include ultrasound-guided biopsy of lymph nodes for stage verification, which can guide decisions regarding the need for neoadjuvant therapy.

Standard ultrasound images are in 2-D, requiring frozen images to display normal and abnormal anatomy. Newer models include 3-D imaging, which capture the anatomy within a cube; this can be manipulated on the unit or on a computer at leisure to reveal anatomy through various cuts along multiple axes or through spinning the cube to allow views from different angles.

▶ Normal Anatomy, Normal Ultrasound

The normal anatomy of the anus can be evaluated through ultrasound with great accuracy. The structures include the anal mucosa, the internal anal sphincter (IAS), the external anal sphincter (EAS), the puborectalis, the perineal body, the seminal vesicles in a man, and any bowel that may fall into a particularly deep cul-de-sac at the level of the upper anal canal.

The anal canal is divided into three general levels, each of which demonstrates different characteristics: upper, mid, and lower. The upper anal canal is marked by the visualization of the puborectalis muscle, which appears as a U-shaped sling surrounding the anus at the superior-most border of the sphincters. Here, the seminal vesicles and occasionally some bowel may also be seen anterior to the anus (Figure 12-1).

The mid-anal canal is best identified by a clear delineation of the IAS and the EAS in the shape of dark and white rings, as well as an inner layer of mucosa containing the hemorrhoidal bundles (Figure 12-2). Any disruption of these rings can be an indication of the abnormalities that would be the source of the patient's complaint. A measurement of the perineal body can be done at this time of the examination by placing a finger against the posterior wall of the vagina to highlight that structure and measuring the distance between that and the anterior mucosa of the anus. Normal thickness of the perineal body is generally considered to be anything greater than 8 or 9 cm.

The distal anal canal is discernible by the loss of the internal anal sphincters, leaving the EAS alone as a distinct

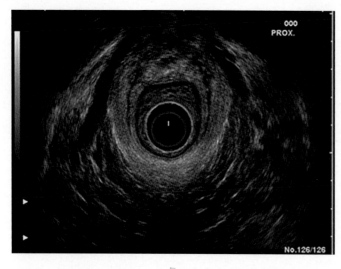

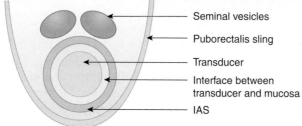

Figure 12-1. Upper anal canal.

structure (Figure 12-3). In the surrounding soft tissues beyond the anal canal and rectum lie the various perianal and perirectal spaces that become significant in the setting of malignancy and infection, but are not usually of much moment in a normal patient.

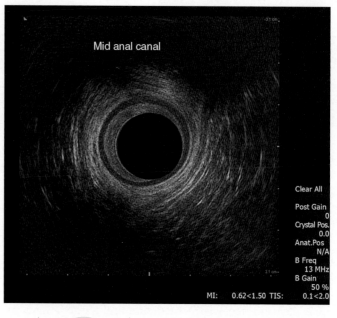

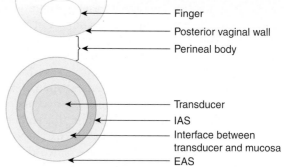

Figure 12-2. Mid-anal canal.

Normal rectal anatomy is also represented by light and dark rings, but the rings now correlate to the different layers of muscle and mucosa (Figure 12-4).[1] The perirectal fat is generally a heterogeneous shade of gray, in which enlarged lymph nodes can be identified by dark, circumscribed spots within the fat. These can sometimes be confused with perirectal vessels, but the vessels can be distinguished by moving the probe and following their linear courses, rather than limited area circumscribed by the outlines of a node.

▶ Scanning Technique for Obtaining These Images

The patient is brought into the office procedure room or endoscopy suite and placed in the left lateral decubitus position. Sedation is not generally necessary, although it is an option for an anxious patient or if a patient has a bulky tumor around which manipulation of an ultrasound probe might be too uncomfortable. The ultrasound unit is set up and the patient's information is entered.

For an anal ultrasound, a 10-MHz transducer is generally used for close-up images; this is attached to the end

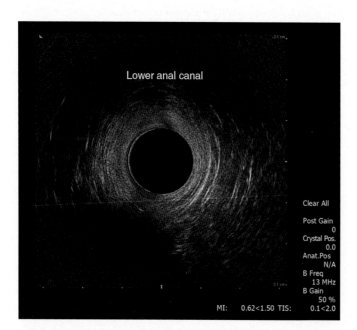

Figure 12-3. Distal anal canal.

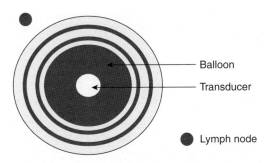

Figure 12-4. Rectal ultrasound. First white line: interface of balloon and mucosa; first dark line: mucosa, muscularis mucosae; second white line: submucosa; second dark line: muscularis propria; third white line: interface of rectum and perirectal fat.

of the ultrasound probe. A small rigid cap is fitted over the transducer and filled with saline. After doing a visual examination of the external anal canal and an initial digital examination, the probe is lubricated and placed into the anal canal. The operator will know when the upper anal canal is reached by identifying the puborectalis sling. Orientation is also achieved by turning the probe until the sling is shown to resemble the letter "U" with the lateral arms reaching upward. The probe is then withdrawn slowly to the mid- and then distal-anal canal, looking for abnormalities. The perineal body in a woman is measured in the manner previously described at the mid-anal canal (Figure 12-5). The 3-D function available on some scanners has the advantage of not needing to withdraw the probe and the ability to manipulate the image in any direction.

Rectal ultrasounds are performed in a slightly different manner. The patient is prepared with an enema prior to the procedure. The 10-MHz transducer is preferred for examination of shallower structures, while the 7-MHz transducer is chosen for deeper, more distant structures. Again, for most purposes, the 10-MHz transducer is generally sufficient. A latex balloon is attached to the probe and inflated with saline, taking care to remove all air bubbles. It is then desufflated prior to insertion. The external anus is visualized and a digital examination performed. A rigid proctoscope is passed transanally and the target lesion examined, taking care to mark distance, size, quadrant, and characteristics. The proctoscope is advanced to a level just proximal to the lesion in order to ensure that the entire lesion can be examined by the ultrasound. The probe is passed through the proctoscope; once the transducer is past the open end of the scope, the scope can be withdrawn slightly for better manipulation. The balloon is then inflated so that the rectal wall is fully distended for optimal contact with the rectal mucosa. The probe is again withdrawn slowly, marking the disruption of the light and dark lines, and looking for any prominent lymph nodes in the surrounding perirectal fat. As with the anal ultrasound, a 3-D module is available to help in creating a block of images that can be examined in an infinite variety of ways after the examination.

▶ Common Findings/Abnormalities

Possibly the most common reason for performing an anal ultrasound is in the workup of fecal incontinence. In conjunction with pudendal nerve latency testing, anal manometry, and defecography, anal ultrasound can confirm structural defects and scarring in the internal and external anal sphincters.[2] The likeliest origin of anal incontinence is sphincter damage after vaginal delivery, often presenting decades after the inciting injury.[3] Sphincter defects should be suspected in a peri- or postmenopausal woman with a history of vaginal delivery, many times complicated by high-birth-weight babies, prolonged labor, use of vacuum or forceps assistance, or episiotomy. Common findings in these patients include anterior scarring or a complete break of the IAS and/or the EAS (Figure 12-6),[4] and thinning of the perineal body (less than 8 mm thickness on digital examination at the mid-anal canal).[5] Some amount

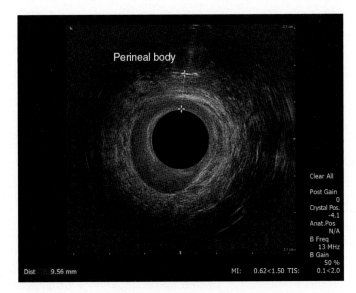

Figure 12-5. Measurement of the perineal body.

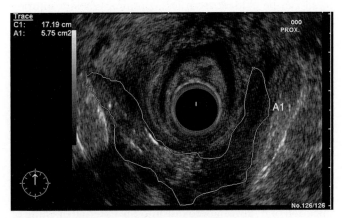

Figure 12-6. Anterior sphincter defect.

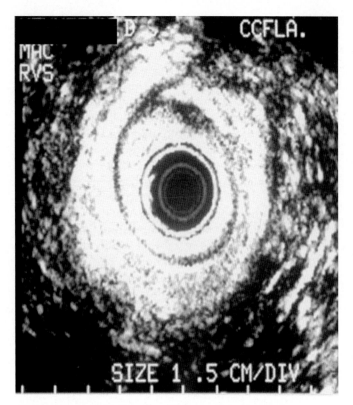

Figure 12-7. "6" sign of overlapping sphincteroplasty.

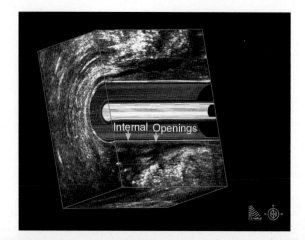

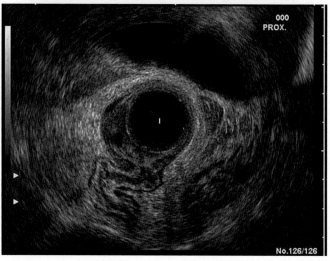

Figure 12-8. Anal fistula.

of anterior scarring, which appears as a break in the rings of tissue with mixed echogenicity, is likely present in many women in the general population; it is unclear what distinguishes those women who are symptomatic from those who are not.[6] However, confirmation of scarring can help delineate surgical options for these patients. Specifically, an overlapping sphincteroplasty is an option for the appropriate patient. In cases of recurrence of symptoms after such an operation, or for follow-up evaluation after this procedure, an ultrasound may be performed. This shows a classic "6" or "reverse 6" sign in an intact repair (Figure 12-7).[7]

Other patients who have fecal incontinence and have no history of traumatic vaginal delivery may have other findings. Multiple or eccentric tears, or scarring, or no scarring at all can be evident from less common types of injuries, limiting the options for surgical intervention. Congenital anomalies can be delineated by ultrasonography and help to determine what structures are absent or aberrant. It can also be useful in identifying occult rectovaginal fistulas, which may mimic or add to the symptoms of fecal incontinence.

Another common use of ultrasound is the evaluation of an anal abscess or anal fistula.[8] Abscess cavities and any fistulous tracts can be seen on ultrasound as dark cavities outlined in white (Figure 12-8).[9] This mode of evaluation is especially useful in tracing complex or high fistula tracts that would be difficult to follow by other methods. The injection of hydrogen peroxide into the external opening of a fistula will make the tract hyperechoic from the bubbling

effect of the fluid from oxygenation and help to distinguish it from other structures in the surrounding tissue.[10]

Anal tumors, both benign and malignant, can be clearly examined with anal ultrasound. Sonographic images can show the relationship of benign tumors to anal anatomy and define tissue planes. Most lesions will be hypoechoic, and ultrasound-guided biopsies may be performed by an advanced operator. Malignant tumors, most commonly squamous cell carcinomas, can be used in pre- and post-treatment staging. While some of the rarer cancers may warrant surgical intervention, the treatment of squamous cell malignancies of the anus is largely radiation. Incomplete response or recurrence can be followed by serial ultrasounds. Staging follows a standard TNM protocol (Tables 12-1 and 12-2) and can be measured either by diameter or by depth of invasion.[11] Staging by ultrasound is labeled by a "u" preceding the standard nomenclature to distinguish it from the final pathologic designation.

Rectal ultrasound is used primarily in staging of rectal malignancies.[12] The first area to evaluate is depth of invasion; staging is similar to the staging used for anal tumors (Table 12-3). Lymph nodes can also be visualized for more accurate preoperative staging.

TABLE 12-1

TNM Staging of Anal Malignancies, by Size of Tumor

Primary Tumor (T)
- TX: Primary tumor cannot be assessed
- T0: No evidence of primary tumor
- Tis: Carcinoma *in situ*
- T1: Tumor 2 cm or less in greatest dimension
- T2: Tumor more than 2 cm but not more than 5 cm in the greatest dimension
- T3: Tumor more than 5 cm in the greatest dimension
- T4: Tumor of any size that invades adjacent organ(s), eg, vagina, urethra, and bladder*

Regional Lymph Nodes (N)
- NX: Regional lymph nodes cannot be assessed
- N0: No regional lymph node metastasis
- N1: Metastasis in perirectal lymph node(s)
- N2: Metastasis in unilateral internal iliac and/or inguinal lymph node(s)
- N3: Metastasis in perirectal and inguinal lymph nodes and/or bilateral internal iliac and/or inguinal lymph nodes

Distant Metastasis (M)
- MX: Distant metastasis cannot be assessed
- M0: No distant metastasis
- M1: Distant metastasis

AJCC Stage Groupings
Stage 0
- Tis, N0, M0

Stage I
- T1, N0, M0

Stage II
- T2, N0, M0
- T3, N0, M0

Stage IIIA
- T1, N1, M0
- T2, N1, M0
- T3, N1, M0
- T4, N0, M0

Stage IIIB
- T4, N1, M0
- Any T, N2, M0
- Any T, N3, M0

Stage IV
- Any T, any N, M1

*Direct invasion of the rectal wall, perirectal skin, subcutaneous tissue, or the sphincter muscle(s) is not classified as T4.

TABLE 12-2

Alternate *u*T Classification by Depth of Invasion

uT1	Confined to submucosa
uT2a	Confined to IAS
uT2b	Through IAS, confined to EAS
uT3	Invades EAS into perianal tissues
uT4	Invades adjacent structures

TABLE 12-3

Staging Classification of Rectal Cancer by Ultrasound

uT0	Confined to mucosa
uT1	Confined to submucosa
uT2	Invades into but not through muscularis propria
uT3	Invades to perirectal fat
uT4	Invades adjacent organs
uN0	No evidence of spread to lymph nodes
uN1	Evidence of spread to lymph nodes

uT0 Lesions

Lesions confined to the mucosa are generally considered to be benign, with little risk of local or distant spread. Fortunately, the more superficial the lesion, the more accurate the ultrasonography is in predicting final staging. Accuracy is from 81% to 96% for uT0 lesions when compared to pathologic staging.[13] The white line that correlates to the submucosa should be intact beneath the lesion in an unbroken fashion. Local excision is acceptable for these tumors, either by transanal excision or by transanal endoscopic microsurgery (TEMS), as there is no need for lymph node excision.

uT1 Lesions

The earliest stages of malignancies fall in the uT1 category. The lesion has invaded the mucosa and submucosa without entering the muscularis propria. On ultrasound, this will look like a mass outlined by an irregular white line and a normal outer black line (Figure 12-9). Any minor breaks in the line of the white muscularis layer indicate a higher T stage. Certain uT1 lesions may be treated locally; a clear lack of abnormal regional lymph nodes, smaller mass

T1 or Villous Adenoma

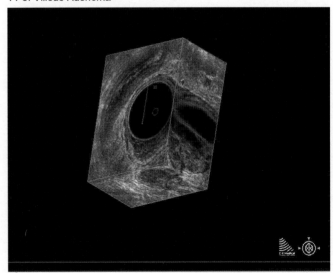

Figure 12-9. uT1 lesion.

T2 Tumor

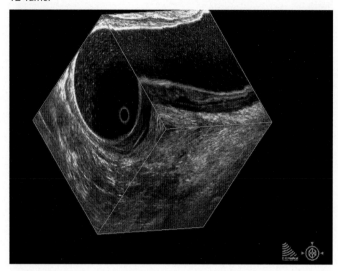

Figure 12-10. uT2 lesion.

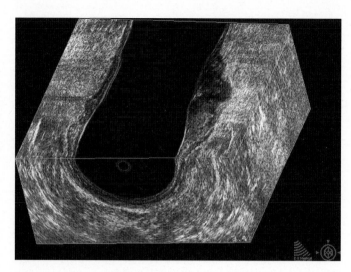

Figure 12-11. uT3 lesion.

size less than 4 cm, less than 1/3 of the circumference, and more distal lesions that would be better amenable to trans-anal procedures are factors to consider when deciding on a treatment plan.

uT2 Lesions

These lesions are important to distinguish from uT1 lesions as more invasive surgical and neoadjuvant therapies may be indicated for the patient. Invasion of the muscularis propria shows up on ultrasound as a disruption of the middle white line and the adjacent black line without a break of the outermost white line that represents perirectal fat (Figure 12-10). Some clinicians may make the distinction in the degree of invasion, deep or early, in order to decide on if neoadjuvant therapy is an appropriate option for the patient.

uT3 Lesions

The observation of invasion into the last white line classifies a lesion to be a uT3 lesion. All the intervening layers are disrupted, and the outline of the mass is generally very irregular or unclear (Figure 12-11). These patients are not candidates for local excision, and usually have neoadjuvant chemoradiation therapy included in their treatment plan. It is very important in these patients to look closely for regional lymph nodes as the likelihood of nodal spread increases dramatically with this depth of invasion.

uT4 Lesions

Invasion into adjacent structures, such as the vagina, uterus, or cervix in women, the prostate or seminal vesicles in men, or the bladder in either gender, qualifies a lesion this advanced to be a uT4 lesion. Typically, these lesions are nonmobile on examination prior to the ultrasound. There is a lack of distinction between the rectum and the sur-

rounding structures. (An example of intact adjacent viscera is shown in Figure 12-12).

▶ Nodal Involvement

The detection of lymph nodes in the perirectal fat is an important clue in determining prognosis for a patient. Accurate preoperative staging helps to determine the need for neoadjuvant therapy, and therefore makes the long-term survival rate easier to determine.

Unfortunately, the accuracy of ultrasound in detecting nodal disease is poorer than that for measuring depth of invasion. Some studies show accuracy to range from as low as 50% to a high of 88%.[14] Most other diagnostic tools are no better, however, with the possible exception of multi-phase MRI or endorectal coil MRI.[15] These have comparable results, but may not be available in all institutions; radiologists with a particular interest in reading these MRI studies are critical for accurate interpretation.

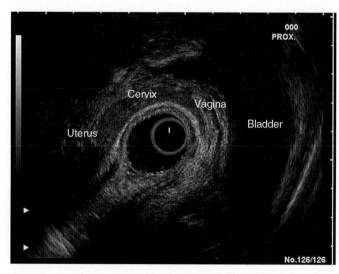

Figure 12-12. Perirectal viscera.

Normal lymph nodes in the mesorectum do not usually appear distinct on endorectal ultrasound. Malignant nodes tend to be large, hypoechoic, and round.[16] Inflammatory nodes, on the other hand, look hyperechoic and irregular. Determining which lymph nodes are truly malignant can be difficult, as size is not a reliable indicator of metastasis, although larger size may indicate a higher likelihood of spread.[17] Also indicative of malignancy is an area of mixed echogenicity, which can be suggestive of lymphovascular invasion.

COMMON PITFALLS

The most difficult aspect of anorectal ultrasound is the dependence on operator skill and interpretation.[18] While most of the target structures that need to be evaluated are close to the transducer, some diseases may fall outside the range of the probe. Using a different frequency transducer may help, although this could sacrifice some accuracy.

Depth of invasion is not always easy to interpret depending on the bulkiness of the tumor. Disruption of the black and white lines at different points versus displacement around the margins of the mass can be difficult to differentiate. Artifact from air bubbles in the balloon around the transducer can also cause shadowing, which can obscure important findings. Lesions more proximal in the rectum can be difficult to evaluate due to angulation of the rectal valves and the rigidity of the probe. Nodes can be confused with vascular structures or other perirectal abnormal lesions.[19]

Anal ultrasounds, generally, are somewhat easier to interpret, with less bulky disease to evaluate. Following fistula tracts can be difficult, especially more complex ones with multiple arms or high courses. Measuring anterior sphincter defects is generally simple, but eccentric or multiple areas of scarring are less obvious.

CLINICAL PEARLS/TIPS

In general, the use of an ultrasound atlas is helpful in refreshing one's mind and reinforcing accurate interpretation of the images obtained. Several are available in print that would serve as supporting references. Also helpful in eliminating variations in analyzing the images is the use of 3-D imagery. These images can be saved and then manipulated in innumerable ways to fully examine pathology, and can always be reexamined at a later date by any number of examiners.

THERAPEUTIC MANEUVERS

The most common procedures done with the anal ultrasound is evaluation of anal fistulas with the assistance of hydrogen peroxide, as described previously in this chapter. It is probably the most useful way available to accurately track complex fistulas and then help decide the best treatment to deal with them.

Another useful tool is ultrasound-guided biopsy of perirectal lymph nodes, which usually requires further training and a probe with the capability to do core biopsies. It has a sensitivity of 71% and a specificity of 89%.[20] Positive findings of metastatic disease justify neoadjuvant therapy for better local disease control.

A newer technique has been described by Drs. Sergio Regadas and Dr. Sthela Murad-Regadas, called echodefecography, using dynamic 3-D ultrasonography.[21] While placing the distal probe at the most proximal end of the anal canal, the patient is instructed to squeeze, relax, then Valsalva while the images are captured and the probe is withdrawn (Figure 12-13). With proper training, the operator can distinguish such pathology as internal intussusceptions, rectocele, grade III enterocele, and anismus in the workup for obstructed defecation.[22] When compared to conventional defecography, echodefecography has similar

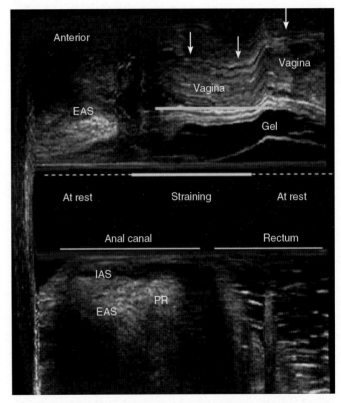

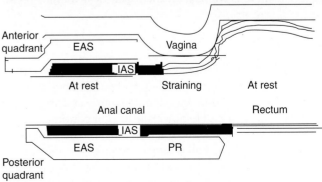

Figure 12-13. Normal echodefecography.

accuracy with regard to rectocele, and may be more sensitive in detecting internal intussusception.[23] It can also be used to measure the puborectalis angle, abnormalities in which can point to a cause for obstructed defecation. The main advantages of this technique over conventional defecography include lack of radiation and better patient tolerance. Due to the limitations of the probe in seeing more distant structures, mild enteroceles or sigmoidoceles may be outside the range of visualization.

CASE STUDIES

▶ **Case 1**

M.O. is a 65-year-old woman with complaint of increasing fecal incontinence. Over the past 3 years, her symptoms progressed from occasional soilage of her underwear to loss of solid stool several times a week. She presents now stating that she never goes out anymore for fear of having an accident and wears a pad constantly. Her stools are generally soft to loose when she loses control, although she occasionally has incontinence of formed or hard stools. She states she cannot feel the passage of gas and has little sensation for when she has bowel movement. In exploring her past medical history she notes that she had two vaginal deliveries, one of which included an episiotomy. Her Wexner score is now 18 out of 20. She is given the appropriate workup during which she has an anal ultrasound. This shows a single, wide, anterior defect of 110 degrees and a perineal body thickness of 5 mm (Figure 12-6). She undergoes an overlapping sphincteroplasty, which she recovers well from. Her postoperative Wexner score improves to 9. One year after her surgery, she returns with worsening symptoms. A repeat anal ultrasound shows slight disruption of the classic "6" sign of her repair. She then undergoes a second overlapping sphincteroplasty with good results.

Discussion

The most common reason for performing anal ultrasound is in the workup for fecal incontinence. It works best in disclosing structural defects that commonly occur from obstetric injuries from several decades earlier. The Wexner fecal incontinence score is useful in tracking improvement or failure of repairs, and postoperative ultrasound can help detect if there is slippage of the repair or if there is recurrence of symptoms.

▶ **Case 2**

P.I. is a 27-year-old man with a 10-year history of Crohn disease, generally well controlled. He has a history of recurrent anal abscesses that drain spontaneously and are treated with oral antibiotics. He notes one area of continual drainage, even without a frank abscess or pain. Examination in the office reveals a small internal opening, but passage of a fistula probe through the external opening is not possible due to discomfort. He is brought to the endoscopy suite for an anal ultrasound. Hydrogen peroxide is injected into

the external opening while the transducer is in place. The images show a high transsphincteric fistula with a small collection at the apex (Figure 12-8). He is brought to the operating room shortly thereafter and a seton is placed through the tract, with some difficulty. Three months later, an ultrasound was repeated to ascertain that the collection had resolved. It had, and he is then scheduled for a placement of an anal fistula plug.

Discussion

In cases of particularly complex anal fistulas, the use of endoanal ultrasound may be very useful in delineating their courses. Patients with Crohn disease have a propensity for eccentric fistula tracts and standard treatments may not be effective. Injection of hydrogen peroxide into the tract during the ultrasound can help to identify any undiagnosed collections. Involvement of a significant portion of the anal sphincters precludes a simple fistulotomy, especially in cases of Crohn, and may help direct staged or more complex repairs.

▶ **Case 3**

I.S. is a 92-year-old woman with a past medical history of pulmonary hypertension and mild aortic stenosis, though very functional and independent, who presents with new-onset rectal bleeding. She is found to have a lower-third rectal mass on colonoscopy. She had not had prior colonoscopies. On digital examination the mass is firm, ulcerated, not very mobile, in the posterior quadrant, and occupies half of the circumference. She has no family history of colon cancer and no obvious risk factors. She is brought to the endoscopy suite and an endorectal ultrasound was performed (Figure 12-11). Her stage at this time is uT3N1. She undergoes neoadjuvant therapy, after which a repeat colonoscopy and ultrasound is performed. Other than scarring, there does not appear to be any residual tumor on the colonoscopy; biopsies show fibrosis but no malignancy. The ultrasound shows some inflammation and scarring, but there is no obvious invasive mass and no enlarged lymph nodes. Due to her advanced age and comorbidities, she decides to opt for continued surveillance rather than undergo a low anterior resection and diverting ileostomy.

Discussion

Endorectal ultrasound is an important tool to stage rectal cancers preoperatively. Since neoadjuvant therapy is an important part of the decisions to be made in the management of rectal cancer, accurate evaluation is important to decide which patients are appropriate for such treatment. In this patient's case, the response of the tumor to the radiation opens up a more conservative option for this elderly lady. While the correct oncologic choice would be a low anterior resection with a coloanal anastomosis and covering ileostomy, such an invasive procedure might worsen her pulmonary and cardiac disease; endoscopic surveillance may be a viable option in her case.

SUGGESTED READINGS

Beynon J, et al. The endosonic appearances of normal colon and rectum. *Dis Colon Rectum.* 1986;29(12):810–813.

Edelman BR, Weiser MR. Endorectal ultrasound: its role in the diagnosis and treatment of rectal cancer. *Clin Colon Rectal Surg.* 2008;21:167–177.

Greene FL, et al. *AJCC Cancer Staging Manual.* 6th ed. New York: Springer; 2002.

Gurland B, Hull T. Transrectal ultrasound, manometry, and pudendal nerve terminal latency studies in the evaluation of sphincter injuries. *Clin Colon Rectal Surg.* 2008;21: 157–166.

Kim DG, Wong WD. Endoluminal ultrasound. In: Wolff BG, et al, ed. *The ASCRS Textbook of Colon and Rectal Surgery.* New York: Springer Science+Business Media; 2007:101–115.

Tjandra JJ, et al. Endoluminal ultrasound is preferable to electromyography in mapping anal sphincteric defects. *Dis Colon Rectum.* 1993;36(7):689–692.

Wu JS. Rectal cancer staging. *Clin Colon Rectal Surg.* 2007;20:148–157.

REFERENCES

1. Beynon J, Foy DMA, Temple LN, et al. The endosonic appearances of normal colon and rectum. *Dis Colon Rectum.* 1986;29(12):810–813.

2. Tjandra JJ, Milson JW, Schroeder T, et al. Endoluminal ultrasound is preferable to electromyography in mapping anal sphincteric defects. *Dis Colon Rectum.* 1993;36(7):689–692.

3. Allen RE, Hosker GL, Smith AR, et al. Pelvic floor damage and childbirth: a neurophysiological study. *Br J Obstet Gynecol.* 1990;97(9):770–779.

4. Burnett SJ, Spence-Jones C, Speakman CT, et al. Unsuspected sphincter damage following childbirth revealed by anal endosonography. *Br J Radiol.* 1991;64(759):225–227.

5. Zetterstrom JP, Mellgren A, Madoff RD, et al. Perineal body measurement improves evaluation of anterior sphincter lesions during endoluminal ultrasonography. *Dis Colon Rectum.* 1998;41(6):705–713.

6. Varma A, Gunn J, Gardiner A, et al. Obstetric anal sphincter injury: prospective evaluation of incidence. *Dis Colon Rectum.* 1999;42(12):1537–1542.

7. Gilliland R, Altomare DF, Moreira H, et al. Pudendal neuropathy is predictive of failure following anterior overlapping sphincteroplasty. *Dis Colon Rectum.* 1998;41(12):1515–1522.

8. Deen KI, Williams JG, Hutchinson R, et al. Fistulas in ano: endoanal ultrasonographic assessment assists decision making for surgery. *Gut.* 1994;35(3):391–394.

9. Law PJ, Talbot RW, Bartram CI, et al. Anal endosonography in the evaluation of perianal sepsis and fistula in ano. *Br J Surg.* 1989;76(7):752–755.

10. Poen AC, Felt-Bersma RJF, Eijsbouts QAJ, et al. Hydrogen peroxide-enhanced transanal ultrasound in the assessment of fistula-in-ano. *Dis Colon Rectum.* 1998;41(9):1147–1152.

11. Greene FL, Page DL, Fleming ID, et al. *AJCC Cancer Staging Manual.* 6th ed. New York: Springer; 2002.

12. Deen KI, Madoff RD, Wong WD. Preoperative staging of rectal neoplasms with endorectal ultrasonography. *Semin Colon Rectal Surg.* 1995;6:78–85.

13. Garcia-Aguilar J, Pollack J, Lee S-H, et al. Accuracy of Endorectal ultrasonography in preoperative staging of rectal tumors. *Dis Colon Rectum.* 2002;45(1):10–15.

14. Kim DG, Madoff RD. Transanal treatment of rectal cancer: ablative methods and open resection. *Semin Surg Oncol.* 1998;15(2):101–113.

15. Beynon J, Mortensen NJ, Foy DM, et al. Preoperative assessment of mesorectal lymph node involvement in rectal cancer. *Br J Surg.* 1989;76(3):276–279.

16. Thaler W, Watzka S, Martin F, et al. Preoperative staging of rectal cancer by endoluminal ultrasound vs. magnetic resonance imaging. Preliminary results of a prospective, comparative study. *Dis Colon Rectum.* 1994;37(12): 1189–1193.

17. Tio TL, Tytgat GN. Endoscopic ultrasonography in analysing peri-intestinal lymph node abnormality. Preliminary results of studies in vitro and in vivo. *Scand J Gastroenterol.* 1986;123(suppl):158–163.

18. Hildebrandt U, Klein T, Feifel G, et al. Endosonography of pararectal lymph nodes. In vitro and in vivo evaluation. *Dis Colon Rectum.* 1990;33(10):863–868.

19. Kruskal JB, Kane RA, Sentovich SM, et al. Pitfalls and sources of error in staging rectal cancer with endorectal US. *Radiographics.* 1997;17(3):609–626.

20. Milson JW, Czyrko C, Hull T, et al. Preoperative biopsy of pararectal lymph nodes in rectal cancer using endoluminal ultrasonography. *Dis Colon Rectum.* 1994;37(4):364–368.

21. Murad-Regadas SM, Regadas FS, Rodrigues LV, et al. A novel three-dimensional dynamic anorectal ultrasonography technique (echo defacography) to assess obstructed defecation, a comparison with defecography. *Surg Endosc.* 2008;22(4):974–979.

22. Murad-Regadas SM, Regadas FS, Rodrigues LV, et al. A novel procedure to assess anismus using three-dimensional dynamic anal ultrasonography. *Colorectal Dis.* 2007;9(2):159–165.

23. Regadas SFP, Haas E, Abbas MA, et al. Prospective multicenter trial comparing echodefecography to defecography in the assessment of anorectal dysfunction in patients with obstructed defecation. *Dis Colon Rectum.* 2011;54(6):686–692.

13

GENITOURINARY ULTRASOUND

JOSEPH A. GRAVERSEN, MOHAMMAD A. HELMY, FARHAN KHAN, ADAM KAPLAN,
COROLLOS S. ABDELSHEHID, PHILLIP MUCKSAVAGE, ACHIM LUSCH, & JAIME LANDMAN

RENAL ULTRASOUND

▶ Clinical Indications

Renal ultrasonography is a commonly employed imaging technique with many useful applications. These include, but are not limited to, evaluation of hydronephrosis, detection and surveillance of nephrolithiasis, characterization of focal renal lesions, and workup of renal failure and hematuria.[1-3] While not without limitations, ultrasound offers many advantages over computed tomography (CT) and magnetic resonance imaging (MRI). Ultrasound does not involve ionizing radiation, which is significantly advantageous in certain populations such as pregnant patients and children. Ultrasound can be used safely in patients with allergies to iodinated contrast agents and in patients with cardiac pacemakers. Ultrasound does not carry a risk of contrast-induced nephropathy or nephrogenic systemic fibrosis, and is not limited by renal function. Imaging guidance by ultrasound is frequently employed in renal biopsies, nephrostomy tube, or ureteral stent placements, and intraoperatively in lesion resection and treatment.

Ultrasound is excellent in detection of hydronephrosis and useful in the workup of hematuria, particularly in low- and medium-risk patients as maintained by the European Society of Urogenital Radiology.[4] In detection and surveillance of nephrolithiasis, ultrasound offers an alternative to CT imaging in more radiosensitive patients and those with body morphology conducive in sonographic imaging. Ultrasound provides a high level of accuracy in characterization of focal masses as solid, cystic, or mixed, and can be utilized in surveillance of focal renal lesions for stability in conjunction with CT and MRI. Doppler imaging can be applied in the evaluation of cystic or solid lesions and in other renal vascular applications such as identifying arteriovenous fistulas or malformations, screening for renal artery stenosis, detection of renal vein thrombosis, and calculation of resistive indices in the workup of obstructive

and medical renal disease. The color comet tail artifact, or "twinkling" artifact, provides additional sensitivity to ultrasound in detection of calcifications, either related to stone disease or complex cystic lesions.

Despite its useful applications, ultrasound possesses many limitations as a modality in renal evaluation. In the setting of acute trauma, ultrasound may not be able to differentiate acute hemorrhage from urine and does not accurately stage the degree of renal injury.[5,6] CT serves as the primary imaging modality of choice following blunt or penetrating trauma, and has the advantage of evaluating adjacent organs and vasculature for concurrent injuries. Ultrasound does not reliably visualize the ureter, thus limiting its evaluation of urolithiasis, an assessment more optimally performed by noncontrast CT imaging.[7]

▶ Normal Anatomy

The kidneys lie in the retroperitoneum surrounded by Gerota fascia and perinephric fat. Each kidney generally weighs 150 g in the males and 135 g in the females. A typical kidney measures 10–12 cm longitudinally, 5 to 7 cm transversely, and 3 cm in the anteroposterior dimension. While the position of the kidney within the retroperitoneum varies by side, degree of inspiration, body position, and anatomic anomalies, the right kidney is usually located 1 to 2 cm lower than the left secondary to inferior displacement by the liver. Anatomically, a normal right kidney can be found in the space between the top of the first lumbar vertebra to the bottom of the third lumbar vertebra, while the left kidney is more superiorly located between the 12th thoracic vertebra and third lumbar vertebra.

The muscles surrounding the kidneys are similar on both sides. The lower two-thirds of the kidneys lie on the psoas muscles posteromedially. This results in the lower pole of the kidney lying anteriorly and laterally relative to the upper pole and rotating the medial aspect of the kidney by approximately 30 degrees. This anatomy is of particular importance while gaining ultrasound-guided percutaneous access to the kidney.

On the right side, the kidney is juxtaposed with a number of structures. The liver lies adjacent to the upper pole both superiorly and anteriorly. The adrenal gland is also encountered in the superomedial aspect of the right kidney. Medially, the duodenum is adjacent to the hilum and hilar structures. The anterior aspect of the lower pole of the kidney is also covered by the hepatic flexure of the colon. On the left side, the spleen and adrenal gland are located at the superior and superior-medial aspects of the upper pole, respectively. The tail of the pancreas and splenic vessels are adjacent medially to the upper pole and renal hilum. Anteriorly the left kidney is covered by the splenic flexure of the colon.

The renal vasculature normally consists of one artery and one vein entering the kidney at the hilum, although occasionally multiple arteries and veins do exist. The renal artery divides into five segmental arteries: an anterior branch, which further subdivides into the apical, upper, middle, and lower segmental arteries, and the posterior branch. Renal arteries are end arteries with no communication between the various branches. The venous structures generally accompany the arteries through the renal parenchyma; however, unlike the arterial system they communicate freely. The left renal vein receives drainage from the adrenal, gonadal, and posterior lumbar veins before crossing midline anterior to the aorta to communicate with the vena cava. No other veins consistently drain into the right renal vein, although occasionally the right gonadal vein may end in the right renal vein instead of its typical drainage into the vena cava.

The renal parenchyma comprises a renal cortex and medulla. The medulla is composed primarily of the collecting ducts, while the cortex houses the majority of the nephrons. Each nephron is associated with an afferent arteriole that enters the glomerulus for filtration to take place. The filtrate from the glomerulus is reabsorbed and concentrated as it passes through the renal tubular system before it finally enters the collecting duct. Multiple collecting ducts make up a pyramid, and the tip of a pyramid is called the papilla. There are generally 7 to 9 papillae within a kidney and each is located within a renal calyx. The minor calyces are connected by infundibulae to form two or three major calyces, which join into the renal pelvis.

The renal pelvis lies posterior to the renal vessels and drains into the ureter. The ureter is generally 22–23-cm long and courses just medial to the psoas muscle in the retroperitoneum. The ureters cross anterior to the common iliac vessels near their bifurcation. The ureters then travel posterior to the gonadal vessels and drain into the bladder.

▶ Normal Appearance on Ultrasound

The normal kidney appears as elliptical on longitudinal views and rounded on transverse views with the renal parenchyma encasing the central renal sinus. The renal

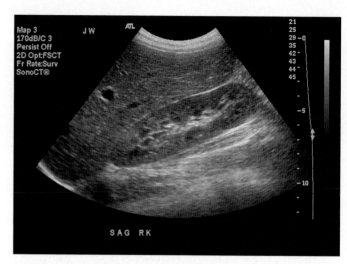

Figure 13-1. Longitudinal image of a normal right kidney. In this image, the liver provides a clear acoustic window for imaging the kidney. The renal sinus fat located in the center of the kidney is clearly distinguished from the renal parenchyma by its hyperechoic echotexture.

cortex is homogeneous and slightly hypoechoic compared to adjacent liver or spleen. The renal sinus is densely echogenic due to its typical fat composition and contains the renal vessels, lymphatics, and renal pelvis. The renal medulla may occasionally be differentiated from the renal cortex as small triangular or rounded hypoechoic structures between the cortex and renal sinus fat. The renal capsule provides a strong acoustic interface with the surrounding perinephric fat providing a distinct demarcation of the renal outline and contour (Figures 13-1 to 13-3).

▶ Scanning Technique

A real-time 2–5-MHz frequency sector or curvilinear transducer is routinely utilized in renal imaging. Each kidney is

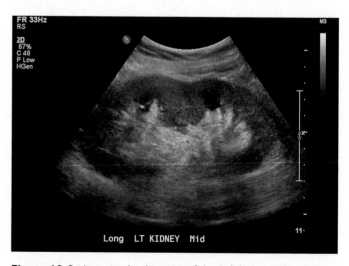

Figure 13-2. Longitudinal image of the left kidney. The gap in the renal outline is the renal hilum. That it is visible indicates that the probe is oriented appropriately to the position of the kidney.

ensuring that the epididymis is well visualized. Long-axis and anteroposterior dimensions of the testicle are measured. The transducer is rotated 90 degrees and imaging resumes in the transverse plane. Each testicle is systematically scanned from superior to inferior poles and measurement of testicular width is documented. An overview image incorporating both testes is helpful in direct comparison of testicular echotexture and homogeneity.

CFD plays an important role in scrotal sonography. Doppler images of each testis and epididymis help in evaluating for abnormally increased or decreased flow, as can be seen in epididymo-orchitis and torsion, respectively. As with gray scale imaging, an overview image incorporating both testes with CFD is helpful in direct comparison of intratesticular flow for assessment of asymmetry and relative hyperemia or ischemia. CFD is also helpful in evaluating peritesticular structures, most often for assessment of varicocele at the superolateral aspect of each hemiscrotum. Dynamic imaging at rest and with Valsalva maneuver in supine and standing positions can be performed to aid in this diagnosis.

▶ Common Findings/Abnormalities

In ultrasound evaluation of the acute scrotum, the two major concerns are testicular torsion and epididymitis/epididymo-orchitis. Clinically, testicular torsion should be suspected when the patient complains of sudden onset of severe, intractable scrotal pain, high-riding testicle, and significant scrotal wall redness and edema (Figure 13-13). On physical examination, the testicle is often exquisitely tender, and there is loss of the cremasteric reflex. Much of the history and many of the physical findings, however, are similar to those seen with epididymo-orchitis, making it difficult to distinguish between these entities. Early after the onset of torsion, gray scale imaging of the testis

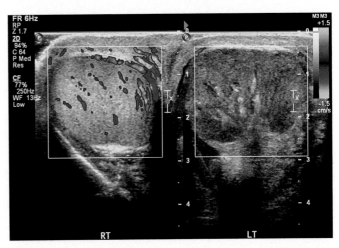

Figure 13-14. CFD of testicular torsion. A hallmark of torsion is loss of blood flow to the testicle. Note that the capsular vessels of the left testicle still demonstrate flow despite an obviously torsed testicle.

is relatively normal. Doppler evaluation becomes essential in documenting diminished or absent flow as a sign of ischemia and torsion. A decrease in testicular echogenicity, loss of normal homogeneous echotexture, and enlargement of the epididymis can begin to appear as early as 6 hours after the onset of ischemia.[39] Over time, the testicle continues to increase in size and becomes more heterogeneous in echotexture and hypoechoic, features that often indicate that the testicle may no longer be surgically salvageable (Figure 13-14).[36]

Pain associated with epididymitis and epididymo-orchitis typically begins more insidiously, worsening over several days. Many patients, however, report a sudden onset of discomfort making it virtually indistinguishable from torsion by history alone. Gray scale imaging usually shows epididymal enlargement and testicular hypoechogenecity.[23] In contrast to testicular torsion, CFD typically demonstrates an increase in testicular and epididymal flow compared to the unaffected side (Figures 13-15 and 13-16).

There are several conditions that can cause painless scrotal enlargement or a palpable mass including malignancies, varicoceles, hydroceles, and spermatoceles/epididymal cysts. Testicular tumors represent 1–2% of all malignancies in men. Among the most important determinants in the evaluation of scrotal masses is location. An intratesticular mass is potentially malignant and often requires subsequent surgical extirpation. In contrast, the vast majority of extratesticular masses are benign and may be observed and followed depending on their appearances.

Germ cell tumors of the testis are divided into two major groups, seminomatous and nonseminomatous (mixed germ cell) tumors. While most intratesticular tumors appear as distinct hypoechoic masses within the parenchyma of the testicle, seminomas tend to be homogenous, while nonseminomatous lesions are often heterogeneous. The difference in appearance is due to varying degrees of hemorrhage, cystic changes, necrosis, and calcifications

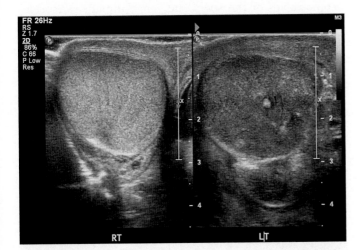

Figure 13-13. Late testicular torsion. In early testicular torsion, there are often no ultrasonographic abnormalities that can be seen with gray scale imaging of the testicle. However, as the necrosis process continues, the echotexture of the testicle becomes heterogeneous as seen in this side-by-side comparison of a normal right testicle and a torsed left testicle.

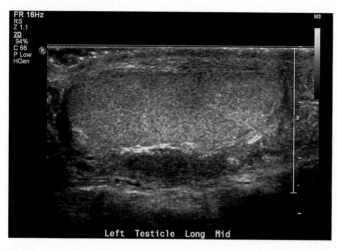

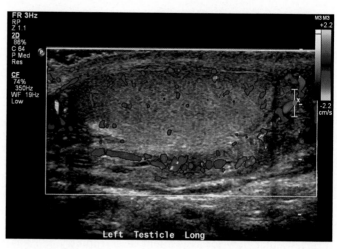

Figures 13-15 and 13-16. In epididymitis, the epididymis becomes inflamed and painful. Often, the inflamed epididymis appears large and thickened (compare to Figure 13-12). The normal epididymis displays little to no flow on CFD. In contrast, the infected/inflamed epididymis displays increased blood flow. Note the normal blood flow within the testicle, differentiating the painful conditions of epididymitis and testicular torsion.

that accompany nonseminomatous tumors. Many benign and non-neoplastic conditions can produce a focal testicular mass and mimic the appearance of malignancy, including hematomas, infarctions, and inflammatory lesions (Figures 13-17 and 13-18).[40-43]

The two major cystic conditions of the scrotum, hydrocele, and epididymal cyst/spermatocele can often be differentiated by careful physical examination and are both generally benign. Hydroceles develop as a result of accumulation of fluid between the layers of the tunica vaginalis. This is due to either communication with the peritoneal cavity via a patent processus vaginalis or an acquired condition. Although most acquired hydroceles can be managed expectantly, they occasionally get very large and require surgical extirpation. Patients with hydroceles too large to allow for an adequate testicular examination should undergo scrotal ultrasound to determine if the hydrocele

is secondary to some underlying testicular malignancy. On ultrasound, hydroceles appear as an anechoic cystic collection that encompasses the testicle (Figures 13-19 and 13-20). Occasionally, hyperechoic cholesterol crystals, blood, septations, or echogenic fluid can be noted in the hydrocele. These findings are suggestive, but not diagnostic, of an underlying inflammatory condition or inciting traumatic event (Figures 13-21 and 13-22).[27] A spermatocele is a benign cystic collection of sperm usually located in the head of the epididymis. An epididymal cyst is a dilated lymphatic structure in the scrotum usually located superior to the testicle. Both lesions are benign and palpably extratesticular. These lesions appear anechoic on ultrasound and are often indistinguishable from one another.

Varicoceles are caused by an abnormal dilation of the pampiniform plexus. This can occur either due to incompetent valves of the spermatic vein (primary varicocele)

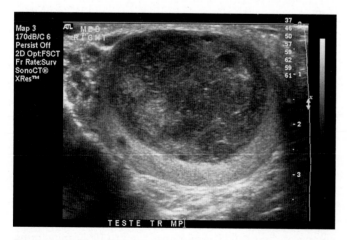

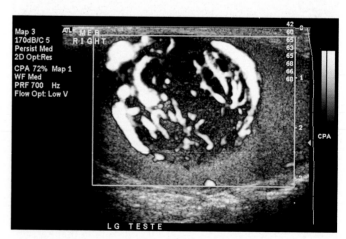

Figures 13-17 and 13-18. Testicular mass. Intratesticular masses are usually indicative of testicular cancer and require surgical extirpation. The mass seen here is typical of a nonseminomatous lesion in that it is heterogeneous with stippled calcifications. The sonolucent areas often correspond to areas of cystic change or necrosis within the mass. As is often the case, the mass demonstrates increased blood flow compared to the normal testicle.

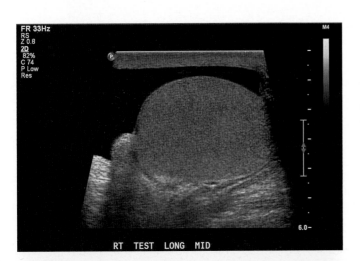

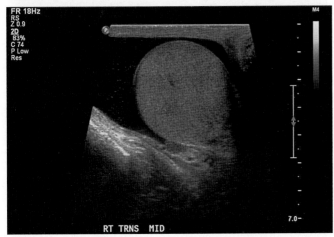

Figures 13-19 and 13-20. Simple hydrocele. When a hydrocele is present, ultrasound of the testicles is often recommended to ensure that there are no underlying abnormalities. Typical of hydroceles, the testicle appears to be "floating" in the fluid. The testicle itself, however, appears normal. In this example of a simple hydrocele, there are no associated septations, or internal echoes suggestive of an underlying process.

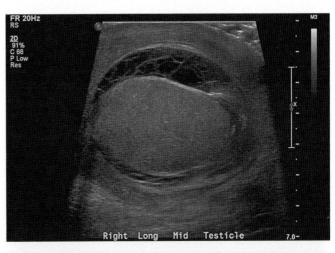

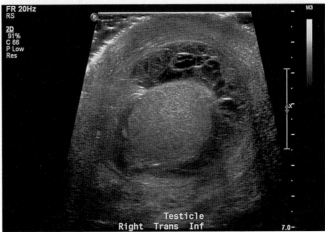

Figures 13-21 and 13-22. Complex hydrocele. In contrast to a simple hydrocele, complex hydroceles demonstrate multiple septations and internal echoes. The presence of a complex hydrocele often, but not always, suggests an inflammatory etiology (epididymitis, orchitis, trauma, malignancy etc).

or from extrinsic compression of the gonadal vein by a mass as it courses through the retroperitoneum (secondary varicocele). Primary varicoceles typically occur on the left side, although bilateral dilatation is not uncommon. A unilateral right varicocele is less common and its isolated presence should prompt evaluation of the retroperitoneum by ultrasound, CT, or MRI to exclude an underlying obstructing or compressing mass. Varicoceles are generally asymptomatic, but should be treated when associated with infertility, scrotal discomfort, or decreased testicular size on the affected side. Varicoceles are characterized by tortuous intrascrotal veins that exceed 2 mm in diameter and demonstrate an increase in flow with Valsalva that lasts longer than 1 second.[44,45] Occasionally, a transient flow increase is noted in patients without a varicocele during Valsalva, but in these instances, flow usually quickly dissipates despite continued straining (Figures 13-23 to 13-25).[22]

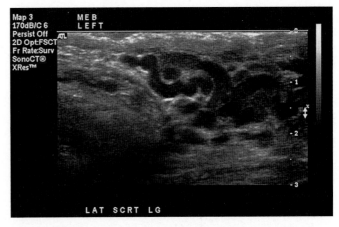

Figure 13-23. Varicocele. Varicoceles are tortuous venous dilations with a diameter greater than 2 mm in size as seen here on gray scale imaging.

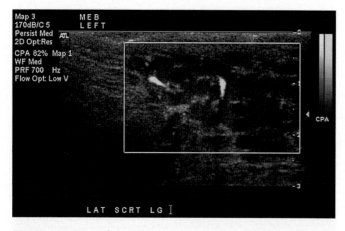 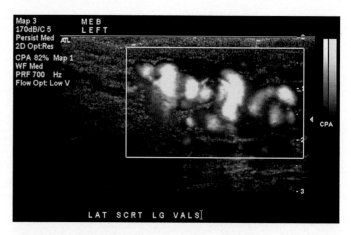

Figures 13-24 and 13-25. Power Doppler of a varicocele. A sustained (>1 sec) increase in blood flow with Valsalva is a characteristic finding of varicoceles. Figure 13-24 demonstrates minimal flow without the Valsalva maneuver, while Figure 13-25 demonstrates a dramatic increase of blood flow after Valsalva.

▶ Common Pitfalls

A common pitfall associated with scrotal ultrasound is loss of proper orientation resulting in an incomplete scan. This occurs in large part due to the similarity of structures bilaterally and relative lack of anatomic landmarks. To avoid this pitfall, the sonographer should develop and adhere to a systematic protocol and method of scanning with appropriate labeling of laterality and location.

In the setting of testicular torsion, scrotal wall and peritesticular hyperemia can be mistaken for intratesticular flow. This pitfall can be prevented by the use of Doppler waveform analysis targeted within the testicular parenchyma to accurately detect or exclude the presence of testicular parenchymal flow. Additionally, simultaneous comparison of both testes is helpful in assessing flow asymmetry. The relative hypoechogenicity of the epididymal body compared to the head may lead to incorrect assessment in evaluation of the region of head–body junction. Oftentimes, particularly on transverse or longitudinal oblique imaging, the partially imaged hypoechoic proximal body may be perceived as an ovoid lesion within the epididymal head. Assessing the continuity of this pseudolesion with the remainder of the epididymal body helps in averting this pitfall.

▶ Clinical Pearls and Tips

In general, the left testicle lies lower than the right. During side-by-side comparisons, it is important to image each testicle at the same point. In order to accomplish this, the transducer can be rotated less than 90 degrees (approximately 60–75 degrees) in the counterclockwise direction so that the midpoints of both testicles are viewed simultaneously. Additionally, scanning in the longitudinal plane on the lateral aspects of each testicle allows for improved visualization of the epididymis.

PROSTATIC ULTRASOUND

▶ Clinical Indications

The two most common indications for prostate ultrasound are for size/shape determinations in the setting of benign prostatic hyperplasia (BPH) and as part of a prostatic biopsy for the diagnosis of prostate cancer. Other less common indications include the evaluation for prostatic abscess, prostatic mapping and seed placement for brachytherapy, and size calculations for determining prostatic specific antigen (PSA) density.

An abnormal digital rectal examination or an elevated PSA alerts the urologist to the possibility of prostate cancer. The first step in diagnosis is to obtain a transrectal ultrasound (TRUS) and biopsy. Prostate biopsies are typically performed with ultrasound guidance using a set template, with additional foci of biopsies performed in areas of any noted abnormalities. As it pertains to BPH, the primary goal of volume and shape calculations is to determine which treatment options are suitable for the patient. The discovery of a large median lobe suggests that minimally invasive office procedures, such as microwave therapy, are likely to fail. Similarly, very large volume prostates are more amenable to an open/robotic approach than to an endoscopic approach.

▶ Normal Anatomy

A chestnut-shaped organ, the prostate is embryologically derived from the urogenital sinus and the mesonephric Wolffian tissue. The prostate is located between the bladder neck and the urogenital diaphragm and envelops the proximal urethra. The prostate is contained within 4 fascial layers: the endopelvic fascia, levator fascia, the prostatic fascia, and posteriorly Denonvilliers' fascia. The ejaculatory ducts extend from the seminal vesicles to the verumontanum where they empty into the prostatic urethra.

The prostate gland is divided into four zonal regions, namely, the transition zone (TZ), the central zone (CZ), the peripheral zone (PZ), and the anterior fibromuscular stroma (AFS).[46] The TZ, also described as the preprostatic region, consists of two lobes extending from bladder neck/base of the prostate to the verumontanum. The TZ mainly surrounds the proximal prostatic urethra. The CZ consists of 25% of the glandular prostate and extends from the central transition zone and envelopes the ejaculatory ducts. In radiology literature, the central zone and transition zone are commonly referred to as the central gland. During the aging process, the TZ is thought to be the primary origin of the adenomas that cause BPH and its sequelae. However, it is likely that BPH involves the entire central gland and not just the TZ. In addition, BPH also involves a TZ enlargement that encroaches on the lumen of the bladder, commonly referred to as the median lobe. The PZ makes up 70% of the prostate and surrounds the prostatic urethra extending to the apex of the prostate. Most prostatic cancers arise from the PZ. The AFS is the sole region in the prostate devoid of glandular tissue. In BPH, the TZ enlarges along with the periurethral gland compressing the anterior AFS, the CZ, and the PZ.

The prostate receives its blood supply from the inferior vesical artery, which branches to also supply the seminal vesicles and the bladder base. The prostate is drained by three veins, which in turn drain into the dorsal vein. The dorsal vein originates from the coalescence of smaller venules that drain the penis.

The prostate has autonomic innervation from both the sympathetic and parasympathetic nervous systems via the pelvic plexus. The pelvic plexus is found on the anterolateral aspect of the rectum directly beneath the prostate. The main erectile component of the plexus forms a neurovascular plate proximally, which coalesces into the two neurovascular bundles. The neurovascular bundles course in close proximity to the prostate between the levator fascia and the prostatic fascia. They penetrate the urogenital diaphragm to innervate the penis and provide erectile function.

▶ Normal Appearance on Ultrasound

In the normal prostate, pathological zonal structures can usually be identified aiding the clinician in detecting potential prostatic abnormalities. The glandular TZ, lying anterior to the CZ and PZ, has a hypoechoic, heterogeneous appearance, while the CZ and the PZ, which lie posteriorly, generally have a hyperechoic homogenous echogenicity (Figures 13-26 and 13-27). BPH affects the appearance of the TZ, which typically becomes more cystic, increasing its heterogeneous appearance. Adenocarcinomas generally tend to affect the CZ (5%) and PZ (70%), creating an increased heterogeneous appearance as well. Unlike cancers that occur in other organs, prostate

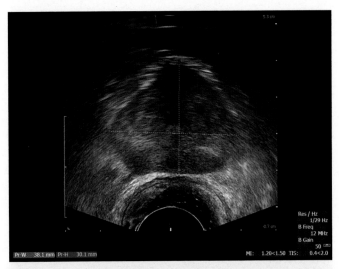

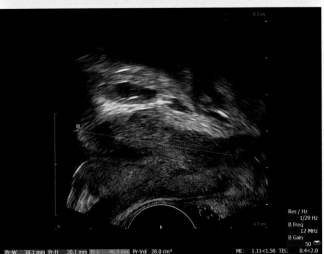

Figures 13-26 and 13-27. Normal transrectal ultrasound in transverse (Figure 13-26) and longitudinal views (Figure 13-27). The peripheral zone is best seen in the transverse image and is characterized by its homogenous, slightly hyperechoic echotexture. The TZ and CZ surround the urethra and are characterized by a more heterogeneous appearance that becomes more prominent in men with BPH.

cancer tends to be multifocal and is often difficult to visualize.[48-50]

In the sagittal plane, the prostatic urethra can be seen traversing the entire gland in the midline. At the base of the prostate, the seminal vesicles appear as symmetric, bilateral saccular structures, each measuring around 1.5–2 cm in width and 2.5–6 cm in length (Figure 13-28). Seminal vesicle width can increase if the examinee has abstained from ejaculations for a prolonged period of time or has an obstruction. In addition, seminal vesicle appearance can be atrophic if the examinee is diabetic or azoospermic.[51]

In the aging population, small prostatic calculi are commonly found incidentally in the urologist's office during a TRUS performed for BPH or prostate cancer.[52] These

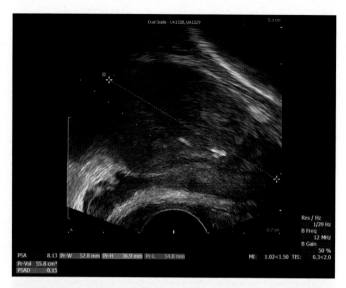

Figure 13-28. Seminal vesicles. The seminal vesicles are an important landmark to identify, especially prior to prostate biopsy. The seminal vesicles are oblong, hypoechoic structures extending from the posterior base of the prostate.

calcifications are often seen in the corpora amylacea zone, which is located between the PZ and the CZ. Although larger calcifications may indicate abnormal pathology, the more commonly seen small stippled calcifications are incidental findings (Figures 13-29 and 13-30).

▶ Scanning Technique

Initially described by Watanabe and colleagues in 1968, TRUS has become an essential part of the armamentarium for examination of the prostate.[47] Gray scale TRUS remains the gold standard for prostate imaging.[48] Lying anterior to the rectum, the prostate lends itself well to ultrasonographic imaging via the transrectal approach. Patients are

typically scanned in both the transverse and sagittal planes with a 5- to 10-MHz probe while in a lateral decubitus position.[49] While critical in evaluating prostate volume, the examiner's experience and ability to delineate between various echodensities is an important aspect of the TRUS examination. Ideally, magnification and gain should be adjusted so that the prostate fills the screen; the peripheral zone is used as a reference point to examine hypo-, hyper-, and isoechoic regions.[48]

The typical endorectal probe is either biplane, multiplane, or end-fire with a frequency range between 6 and 8 MHz.[8,53] If a transrectal biopsy is to be performed, the sonographer should be familiar with biopsy gun targeting and usage. Furthermore, the patient should be treated prophylactically with either a single dose or alternatively a 3-day course of antibiotics, typically ciprofloxacin.[54-58] Despite the lack of consensus, the current standard is to have the patient perform a rectal enema on the morning prior to biopsy. While rectal preparation may not necessarily prevent postbiopsy bacteremia/sepsis, it does improve visualization of the prostate and possibly even analgesia due to improved accuracy of local anesthesia injection.[53,49-61]

The transrectal ultrasound is typically an office procedure performed under local anesthesia only. The patient is positioned in the left lateral decubitus position with the knees tucked into the chest. All prostate examinations should begin by performing a digital rectal examination of the prostate. Not only does this give the urologist a better understanding of the prostatic anatomy including abnormal nodules, but it also helps lubricate the anus and rectum and prepare the patient for probe insertion. The probe is inserted into the rectum and the prostate is initially scanned, first transversely then sagittally, taking note of any hypoechoic lesions and dense calcifications. The prostate is then measured in three dimensions for volume

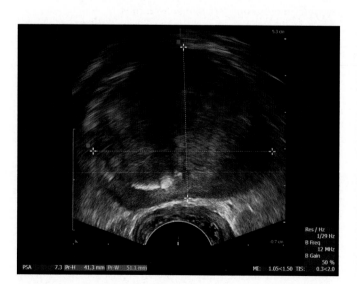

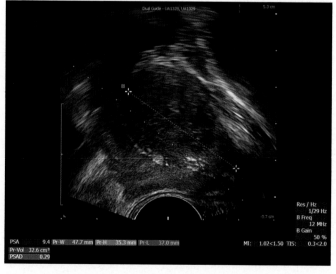

Figures 13-29 and 13-30. Prostatic calcifications. Stippled calcifications especially along the corpora amylacea are commonly seen and considered normal.

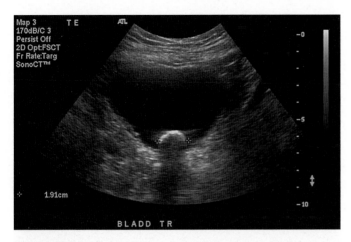

Figure 13-31. Transabdominal ultrasound of the bladder. Transabdominal ultrasound of the bladder allows for bladder wall thickness, and postvoid residual determinations along with prostate and bladder stone size measurements. In this image, a bladder stone can be seen with its characteristic hyperechoic interface and shadowing effect.

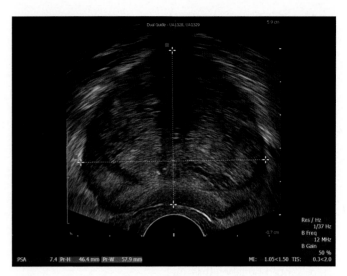

Figure 13-32. Benign prostatic hyperplasia. The TZ and CZ in benign prostatic hyperplasia become significantly enlarged with an increase in heterogeneity. Small adenomas appear hyperechoic.

determination. If biopsy is to be performed, tissue should first be obtained from any previously palpated nodules or any hypoechoic lesions identified during the initial scan. Standard sextant biopsy is then performed by obtaining 2 cores from the peripheral zone in each prostate sextant (right and left, apical, mid, and base).

Transabdominal (TA) ultrasound evaluation of the pelvis can be performed to evaluate the prostate gland and urinary bladder. TA imaging of the prostate gland can allow for size and volume determinations in patients who do not undergo TRUS. The distended urinary bladder serves as an acoustic window for visualization of the prostate gland and seminal vesicles by TA approach. Encroachment of the median lobe of the prostate gland by TZ enlargement on the urinary bladder base can readily be detected. During this evaluation, urinary bladder volume measurements can be assessed pre- and postvoiding to determine postvoid residual volumes. The examination may reveal bladder wall thickening and trabeculation that can result from chronic outlet obstruction by an enlarged prostate gland. Ureteral jets can be assessed and may help in localizing the ureteral openings relative to an enlarged prostate gland. Distal hydroureter can sometimes be observed if there is obstructive mass effect at the ureterovesical junction. TA imaging of the urinary bladder can detect mural irregularities, focal masses, stones, and diverticula, and may help direct subsequent cystoscopic evaluation (Figure 13-31).

COMMON FINDINGS/ABNORMALITIES

Unfortunately, prostatic ultrasound demonstrates few pathognomonic abnormalities. In benign prostatic hyperplasia, the transition zone of the prostate can often appear diffusely enlarged and demonstrate subtle internal

echoes caused by small adenomas (Figure 13-32).[9] Prostate cancer, especially in the early stage, demonstrates few characteristic findings on ultrasound. Previous studies have suggested that prostate cancer can appear as a distinct hypoechoic lesion, particularly in the peripheral zone of the prostate, or rarely as a hyperechoic lesion (Figure 13-33).[62] However, even with modern high-frequency transrectal probes, almost half of all histologically confirmed prostate cancers are indistinguishable from normal adjacent tissue.[63] As such, diagnostic ultrasound of the prostate provides little benefit over that of template needle biopsy.[64,65]

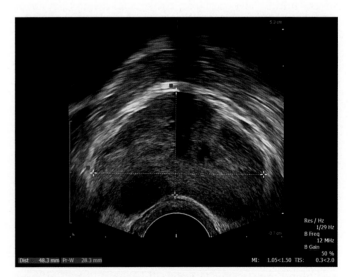

Figure 13-33. Prostate cancer. Classically, prostate cancer is described as hypoechoic nodules in the peripheral zone as seen here. In reality, prostate cancer is often multifocal and cannot be distinguished from adjacent normal prostate.

COMMON PITFALLS

Transrectal ultrasound and biopsy can be traumatic to the patient and proper preparation is key. Although previous studies on the benefits of prebiopsy rectal enemas have demonstrated mixed results, stool within the rectal vault obscures visualization of the prostate, prolonging the procedure and decreasing biopsy accuracy. Furthermore, to improve the sensitivity of prostate biopsy, the peripheral zones of the prostate should be targeted, since most prostate cancers arise from this area. However, it is important to recognize that when obtaining tissue, laterality can often be confused. For example, with the patient in the left lateral decubitus position, rotating the handle of the probe downward (toward the patient's left side) visualizes the opposite side of the prostate (right side) and biopsies taken there should be labeled as such.

CLINICAL PEARLS AND TIPS

When using local anesthesia, appropriate injection in the midline near the base of the seminal vesicles provides the greatest nerve block. The appropriate technique is to identify the seminal vesicles, and then to retract the probe until their junction with the prostate can be visualized. The needle is then advanced into the space between the rectal wall and the prostate, and lidocaine or other anesthetic is injected into that space. When the needle is in the appropriate plane, the injectate will visibly "hydrodissect" the prostate away from the rectal wall. More laterally targeted injections can also be performed, but it is the midline injection that appears to be the most effective.

CASE STUDY 1

A 65-year-old man with coronary artery disease, diabetes, severe mitral valve prolapse, stroke, and a long history of urolithiasis, status post bilateral, open pyelolithotomies in the 1970s, and multiple prior bilateral endoscopic procedures presented with a significant bilateral stone burden. Two months ago, at an outside facility, he underwent a right percutaneous nephrolithotomy (PCNL) via lower pole access, which was terminated early due to bleeding. He was scheduled for a repeat right endoscopic-assisted PCNL for removal of residual stone (Figure 13-34). A ureteroscope was passed via a 12/14 55 cm access sheath into the renal pelvis. Lower pole access was unsuccessful, so instead, upper pole access was obtained above the 12th rib. Approximately 1.5 cm of stone burden was removed before the procedure was prematurely aborted due to hemodynamic instability. A ureteral stent and nephrostomy tube were left in place.

Throughout his postoperative course, he had persistent gross hematuria and required continuous bladder irrigation and blood transfusions. A renal ultrasound with duplex on postoperative day 5 demonstrated residual hydronephrosis (Figure 13-35) and a lower pole cystic lesion not previously noted on the computed tomography scan (Figure 13-36).

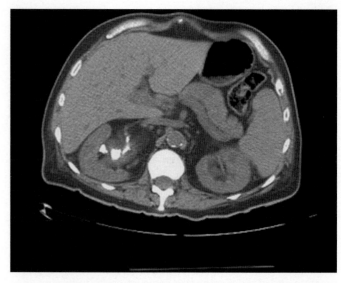

Figure 13-34. Noncontrast computed tomography (CT) scan of the abdomen demonstrating a large stone burden in the right kidney.

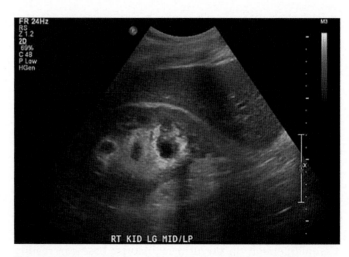

Figure 13-35. Postoperative ultrasound demonstrating residual hydronephrosis.

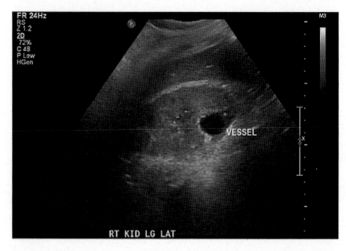

Figure 13-36. Cystic lesion of the renal parenchyma not previously noted on CT scan.

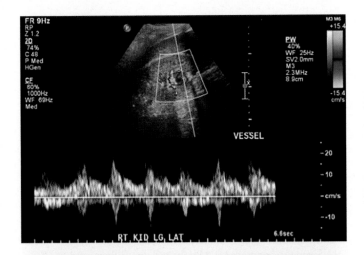

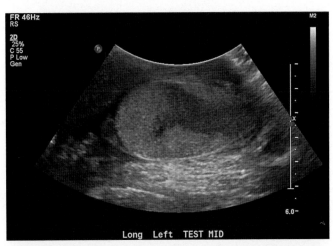

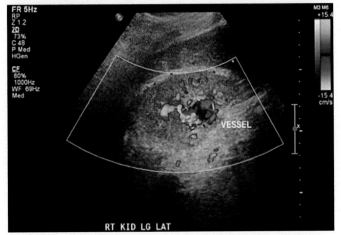

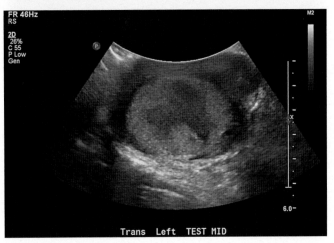

Figures 13-37 and 13-38. Color flow Doppler of the cystic lesion demonstrating mixed/turbulent flow consistent with a pseudoaneurysm.

Figures 13-39 and 13-40. Longitudinal and transverse images of a hypoechoic lesion consistent with an intratesticular hematoma of the left testicle.

CFD was performed and identified mixed, turbulent flow within the cystic lesion, confirming the finding of a pseudoaneurysm (Figures 13-37 and 13-38). The pseudoaneurysm was subsequently embolized, and the hematuria resolved within 12 hours of embolization. The patient recovered and was discharged on hospital day of stay 10.

CASE STUDY 2

A 34-year-old male presented to the emergency room after being struck by a car while on a motorcycle. The patient denied loss of consciousness or head trauma, but complained of pain in the bilateral groin, right hand and wrist, and right knee. The patient otherwise had no past medical or surgical history. The physical examination demonstrated a right wrist deformity consistent with a dislocation, and very firm, exquisitely tender testicles bilaterally. Radiographic workup verified the presence of a right wrist dislocation and also identified a right tibial fracture for which orthopedic surgery was consulted. On scrotal ultrasound, a left-sided intra-testicular mass consistent with a hematoma was identified (Figures 13-39 and 13-40). The right

testicle was grossly abnormal demonstrating significant heterogeneity, loss of normal contour with an inability to completely visualize the tunica albuginea, and the presence of a hematocele (Figures 13-41 and 13-42).

Due to the findings on the testicular ultrasound, the patient was brought to the operating room for repair of a suspected right testicular rupture. The scrotum was explored and both testicles were inspected. The left testicle and spermatic cord appeared intact and were returned to the left hemiscrotum. The right testicle was noted to have an isolated rupture of the testicle with protuberant seminiferous tubules, but otherwise looked viable. The testicle was extensively debrided and the tunica albuginea reapproximated. Over the ensuing 24–48 hours, the patient's testicular discomfort improved and the patient was discharged to home on hospital day of stay 6.

CONCLUSION

Genitourinary ultrasound is uniquely suited for evaluating testicular and prostatic disorders, and is a key element in the evaluation of renal and bladder pathology. It offers the advantages of an excellent safety profile, rapid

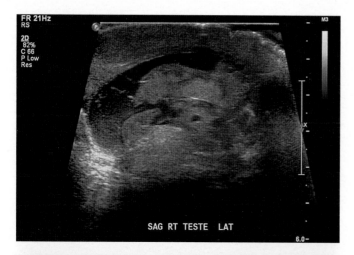

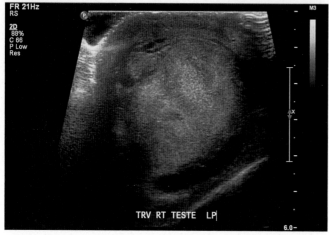

Figures 13-41 and 13-42. The testicle demonstrates loss of normal contour with an inability to demonstrate the continuity of the tunica albuginea, testicular heterogeneity, and a hematocele, all consistent with the diagnosis of testicular rupture.

and reproducible results, and a high sensitivity and specificity for certain urological disorders. Furthermore, the ability to evaluate in real time, using both gray scale and CFD or power Doppler imaging, provides insight into the affecting pathology that is not afforded by other imaging modalities. When judiciously employed, ultrasound has the capability of rapidly providing an immediate diagnosis or can suggest whether further testing is indicated. Having an understanding of the limitations of this modality in the genitourinary system is paramount to avoiding a missed or erroneous diagnosis. However, when coupled with sound clinical judgment, ultrasound is an irreplaceable element in the workup of most genitourinary disorders.

REFERENCES

1. Teichman JM. Clinical practice. Acute renal colic from ureteral calculus. *N Engl J Med*. 2004;350:2422–2423.
2. Ripolles T, Agramunt M, Errando J, et al. Suspected ureteral colic: plain film and sonography vs. unenhanced helical CT. A prospective study in 66 patients. *Eur Radiol*. 2004;14:129–136.
3. O'Connor OJ, Fitzgerald E, Maher MM. Imaging of hematuria. *AJR Am J Roentgenol*. 2010:263–267.
4. Van Der Molen AJ, Cowan NC, Mueller-Lisse UG, et al. CT urography working group of the European Society of Urogenital Radiology (ESUR). CT urography: definition, indications and techniques: a guideline for clinical practice. *Eur Radiol*. 2008;18:4–17.
5. Kuan JK, Porter J, Wessells H. Imaging for Genitourinary Trauma. *AUA Update Series*. 2006;25. Lesson 4.
6. Perry M, Porte M, Urwin G. Limitations of ultrasound evaluation in acute closed renal trauma. *JR Coll Surg Edinb*. 1997;42:420.
7. Koelliker SL, Cronan JJ. Acute urinary tract obstruction: imaging update. *Urol Clin North Am*. 1997;24:571.
8. McAchran SE, Dogra V, Resnick MI. Office urologic ultrasound. *Urol Clin North Am*. 2005;32:337–352.
9. Spirnak J, Resnick MI. Ultrasound. In: Gillenwater JY, Grayhack JT, Howards SS, Mitchell ME, eds. *Adult and Pediatric Urology*. 4th ed. Philadelphia: Lippincott Williams and Wilkins; 2002:123–150.
10. Pollack HM, Banner MP, Arger PH, et al. The accuracy of gray-scale renal ultrasonography in differentiating cystic neoplasms from benign cysts. *Radiology*. 1982;143:741–745.
11. Jamis-Dow CA, Choyke PL, Jennings SB, et al. Small (< or = 3-cm) renal masses: detection with CT versus US and pathologic correlation. *Radiology*. 1996;198:785–788.
12. Rahmouni A, Bargoin R, Herment A, Bargoin N, Vasile N. Color Doppler twinkling artifact in hyperechoic regions. *Radiology*. 1996;199:269–271.
13. Chelfouh N, Grenier N, Higueret D, et al. Characterization of urinary calculi: in vitro study of "twinkling artifact" revealed by color-flow sonography. *AJR*. 1998;171:1055–1060.
14. Kamaya A, Tuthill T, Rubin JM. Twinkling artifact on color Doppler sonography: dependence on machine parameters and underlying cause. *AJR*. 2003;180:215–222.
15. Lee JL, Kim SH, Cho JY, Han D. Color and power Doppler twinkling artifacts from urinary stones: clinical observations and phantom studies. *AJR*. 2001;176:1441–1445.
16. Carroll BA, Gross DM. High frequency scrotal ultrasonography. *AJR Am J Roentgenol*. 1983;140:511–515.
17. Hricak H, Filly RA. Sonography of the scrotum. *Invest Radiol*. 1983;18:112–121.
18. Krone KD, Carroll BA. Scrotal ultrasound. *Radiol Clin North Am*. 1985;23:121–139.
19. Rifkin MD, Kurtz AB, Past ME, et al. The sonographic diagnosis of focal and infiltrating intrascrotal lesions. *Urol Radiol*. 1984;6:20–26.
20. Vick W, Bird KJ, Rosenfield AT, et al. Ultrasound of scrotal contents. *Urol Radiol*. 1982;4:147–153.
21. Burks DD, Markey BJ, Burkhard TK, et al. Suspected testicular torsion and ischemia: evaluation with color Doppler ultrasnography. *Radiology*. 1990;175:815–821.
22. Horstman WG, Middleton WD, Melson GL, Siegel BA. Color Doppler US of the scrotum. *Radiographics*. 1991;11:941–957.
23. Horstman WG, Middleton WD, Melson GL. Scrotal inflammatory disease: color Doppler ultrasound findings. *Radiology*. 1991;179:55–59.
24. Learner RM, Mvorach RA, Hulbert WC, et al. Color Doppler ultrasound in the evaluation of acute scrotal disease. *Radiology*. 1990;176:355–358.

25. Middleton WD, Melson GL. Testicular ischemia: color Doppler sonographic findings in five patients. *AJR Am J Roentgenol.* 1990;152:1237–1239.

26. Ralls PW, Jensen MC, Lee KP, et al. Color Doppler sonography in acute epididymitis and orchitis. *J Clin Ultrasound.* 1990;18:282–286.

27. Gilbert BR. Office scrotal ultrasound. Part II: scanning protocol, normal examination. Indications and practice management concerns. *AUA Update Series.* 2008;27. Lesson 2.

28. Dogra V, Bhatt S. Acute painful scrotum. *Radiol Clin N Am.* 2004;42:349.

29. Bhandary P, Abbitt PL, Watson L. Ultrasound diagnosis of traumatic testicular rupture. *J Clin Ultrasound.* 1992;20:346.

30. Dogra VS, Gottlieb RH, Oka M. Sonography of the scrotum. *Radiology.* 2003;227:18.

31. Dogra VS, Bhatt S. Categorical course in diagnostic radiology: acute scrotal pain: imaging evaluation for a more specific diagnosis. Edited by P Ramchandani. Oak Brook, IL: Radiological Society of North America: Genitourinary Radiology; 2006:255–270.

32. Herbener TE. Ultrasound in the assessment of the acute scrotum. *J Clin Ultrasound.* 1996;24:405.

33. Gilbert BR. Office scrotal ultrasound. Part I: scanning protocol, normal examination. Indications and practice management concerns. *AUA Update Series.* 2008;27. Lesson 1.

34. Horstman WG. Scrotal imaging. *Urol Clin North Am.* 1997;24:653–671.

35. Owen CA, Winter T 3rd. Color Doppler imaging of the scrotum. *SDMS-JDMS.* 2006;22:221.

36. Middleton WD, Thorne DA, Melson GL. Color Doppler ultrasound of the normal testis. *AJR Am J Roentgenol.* 1989;152:293–297.

37. Bird K, Rosenfield AT, Taylor KJW. Ultrasonography in testicular torsion. *Radiology.* 1983;147:527–534.

38. Benson CB, Doubilet PM, Richie JP. Sonography of the male genital tract. *AJR Am J Roentgenol.* 1989;153: 705–713.

39. Rifkin MD, Kurtz AB, Pasto ME, et al. Diagnostic capabilities of high-resolution scrotal ultrasonography. Prospective evaluation. *J Ultrasound Med.* 1985;4:13–19.

40. Arger PH, Mulher CB, Coleman BG, et al. Prospective analysis of the value of scrotal ultrasound. *Radiology.* 1981;141:763–768.

41. Fournier GR, Laing FC, Jeffrey RB, Macanninch JW. High resolution scrotal ultrasonography: a highly sensitive but non-specific diagnostic technique. *J Urol.* 1985;134:490–493.

42. Schwerk WB, Scherk WN, Rodeck G. Testicular tumors: prospective analysis of real time US patterns and abdominal staging. *Radiology.* 1987;164:369–374.

43. Tackett RE, Ling D, Catalona WJ, Melson GL. High resolution sonography in diagnosing testicular neoplasms: clinical significance of false positive scans. *J Urol.* 1986;135:494–496.

44. Rifkin MD, Foy PN, Kurtz AB, et al. The role of diagnostic ultrasonography in varicocele evaluation. *J Ultrasound Med.* 1983;2:271–275.

45. Wolverson MK, Houttuin E, Heiberg E, et al. High resolution real-time ultrasonography of scrotal varicocele. 1983;141:775–779.

46. McNeal JE. The zonal anatomy of the prostate. *Prostate.* 1981;2:35–49.

47. Watanabe H, Kato H, Kato T, et al. Diagnostic application of the ultrasonotomography for the prostate. *Jpn J Urol.* 1968;59:273–279.

48. Linden RA, Halpern EJ. Advances in transrectal ultrasound imaging of the prostate. *Semi Ultrasound CT MR.* 28(4):249–257.

49. Kossoff G. Basic physics and imaging characteristics of ultrasound. *World J Surg.* 2000;24:134–142.

50. Byar DP, Mostofi FK. Carcinoma of the prostate: evaluation of certain pathologic features in 208 radical prostatectomies. *Cancer.* 1972;30:5–13.

51. Purohit RS, Wu DS, Shinohara K, Turek PJ. A prospective comparison of 3 diagnostic methods to evaluate ejaculatory duct obstruction. *J Urol.* 2004;171:232–235.

52. Shoskes DA, Lee CT, Murphy D, et al. Incidence and significance of prostatic stones in men with chronic prostatitis/chronic pelvic pain syndrome. *Urology.* 2007;70:235–238.

53. Hemani ML, Taneja SS. Prostate biopsy: contemporary ultrasound guided indications, techniques and future directions. *AUA Update Series.* 2009;28. Lesson 22.

54. Wolf J, Bennett C, Dmochowski R, et al. Best practice policy statement on urologic surgery antimicrobial prophylaxis. *J Urol.* 2008;179:1379.

55. Kapoor D, Klimberg G, Malek J, et al. Single-dose ciprofloxacin versus placebo for prophylaxis during transrectal prostate biopsy. *Urology.* 1998;52:552.

56. Aron M, Rajeev T, Gupta N. Antimicrobial prophylaxis for transrectal needle biopsy of the prostate: a randomized controlled study. *BJU Int.* 2000;85:682.

57. Sabbagh R, McCormack M, Peloquin F, et al. A prospective randomized trial of 1-day versus 3-day antimicrobial prophylaxis for transrectal ultrasound guided prostate biopsy. *Can J Urol.* 2004;11:2216.

58. Shigemura K, Tanaka K, Yasuda M, et al. Efficacy of 1-day prophylaxis medication with fluoroquinolone for prostate biopsy. *World J Urol.* 2005;23:356.

59. Carey J, Korman H. Transrectal ultrasound guided biopsy of the prostate: do enemas decrease clinically significant complications? *J Urol.* 2001;166:82.

60. Jeon S, Woo S, Hyun J, et al. Bisacodyl rectal preparation can decrease infectious complications of transrectal ultrasound-guided prostate biopsy. *Urology.* 2003;62:461.

61. Lindert K, Kabalin J, Terris M. Bacteremia and bacteriuria after transrectal ultrasound guided prostate biopsy. *J Urol.* 2000;164:76.

62. Shinohara K, Wheeler TM, Scardino PT. The appearance of prostate cancer on transrectal ultrasonography: correlation of imaging and pathological examinations. *J Urol.* 1989;142:76.

63. Scherr DS, Eastham J, Ohori M, et al. Prostate biopsy techniques and indications: when, where, and how? *Semin Urol Oncol.* 2002;20:18.

64. Klein EA, Zippe CD. Editorial: transrectal ultrasound guided prostate biopsy-defining a new standard. *J Urol.* 2000;163:179.

65. McAchrin SE, Dogra VS, Resnick MI. Office-based ultrasound for urologists. Part II: prostate, scrotum, penis, urethra and office standards. *AUA Update Series.* 2004;23. Lesson 29.

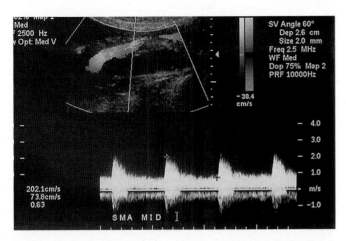

Figure 14-6. Mid SMA with PSV 287 vs aorta with PSV 76, nonfed.

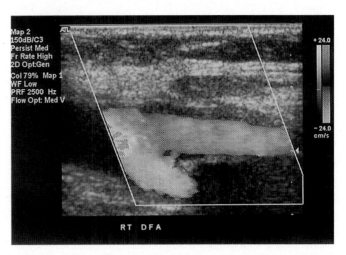

Figure 14-7. The superficial femoral–popliteal bifurcation 001.

addition, a thorough understanding of the anatomic variations is necessary in order to recognize anomalous anatomy, which may be present in up to 20% of patients.

Aorta and iliac arteries

Again, while not as important as in the evaluation of the smaller vessels, an overnight fast is desirable in order to reduce bowel gas. Once again the 3-MHz transducer is used, and while lateral windows can be necessary, a midline approach is usually adequate. Similar to the renal study, the aorta is insonated just below the xiphoid. The study then proceeds to the bilateral inguinal creases. For severe aortic and iliac stenosis no strict criteria correlate to a physiologic effect of stenosis. B-mode imaging takes on a larger role in these anatomic beds, as diameter (ie, aneurysm) matters more in many cases than stenosis. For the aneurysmal vessel the cross-sectional area of the vessels is evaluated with great care in the correct orientation to ensure appropriate sizing of the vessel. To aid in the potential decision for endovascular repair, the distance between the lowest renal artery and the dilation of the aorta should be measured.

Peripheral Vessels and Arteriovenous Grafts/Fistulas

The 7- to 7.5-MHz transducer is typically used to study these peripheral vessels. As the vessels get smaller (such as the tibial arteries), color flow imaging becomes much more useful. In the distal arterial beds, technical adequacy of the examination for vessel anatomic lesion identification exceeds 90%.[18]

Femoral artery

This artery is examined above the groin crease, as the inguinal ligament is defined by the pubic tubercle and the anterior superior iliac crest, which is usually above the groin crease. The end of the common femoral artery is defined as the point where the profunda femoris originates and bifurcates to become the superficial femoral artery (Figure 14-7).

Superficial femoral artery/popliteal artery

The probe can be placed medially in the thigh, in the groove between the quadriceps and the adductor muscles. For the popliteal artery the probe can be placed medially or posteriorly. From a medial approach, flexion of the knee and mild external rotation of the leg facilitate visualization of the artery.

Surgically created arteriovenous fistula

This study is designed to assess the location and any abnormality in a hemodialysis access. In these settings, it is paramount to understand the anatomic configuration of the access. In order to understand the anatomy, one should find the arterial to conduit (vein or graft) anastomosis first; this will be an end-conduit to side-artery configuration in almost all cases. It can be difficult to insonate this area at 60 degrees to the angle of flow due to the configuration, but the area can also be recognized by its high flow and turbulence. Once the origin of the arterial inflow is found, the conduit is traced toward its venous outflow. The initial evaluation of the fistula for diameter and stenosis is performed with gray scale imaging. Once completed, color and spectral Doppler are used for further characterization. The PSV is obtained at the anastomosis and in the artery 2 cm proximal to the anastomosis. The vein graft needs to be insonated along in its entire course, examining both sagittal velocity images and cross-sectional images, which may delineate clot burden and/or aneurysmal dilations. The two most likely sites of stenosis are the arterial anastomosis and, if a graft is used, the anastomosis to the outflow vein.

Any visible narrowing of the access on B-mode image should be assessed with velocity criteria, and any color flow aliasing should be assessed carefully as well. Aliasing is a form of artifact that occurs during spectral analysis, where the spectrum is "wrapped" around the screen so that the top of the waveform is seen at the bottom. This problem can be corrected by increasing the pulse repetition frequency

(PRF) (aliasing occurs when the highest Doppler shift is greater than half the PRF), increasing the Doppler angle, shifting the baseline, lowering the emitted frequency, or using a continuous wave device. If a narrowing is found, the velocity at the narrowing is compared to the velocity 2 cm distal (within the access) from the narrowing. The direction of flow distal to the anastomosis should be assessed for directionality. Distal artery steal is found in 20% of AV access, although it is usually asymptomatic.[19] Though hard to detect with ultrasound, in some cases of steal reversal of flow in the artery distal to the conduit anastomosis can be seen during diastole.

Somewhere between 28% and 53% of surgically created AVFs fail to mature.[20] If an AVF does not appear to be maturing four weeks after creation, ultrasound may be performed to determine the underlying cause. The above criteria should be measured as well as volumetric blood flow in the midportion of the draining vein. A portion of the vein that is straight, nontapering, and nonturbulent is selected; a time-averaged PSV (over 3–4 cardiac cycles) is obtained. The area of the access is obtained using the B-mode function; then by multiplying the cross-sectional area with the velocity, one obtains the volume of flow. For accurate determination of flow rates a 9- to 15-MHz transducer is necessary, preferably a linear array transducer. Venous side branches are identified, and their size and the distance from the anastomosis are assessed. Such veins can be ligated to help a nonfunctioning access to mature.[21]

▶ Venous Studies

Evaluation for deep venous thrombosis

The most commonly performed vascular ultrasound study is the "rule out DVT" study. The fundamental purpose of this study is to determine if the patient has a potentially life-threatening condition, namely, thrombosis of the lower extremity vessels. The procedure consists of compressing the popliteal, superficial femoral, and common femoral veins, ensuring that the vein is fully compressible (Figure 14-8) and that it reforms normally with no evidence of obstructive clot (Figure 14-9). The addition of normal respiratory movement within the vessel is an indicator that the proximal veins are patent.

Complete examination involves interrogation of the lower extremity from the inferior vena cava to the tibial veins. At each position, the technologist must assay the vein for venous compressibility and the presence of echogenic thrombus with B-mode imaging; venous flow characteristics are assessed to determine proximal occlusion. The deep veins should be interrogated in both transverse and longitudinal views. Compression maneuvers are performed in the transverse view every 1–2 cm from the inguinal ligament to the calf. If the vessel walls coapt completely with gentle pressure, thrombosis can be excluded. Longitudinal views are then obtained, evaluating both spectral Doppler images and color flow images. Color flow is helpful

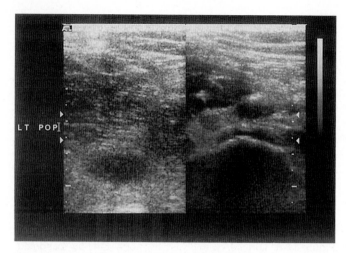

Figure 14-8. Fully compressible popliteal vein.

in identifying partial vessel occlusion of acute echolucent thrombus.

The head of the bed should be elevated approximately 20 degrees in reverse Trendelenberg to facilitate venous filling. The examination starts at the level of the umbilicus, ideally, where Doppler flow evaluation of the iliac veins can be achieved. Although compressibility is limited secondary to the abdominal wall, bowel gas, and patient discomfort, in a thin and compliant patient one can try compression maneuvers. Once at the inguinal ligament, the origin of the greater saphenous and profunda femoris vein can be identified by holding the probe transversely to the vessels' course. The superficial femoral vein is best examined with the leg slightly flexed and abducted, while the superficial femoral vein in the abductor canal may be noncompressible. Color flow is used to assess for duplicate superficial femoral veins that are common.[22] While the popliteal vein is best examined with the patient prone, most technologists just move the probe posteriorly to the popliteal fossa to allow for patient comfort.

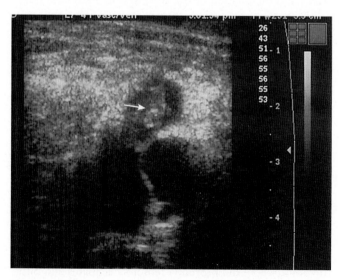

Figure 14-9. Noncompressible deep vein thrombosis.

TABLE 14-1		
Etiologic, Anatomic, and Pathophysiologic Venous Criteria		
Etiologic Classification	**Anatomic Classification**	**Pathophysiologic Classification**
Ec: Congenital	As: Superficial veins	Pr: Reflux
Ep: Primary	Ap: Perforator veins	Po: Obstructive
Es: Secondary (post-thrombotic)	Ad: Deep veins	Pr,o: Reflux and obstruction
En: No venous cause identified	An: No venous location identified	Pn: No venous pathophysiology identified

However, once the popliteal vein is assessed, it is much easier to assay the infrageniculate veins in the prone position. Many technologists keep the patient sitting, though, which is not only more comfortable for the patient but facilitates venous filling.[23] The paired posterior tibial veins are identified adjacent to the posterior tibial artery at the groove between the medial malleolus and the Achilles tendon and are then followed cephalad. The paired peroneal veins are identified along the medial border of the fibula, again abutting the centrally located peroneal artery. If thrombus or a postphlebitic state is present proximally these distal veins may be quite distended and prominent. Similarly, the gastrocnemius and more notably soleal veins may be distended in the presence of infrageniculate vein thrombosis. For a complete examination both the peroneal and the posterior tibial veins need to be assessed. Isolated calf vein thrombosis most often involves the peroneal veins, followed by the posterior tibial veins, while isolated anterior tibial vein thrombosis is very rare.[24]

The upper extremity veins and the thoracic inlet examination are performed with the patient supine, with the neck turned to the contralateral side. The upper extremity is abducted to facilitate access to the axilla. First the internal jugular vein is identified in the neck and followed into the mediastinum to identify the medial subclavian and innominate veins, which are insonated from a supraclavicular window. The probe is then moved to the infraclavicular lateral window to image the lateral subclavian and axillary veins. While with patience and in the right body habitus the entire subclavian vein can be seen, overlying bone and muscle prevent the use of compression as a mode of fully evaluating these vessels in most cases. Therefore, color flow Doppler and appropriate variation with respiration are very helpful in assessing patency. The examination can then proceed down the arm to evaluate the axillary, paired brachial, basilic, and cephalic veins. If need be, the paired radial and ulnar veins in the forearm can also be assessed.

Evaluation of chronic venous disease

In the evaluation of chronic venous disease, the author feels it is best to separate the problem into the components of venous disease as outlined in the CEAP classification scheme.[25] While the (C)linical classification portion is very helpful to the clinician, for the ultrasonographer it is (E)tiology, (A)natomic, and (P)athophysiologic classification systems (Table 14-1) that allow the individuals using ultrasound to determine the cause of the disease, and to place the appropriate weight on their findings. Fundamentally, when assessing the patient with chronic disease one wants to determine where (anatomic classification), what (pathophysiologic classification), and why (etiologic classification).

Chronic deep venous disease

Duplex ultrasound is well suited to visualize partial and complete anatomic obstruction of the deep and superficial venous system. In addition, it can assay valve closure times and characterize direction and duration of flow in the deep, superficial, and perforating venous systems. In general, the initial assessment of the patient with chronic venous disease is carried out as described in the section on assessing for DVT. However, there are many added maneuvers to aid in the diagnosis.

Valve closure is a passive event, which is initiated by the reversal of flow. This occurs as the venous pressure grade is reversed; therefore, there is a short period of physiologic reflux until the gradient is sufficient to result in valve closure. Valve closure, in part, depends upon flow velocity; at reversed flow velocities greater than 30 cm/s, valve closure will occur as rapidly as 100 m/s; at velocities less than 30 cm/s, valve closure can take significantly longer. Therefore, the determination of valvular incompetence requires that pathologic reversal of flow be reproduced. In addition, since clinically relevant reflux occurs during calf muscle contraction and relaxation while standing, tests to elicit valvular incompetence should mimic this condition. In the supine position, the combination of Valsalva and manual compression has been noted to be 88% sensitive and 93% specific for detecting reflux in the SFV.[26] Therefore, the patient is best tested in the standing position,[27] and rapid inflation and deflation pneumatic cuffs should be used. Rapid distal cuff deflation simulates calf muscle relaxation and is the most reproducible method for eliciting valve closure. Pressures of 80 mm Hg in the thigh, 100 mm Hg in the calf, and 120 mm Hg in the foot with 3 seconds of inflation time and 0.3 seconds of deflation time have been shown to be appropriate.[28] Using these techniques, both the deep and the superficial systems can be assessed. In the supine position, Valsalva and manual compression

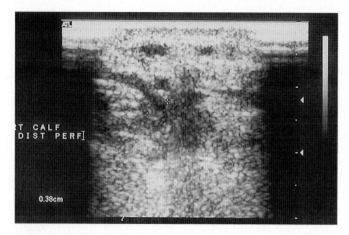

Figure 14-10. Perforating vein.

have been noted to be 67% sensitive, while 100% specific for detecting superficial reflux.[26] When assessing the superficial system, not only should valvular reflux times be reported, but GSV diameter should be reported at the junction with the CFV, mid thigh, and distal thigh, and duplications of the GSV should be reported as well. When assaying the short saphenous vein (SSV), reflux times in addition to diameters should be reported.

Perforator disease

The perforating veins are evaluated while standing, and can be seen along the course of the superficial femoral vein in the distal thigh. In the distal calf, perforating veins are evaluated along the posterior tibial veins. Usually, one to six perforating veins can be found, and the veins are traceable as they penetrate the fascia between the superficial and deep venous compartments (Figure 14-10). These veins are variable in location and may occur anywhere along the medial calf; the most common locations are just below the malleolus, 15 to 19 cm and 30 to 34 cm proximally.[27,28] Flow in nonpathologic perforators is only from superficial to deep, and occurs during distal compression of the foot or calf. Any bidirectional or reversal of flow during the relaxation phase after compression is consistent with pathology.[27] Duplex ultrasound for perforators has been noted to be 82% sensitive and 100% specific when compared to surgical findings.[29]

COMMON FINDINGS/ABNORMALITES

▶ Arterial Studies

Extracranial carotid artery

In this author's opinion, probably more has been written about the findings and interpretation of carotid studies than any other vascular ultrasound procedure. The carotid artery study needs to include the PSV and EDV within the tightest portion of the carotid. The original University of Washington study focused on frequency shift where angle-adjusted velocities were 4 kHz=125 cm/s, and 4.5 kHz=140 cm/s (Table 14-2). The CCA velocity is noted as many grading scales use a ratio of ICA:CCA velocity to aid in determining the degree of stenosis (Table 14-3).[30] The degree of plaque and the characteristics of the plaque should be commented upon, in addition to any unusual anatomy; twists, kinks, and loops should be documented. The amount of plaque should clearly be described, as the carotid bulb can be dilated and therefore a significant amount of plaque can be present with low velocities. Waveforms that are consistent with proximal stenosis should also be noted. A finding of the pathognomonic "string of pearls" or "chain of lakes" appearance of fibromuscular dysplasia must be documented, especially if the patient is a middle-aged female.

TABLE 14-3				
Carotid Stenosis Ultrasound Criteria – Consensus Document				
Degree of Stenosis	**ICA PSV(cm/s)**	**Plaque Estimate**	**ICA/CCA PSV Ratio**	**ICA EDV (cm/s)**
Nl	<125	None	<2.0	<40
<50	<125	<50	<2.0	<40
50–69	125–230	=50	2.0–4.0	40–100
>70	>230	>50	>4.0	>100
Near occlusion	High, low, and undetectable	Visible	Variable	Variable
Total occlusion	Undetectable	Visible, no lumen	NA	NA

In the mid 1990s debate around two pivotal carotid artery surgery trials, the North American Symptomatic Carotid Endarterectomy Trial (NASCET) and the Asymptomatic Carotid Artery Surgery (ACAS), defined a new convention for the radiographic method of determining stenosis. Since ultrasound is still compared to contrast arteriography, it is necessary to understand what portion of the carotid is defined as "normal" against which the percentage of stenosis is determined. The narrowest portion of the lumen is now compared to the "normal" appearing distal internal carotid artery, while historically the stenotic area was compared to the bulb of the carotid to determine the percentage of stenosis.[33,34]

Contralateral ICA stenosis/occlusion can result in very significant compensatory flow increases in the ipsilateral CCA/ICA. Therefore, in patients with a contralateral occlusion PSV-based stenosis criteria may be artificially elevated. No strict grading scales have been devised for this situation. The author recommends using CCA:ICA ratio and B-mode imaging in addition to EDV ratios in this situation. Also, in the setting of bilateral high-grade stenosis, repeat of the contralateral carotid ultrasound is necessary after ipsilateral carotid revascularization, as the decreased need for compensatory flow may downgrade the measured level of stenosis.

Postcarotid intervention studies are performed on a scheduled basis by most centers. This usually follows a schedule of 1 month, 3 months, 6 months, and 1 year post intervention. Classically, it is agreed that technical errors will be noticed at the 1-month ultrasound, accounting for this relatively short follow-up interval. Neointimal hyperplasia can cause restenosis at up to 2 years; and after 2 years, recurrent disease is recognized as the cause of restenosis. Most labs use their standardized velocity criteria to evaluate postoperative restenosis. However, with the addition of carotid stenting, whether of questionable utility or not, the criteria for restenosis needed to be modified in the cohort that undergo stenting. In addition, since this group did not have an atheroreductive procedure, carotid duplex is recommended previous to and 24 hours after placement of the stent in order to establish baseline PSV data for the ICA and CCA. Otherwise, the patient should follow the same schedule as above,; if there is an increase in PSV of 80% in the stented segment, an 80% increase in the ICA:CCA ratio, or the finding in Table 14-4, the patient should undergo further radiographic reimaging, usually contrast arteriography.[35,36]

TABLE 14-4

Recommended Postcarotid Stent Criteria

Restenosis	Absolute PSV	ICA:CCA Ratio
≤20%	<150 cm/s	<2.15
≥50%	≥220 cm/s	>2.70
≥80%	≥340 cm/s	>4.15

TABLE 14-5

St Luke's-Roosevelt Carotid Stenosis Criteria

Degree of Stenosis	Velocity Criteria
<40%	PSV <125 cm/s
40–59%	PSV 125 to 199 cm/s
60–79%	PSV 200 to 299 cm/s and EDV <100 cm/s
80–99%	PSV >300 cm/sec or EDV >100 cm/s
All studies have comment on plaque quantity	Spectral analysis is evaluated as well

Each Intersocietal Commission for the Accreditation of Vascular Laboratories (ICAVL) accredited laboratory needs to validate its own findings, with both angiographic (CT, MRA, and traditional) and operative findings. This is a locally developed system in which the literature is a significant help, but since the specificity and the sensitivity of this test cannot be overemphasized, it must be each laboratory's internal quality assurance program that determines the criteria for reporting stenosis (Table 14-5). One of the other factors effecting the sensitivity and specificity of this test is the actual ultrasound machine used; both the software and the hardware create subtle but real differences in the exact velocity criteria. In general, accredited centers publish sensitivity, specificity, and accuracy data of slightly greater than 90%.[31,32]

Brachiocephalic arteries

The finding one is looking for in pathology of the great vessels is a two-fold change in PSV. In addition, poststenotic turbulence and spectral broadening are paramount to discerning subtle disturbances in flow. Obviously a nonpulsatile waveform is pathognomonic for significant stenosis.

Vertebral arteries

Due to location and resolution it is difficult to see subtle vertebral artery disease especially at the origin of the vessel. Therefore, surrogate markers are used to identify vertebral artery disease. The finding of reversal of flow in the vertebral artery correlates to anatomic subclavian steal, while a stronger signal in one vertebral artery correlates to contralateral occlusion, contralateral subclavian steal, or significant carotid disease.

Transcranial Doppler

The velocity in this bed is reported as a mean velocity, not as angle-corrected velocity. This is, in large part, due to the inability to obtain angle-appropriate windows, and mean velocity is less dependent upon the correct angle of insonation. The range of the normal velocity in the MCA is between 30 and 80 cm/s, while vasospasm or stenosis correlates with velocities of 120 cm/s. Using a ratio of the mean velocity in the MCA:distal extracranial ICA can help

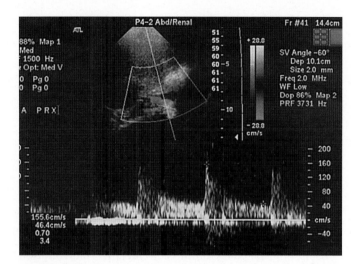

Figure 14-11. Renal artery with RAR 1.8.

distinguish vasospasm from hyperemia when MCA velocities are elevated.[37]

At the present time, TCD for the surgeon appears to be used primarily in the setting of carotid stenting and protection devices. This is due to the efficacy of ultrasound to detect emboli and record their frequency.[38] A contemporary area of interest is the use of TCD to predict post-carotid endarterectomy hyperperfusion syndrome, which appears to correlate with approximately a 100% increase in MCA velocity.[39]

▶ **Aorta and Abdominal Visceral Arteries**

Renal arteries

In general, normal renal arteries exhibit low-resistance Doppler waveforms (Figure 14-11). As Kohler first described, we use the renal-aortic ratio (RAR), or the mid-aortic PSV: to renal artery PSV, as the diagnostic criterion to determine potentially significant renal artery stenosis.[40] An RAR >3.5 has been noted to correlate to a >60% diameter reduction (Figure 14-12). If this criterion is used,

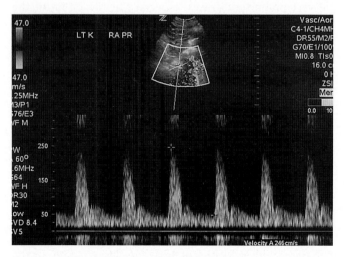

Figure 14-12. Significant renal artery stenosis.

TABLE 14-6		
University of Washington Renal Artery Stenosis Criteria		
Degree of RA Stenosis	**PSV**	**RAR**
Normal	<180 cm/s AND	<3.5
<60%	>180 cm/s BUT	<3.5
>60%	<>180 cm/s BUT	>3.5

there is a sensitivity of 91% and a specificity of 95%.[40] Not routinely used but of significance is the end diastolic ratio (EDR), which is the ratio of end diastolic frequency to peak systolic frequency.[41] The EDR is lower in patients with end-stage renal parenchymal disease.

Some authors have used the PSV of 200 cm/s as a marker of >60% stenosis, which was not chosen for a particular clinical significance but as a radiographic correlation.[42] The same researchers found that the sensitivity of renal artery ultrasound was only 67% if multiple renal arteries were present. Based on numerous studies the University of Washington group recommends criteria as outlined in Table 14-6. The Cleveland Clinic group prospectively tested an algorithm that included a PSV >200 cm/s or a RAR >3.5 as a criteria for renal artery stenosis >60%.[43] These criteria had a sensitivity of 98%, specificity of 98%, positive predictive value of 99%, and a negative predictive value of 97%. It should be noted that the same ratio and velocity criteria can be used after revascularization, without significant modification.[44,45]

Mesenteric arteries

The finding of a velocity of 275 cm/s has been identified as being consistent with a >70% stenosis.[46,47] Others have noted an EDV >45 cm/s to be consistent with a >50% stenosis of the SMA.[48] This single PSV had a sensitivity of 89% and a specificity of 92%, while the EDV had a sensitivity of 100% and a specificity of 92%. The celiac artery has a slightly lower stenosis threshold at a PSV >200 cm/s, with an EDV of >55 cm/s.[49] Due to the rich collateral flow to the celiac axis, a single PSV or EDV is very hard to correlate with a significant stenosis. However, it has been noted reliably that retrograde flow in the hepatic artery is consistent with high-grade celiac stenosis or occlusion.[50]

Aorta and iliac arteries

In general, the peripheral arterial criteria used to define stenosis is a 100% increase in PSV, or otherwise a PSV ratio of 2, when comparing the area of stenosis to the proximal artery. This finding correlates to a >50% stenosis, and better accuracy has been noted at higher ratios.[51,52,53] At this point in time most authors use the following categories: patient without significant stenosis, patient with a stenosis ≥50%, or occluded.[54] In the proximal vascular beds sensitivities from 81% to 91% have been reported, and specificities from 90% to 99% have been noted when comparing duplex ultrasound with contrast angiography.[55-68]

Duplex evaluation of endovascular aneurysm repair

For preoperative imaging of the aorta, prior to placing an endograft, a helical CT scan is the study of choice. However, after the endograft is in place follow-up imaging is mandatory. The gold standard has been CT scan as well. However, the cost and the large amount of ionizing radiation associated with annual CT scan is causing investigators to assess Duplex ultrasound as a modality to monitor for endoleak and aneurysm shrinkage. Currently it is thought that between 15% and 25% of patients undergoing EVAR will experience an endoleak. Type I endoleaks, which are the most serious, are characterized by arterial flow outside the graft and aneurysmal enlargement. Retrograde branch flow endoleaks are categorized as Type II (Figure 14-13) and may be from the lumbar arteries or inferior mesenteric artery. Investigators have characterized Type II endoleaks with duplex as biphasic (high resistance) or monophasic (bi-directional). Biphasic endoleaks are more likely to thrombose without intervention, whereas monophasic endoleaks require intervention.[56,57] While the use of ultrasonic contrast agents has increased the sensitivity of duplex to 100%, contrast-enhanced color Doppler has also improved the diagnostic accuracy.[58] At present this technique is supplanting traditional CT scan with contrast ultrasound at many centers.

Peripheral vessels

Performing a comprehensive scan of the entire arterial tree from the aorta to the pedal vessels takes easily over an hour. However, it has been noted that Duplex ultrasound may be able to provide enough data upon which to base a distal revascularization in 83% of cases.[55] When EDV and transverse imaging of the arteries are added, duplex is 88% specific.[59] Other authors have reported up to 100% predictive success for planning fem-crural bypasses.[60] It is worth noting that duplex scanning has been shown to be able to distinguish distal disease even when there is multi-level proximal disease.[61] Distal vessels can be hard to assess, especially the peroneal artery. In addition, heavy calcification can hamper distal small vessel imaging. Due to the time requirements, the author currently reserves this technique to assess inframalleolar vessels that are difficult to see on arteriogram.

Arterial bypass graft surveillance

This type of study is usually undertaken 1, 3, and 6 months post bypass and then on an annual basis. By being able to diagnose and intervene in a distal bypass prior to its failure, we can keep most grafts open with a generally recognized primary assisted patency at 5 years of 80% to 85%. This represents an improvement in patency at 3 to 5 years of approximately 20%.[62] Unfortunately, only about one third of failing grafts can be recognized on history and physical examination.[63] The finding of a PSV <45 cm/s anywhere in the bypass and the absence of diastolic forward flow

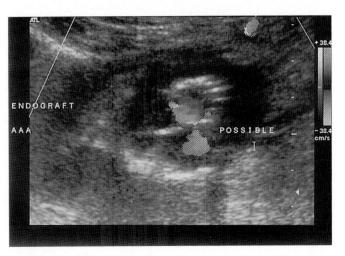

Figure 14-13. Aortic Type 2 endoleak-lumbar color flow blush.

are predictive of impending graft failure.[64] The specific site to intervene can be diagnosed by a PSV ratio of 3.4 to 4.0, the author uses the ratio of 4.0 (Figure 14-14A and 14-14B).[65] Other authors advocate ratios in conjunction with PSV >300 cm/s as indicators of the correct location to intervene.[66]

Surgically created arteriovenous fistula

Since AV fistulas are very high-flow systems, they can be difficult to assess solely with duplex. In a vein, a PSV ratio (anastomosis:artery 2 cm proximal to anastomosis) greater than 3:1 is thought to represent a diameter reduction greater than 50%,[67,68] while in a graft a PSV ratio of 2:1 is necessary to define a 50% stenosis, and a 3:1 ratio is consistent with a 75% stenosis.[69,70] This author reviews the B-mode image carefully to ensure that the diameter of the anastomosis is equal to or greater than the inflow artery. It should be noted that a small outflow vessel and/or an acute anastomotic angle can create an artificially elevated velocity. An intra-access stenosis of 50% or greater is suggested by a stenosis:2 cm distal stenosis PSV ratio of 2:1.[71] A 4-mm vein with at least 500 mL/min of flow should allow for adequate hemodialysis access, although depth of the vein from the skin needs to be assessed as well.[72]

▶ Venous Studies

Evaluation for deep venous thrombosis

The diagnostic criteria for DVT include an evaluation of venous compressibility, intraluminal echoes, venous flow characteristics, and differential filling of the vessel in color Duplex (Table 14-7). The inability to compress the vein is the most commonly used criterion to define DVT. The vein may well appear dilated with echogenic thrombus present. However, acute thrombus is usually less echogenic than old thrombus, and is visible in acute DVTs as low as 50% of the time.[73,23,74] Spectral analysis and color flow interpretation can aid in the diagnosis. Above the popliteal vein, normal venous flow is spontaneous and varies with

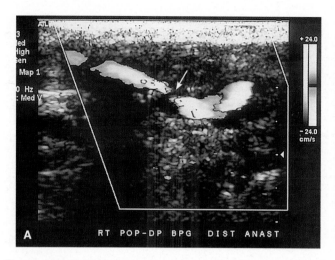
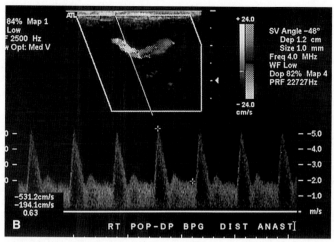

Figure 14-14. (A) Color image of femoral to dorsalis pedis bypass; **(B)** High-grade stenosis by velocity.

respiration, augments with distal compression, and diminishes with Valsalva. In the calf spontaneous flow may be absent; however, flow should augment in the tibioperoneal veins distal compression.

Proximal obstruction is suggested by continuous flow signals without respiratory variation, lack of augmentation with release proximal compression, and continuous flow during Valsalva. Distal obstruction is suggested by diminished or absent augmentation with distal compression. Color flow can be helpful in areas where compression is limited, and the examiner should note that the entire proximal vein (popliteal and above) should completely fill with color flow in the normal vein.

Upper extremity veins are affected to a greater extent by cardiac and respiratory variability. Flow is completely stopped or severely limited during the Valsalva maneuver while vein diameter increases. The internal jugular vein is assessed by criteria similar to lower extremity veins. However, due to the musculoskeletal encumbrances, the subclavian vein is assessed using indirect flow criteria: complete color filling of the lumen, normal respiratory variation, and cardiac pulsatility of the Doppler signal. Thrombosis is suggested by direct visualization of thrombus, absent or incomplete color filling of the lumen, and an absent diameter response to rapid inspiration.[75,76]

While noncompressibility remains the cornerstone, it is not the most sensitive method to detect DVT in all beds. Noncompressibility is the most objective of the criteria, though, and has a 100% interobserver agreement.[77] If one compares B-mode incompressibility, visualization of thrombus, absence of spontaneous flow, and absence of phasic flow, only the absence of phasic flow has both a sensitivity and specificity greater than 90%.[74] Sensitivity is significantly improved when criteria are used in combination; sensitivity approaches 95% and specificity 83% when thrombus visualization and absence of variation of flow with respiration are evaluated together.[74] In some patients free-floating thrombus is seen, defined as color flow surrounding a filling defect; in addition, like other authors, we prefer to include movement of the unattached segment within the flow stream as part of the criteria of the definition.[78,79,80] It is probably useful to re-image these patients 7 days after diagnosis, as in one study 55% of these patients had demonstrated attachment of their free-floating tail, 24% showed partial or complete resolution, 9% showed an increase in size of their thrombus, and 12% had no change in their characteristics.[81]

The differentiation between chronic and acute DVT remains a difficult dilemma, but one of key importance as the different diagnoses warrant different treatments. While many patients experience early recanalization, 50% of compression studies remain abnormal at 6 months, and around 25% of patients at one year after diagnosis.[82,83] There are some key generalizations about thrombus as it ages that are helpful in determining thrombus chronicity, as thrombus appears more echogenic and more heterogeneous as it ages, and the acute thrombus causes dilation of the vessel while chronic thrombus causes contraction (Figure 14-15).[82,84]

Like other authors we advocate a DVT study 6 months after the initial diagnosis to have a baseline study on which to base assessments of recurrent episodes.[82,83,85] This allows the ultrasonographer to have objective data on which to compare repeat ultrasound examinations in the patient

TABLE 14-7	
Ultrasound Criteria for Acute DVT	
Diagnostic Criteria	**Adjunctive Criteria**
Non-compressibility of veins	Dilated vein <50% increase in diameter with valsalva
Echonenic thrombus	
Diminished/Absent venous flow	Non-visualization of venous valves
Absence of respiratory phasicity	
Absent or incomplete color filling	

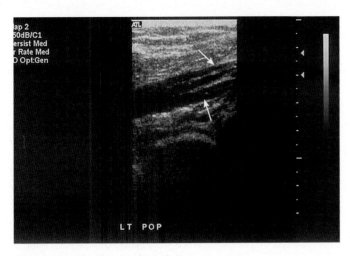

Figure 14-15. Chronic thrombus.

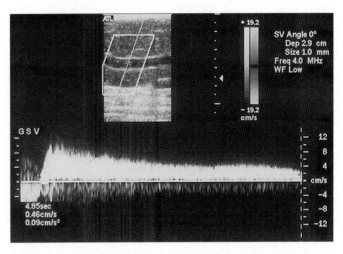

Figure 14-16. Retrograde flow greater than 4 seconds.

with recurrent symptoms. On these repeat studies, a 2 mm or greater increase in compressed thrombus thickness has correlated to a 100% sensitivity and specificity for recurrent DVT.[83]

Evaluation of chronic venous disease

When assessing for chronic disease one has to consider both obstructive and reflux components. Obstructive components are determined by the methods outlined above. Chronic obstructive disease is recognized in the deep and superficial systems as noted in Table 14-8. However, reflux components in both the deep and superficial systems are evaluated by assessing valve closure times. The duration of retrograde flow is best seen with spectral analysis (Figure 14-16). Ninety five percent of normal

valves will close in 0.5 seconds of appropriate reversal of flow.[86] As stated earlier, the method to obtain this reversal of flow is somewhat controversial. Most laboratories use 2.0 seconds as the threshold for significant reflux, as this allows for complete separation of those with pathological valve processes.[87]

It should be noted that the dynamics of venous return are probably better understood with direct pressure measurements than with ultrasound alone. Only 80% of patients with abnormal common femoral or popliteal venous ultrasounds were found to have abnormal direct venous pressures.[88] The best method of quantifying global limb reflux is probably one based upon either the axial extent or segmental distribution of reflux.[89] Valve closure times in individual venous segments correlate poorly with reflux volume.[90] However, peak reflux volume flows above 10 mL/s correlate to a cohort of patients in which 66% have lipodermatosclerosis.[90] Much like lower extremity arterial assessment, the best method of assessment of chronic venous insufficiency is probably one that involves two complementary tests, one physiologic and one anatomic, based upon the patient's symptomatology.

COMMON PITFALLS

Notable variation in measurements has been observed across ultrasound device manufacturers. In all vascular beds, different machines, which may have very similar gray scale capabilities, often have different internal software computational methods. In one study, while somewhat historic, only 21% of machines tested achieved "excellent sensitivity" (≥80%) when assessing carotid stenosis.[91] This again underscores the need for local quality control and validation.

In the diagnosis of DVT, there will be some indeterminate studies. Most reports cite a 1% to 6% rate of limited diagnostic results for proximal DVT.[92,93] Often it is anatomic features that limit visualization; obesity and difficult insonation windows such as the thoracic and pelvic inlets can hinder complete visualization. Overlying bowel

TABLE 14-8

Ultrasound Characteristics of Acute vs Chronic Obstructive Venous Occlusion

Diagnostic Criteria	Acute Thrombus	Chronic Thrombus
Incompressibility	Yes-but soft	Yes-but firm
Vein diameter	Dilated	Contracted
Echogenicity	Echolucent	Echonenic
Heterogeneity	Homonenous	Heterogeneous
Color luminal appearance/Flow channel	Smooth/ laminar	RouRh/multiple
Collaterals	None	Many
Free floating tail	Present	Absent
Incompressibility	Yes-but soft	Yes-but firm
Vein diameter	Dilated	Contracted
Echogenicity	Echolucent	Echogenic
Heterogeneity	Homogenous	Heterogeneous
Color luminal appearance/ Flow channel	Smooth/laminar	Rough/multiple
Collaterals	None	Many
Free floating tail	Present	Absent

gas certainly limits visualization of the inferior vena cava and the iliac veins. Furthermore, large calf size and edema can greatly attenuate ultrasound imaging of the tibial veins. Since vascular ultrasound is inherently operator-dependent, the other pitfalls really have to do with things that distract the operator: being rushed, being preoccupied, and not understanding the underlying pathophysiology or anatomy.

CLINICAL PEARLS/TIPS

For the most part blood behaves as a Newtonian fluid, although due to particulate size in vessels less than 1 mm blood is non-Newtonian. The Newtonian characteristics at a stenosis lead to the pathognomonic prestenotic, stenotic, and poststenotic patterns that are observed. Blood forms a velocity gradient across the vessel lumen as it moves. Thus, once the blood enters a stenosis, it increases its velocity while maintaining a linear flow profile. But when the narrow high-velocity stream enters the dilated (poststenotic) segment of the vessel, it becomes unstable. There is a central jet with adjacent flow reversals and eddy currents. As flow continues past the stenosis, the stream stabilizes again. Then again, this theory is predicated upon the vessel being straight and the lesion (narrowing) being symmetrical. In truth, while the fluid behaves in a Newtonian fashion, its conduit (the vessel) is irregular, as is the lesion. Therefore, high-velocity blood will veer away from the axis of the vessel, much like a tractor trailer on a curvy road. This is in addition to the fact that the flow jet is most likely not down the axis of the vessel. It is therefore incumbent upon the ultrasonographer to assess the correct flow pattern and align the axis of insonation appropriately.

THERAPEUTIC MANEUVERS/ULTRASOUND-GUIDED PROCEDURES

▶ Intraoperative Studies

Small footprint high-frequency probes allow for the intraoperative assessment of vascular repairs. These are of the most use in small-diameter, technically challenging repairs such as carotid endarterectomy and distal tibial anastomoses. Technical errors such as residual flaps, suture line stricture, and plaque dissection can be identified by this technique. Most clinicians use a minimum of continuous wave Doppler ultrasound to assess flow at the end of endarterectomy and bypass. While this technique allows for the assessment of flow and augmentation, for those who desire anatomic information, a completion arteriogram, while cumbersome, has been the norm.

Ease of use and high resolution have made small, linear array 7- to 10-MHz probes attractive. However, data interpretation is less clear. In the carotid artery residual flaps less than 2 mm can safely be left in place, but flaps of 3 mm or greater may require reintervention. In addition, PSV at the distal anastomosis of >200 cm/s may also require reintervention.[94,95]

In the case of the distal bypass, the entire bypass is scanned from the proximal through the distal anastomosis. Measurements of PSV and ratios at the lesion divided by proximal velocity are used as criteria to assess for graft/anastomotic defects. In one study intraoperative PSV <25 cm/s was consistent with graft abnormalities. If a velocity ratio of 2:1 was noted, the area was more closely scrutinized, and underwent revision if an area exhibited a PSV >180 cm/s and velocity ratio >2.5. In patients with impaired outflow, defined as PSV <45 cm/s, postoperative anticoagulation was given.[96] Following these criteria, there was a 15% intraoperative revision rate, but only a 2.5% 30-day revision rate.

▶ Pseudoaneurysm Compression/Injection

Pseudoaneurysms are noted to occur 0.05% to 0.8% after diagnostic procedures and 0.4% to 3% after therapeutic intervention.[97] In 1991 ultrasound-guided compression replaced surgical correction as the initial therapy for PSA. However, this technique, which requires gray scale verified occlusion of the PSA while allowing flow through the common femoral artery to promote thrombosis, can require up to 90 minutes of compression, which is uncomfortable for the patient and very time-consuming for the laboratory. While efficacy rates have been noted to be between 66% and 94%, recurrences occur frequently especially in patients on anticoagulation.[98]

For the above reasons simple compression has been replaced with thrombin injection. In this technique, 500 units of thrombin (0.5 to 1.0 mL of 1000 units/mL) is injected under ultrasound guidance along the wall of the aneurysm furthest away from the connection to the artery, while the arterial neck is being compressed.[99,100] This was noted to be 97% effective in simple aneurysms and 61% effective in complex aneurysms. Certain anatomic findings preclude this procedure, such as multilobed aneurysms that may require multiple or repeat injections, and aneurysms with short wide necks that can allow thrombin to enter the arterial circulation resulting in distal thrombosis. Both of these variants will often require surgical repair.

▶ Arteriovenous Access Interventions

Percutaneous interventions for arteriovenous access have been on the rise, and these are primarily done with the aid of fluoroscopic guidance.[101] The high cost of fluoroscopic units, the exposure of the patient and the clinician to ionizing radiation, and the use of sedation make these procedures less attractive. Recently a growing body of literature has supported the use of Duplex ultrasound to intervene on hemodialysis access, for both salvage and maturation procedures.[102,103]

By using Duplex ultrasound one can directly measure the size of the balloon and stent that may be needed for the intervention. Duplex's unique ability to measure diameter, flow velocity, and volume of flow makes it a strong tool in guiding interventions. In addition, these procedures can be done completely under local anesthesia

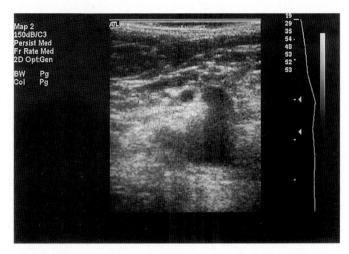

Figure 14-17. Greater saphenous/common femoral vein junction in coronal view.

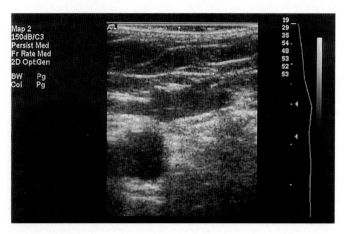

Figure 14-18. 5-French sheath tip in GSV distal to superficial inferior epigastric vein.

in a procedure suite. The choice of balloon can be made by measuring the vessel diameter adjacent to the stenotic area and oversizing by 1–2 mm. Following the angioplasty/stenting, volume flow measurements can be made in a nontortuous segment of the access. Fox et al recommend that this be done prior to placement of the introducer, immediately after the intervention and removal of the introducer.[103] Technical success has been reported in 98.2% of cases, with a complication rate of 8.5%. In AV access undergoing PTA median volume flow was noted to increase from 210 mL/min to 485 mL/min, while in those AVF/AVG undergoing salvage median VF increased from 472 mL/min to 950 mL/min.

▶ Endovenous Ablation Procedures

For several reasons, some based upon efficacy, some on patient comfort, and some on financial considerations, laser or radiofrequency ablation of the greater saphenous vein (GSV) has largely replaced operative stripping as the procedure of choice for superficial reflux.[104,105,106] This entire procedure, whether using laser or radiofrequency, is completely reliant upon B-mode imaging of the GSV. At the time of the procedure the GSV is imaged using a 7-MHz probe from its junction with the common femoral vein (CFV), which has a characteristic "Mickey Mouse" appearance on cross section (Figure 14-17), to the above knee crease. The GSV is visualized transversely at the popliteal crease to allow for access with a micropuncture sheath. The j wire is visualized passing up the GSV to the junction with the CFV. This is followed by the 5-French sheath to just 1 cm distal to the origin of the superficial inferior epigastric vein (SIEV); then the energy delivery device is passed inside the sheath to be just distal to the SIEV (Figure 14-18), between 1 and 3 cm distal to the CFV/GSV junction. After this, the sheath/vein complex is visualized transversely to allow for evaluation of the tumescent anesthetic solution. Postprocedure insonation of the GSV is not done as it has little correlation with outcome, and is

difficult to interpret. Ablation is associated with a 94% or better success rate. Thrombus can protrude into the lumen of the GSV in 2.3% of patients.[107] In order to assess efficacy of the procedure and initiate anticoagulation therapy if a clot was found, a follow-up ultrasound is usually performed on postprocedure days 2–6, and at 6 weeks post procedure.

CASE STUDIES

▶ Carotid Stenosis

A 58-year-old male, who had smoked for 30 years presented with a left-sided bruit. He underwent carotid duplex (Figure 14-19); PSV was 394.4 cm/s EDV 90.2 cm/s. He underwent an uneventful carotid endarterectomy with Dacron patch repair. At his 1-month study he was seen to be free of disease and his patch is visible (Figure 14-20), PSV 78 cm/s; EDV 44.4 cm/s.

▶ Aortic Aneurysm

A 66-year-old male was followed for 3 years with aortic ultrasound until his abdominal aortic dilation reached 5.5 cm in diameter (Figure 14-21). He underwent a successful endovascular aneurysm repair. His 1-year ultrasound is seen with endostent clearly seen (Figure 14-22).

▶ Postphlebitic Syndrome

A 29-year-old female is now 2 years status post gastric bypass surgery. The patient has a history of right popliteal deep venous thrombosis 4 years ago. She presents with ongoing swelling of the right foot and ankle with generalized pain. A B-mode image shows "webbing" in the right popliteal vein (Figure 14-23). She then underwent an ascending venogram from her posterior tibial vein, which confirmed the venous pathology prior to venoplasty (Figure 14-24).

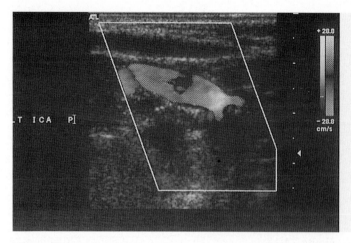
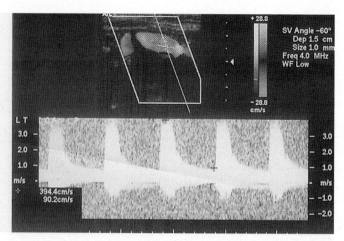

Figure 14-19. Carotid lesion with concerning color image high EDV.

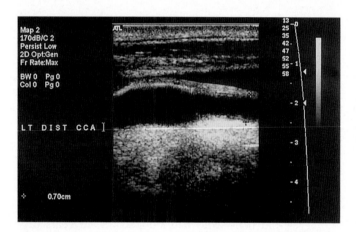

Figure 14-20. After carotid endarterectomy with dilation of patch.

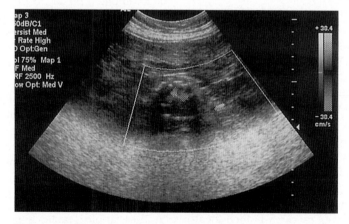

Figure 14-21. Abdominal aortic aneurysm, transverse image.

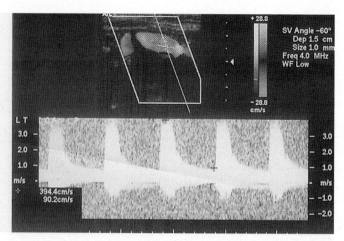

Figure 14-22. Endograft sitting within the aortic aneurysm.

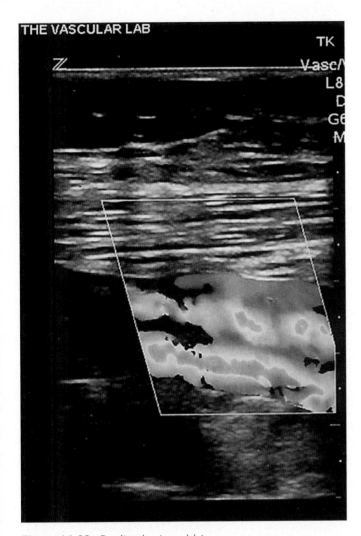

Figure 14-23. Popliteal vein webbing.

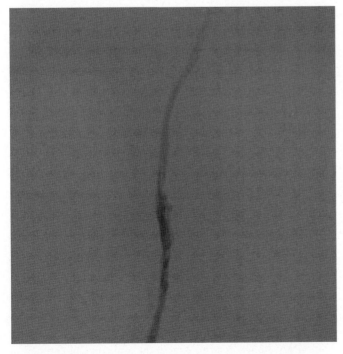

Figure 14-24. Ascending venogram with popliteal webbing.

SUGGESTED READINGS

Kremkau FW. Principals and pitfalls of real time color flow imaging. In: Berstein EF (ed). *Vascular Diagnosis*. St Louis: Mosby-Year Book; 1993.

ACR-AIUM Practice Guideline for the Performance of Vascular Ultrasound for Postoperative Assessment of Dialysis Access. 1–6.

SVU Vascular Technology Professional Performance Guidelines: Mesenteric/Splanchnic Artery Duplex Imaging.

Mattos MA Hodgson KJ, Faught WE, et al. Carotid endarterectomy without angiography: is color flow duplex scanning insufficient? *Surgery*. 1994;116:776.

Cogo A, Lensing AWA, Prandoni P, et al. Comparison of real time B-mode ultrasonography and Doppler ultrasound with contrast venography in the diagnosis of venous thrombosis is symptomatic outpatients. *Thromb Haemost*. 1993;70:404.

REFERENCES

1. Blackshear WM, Phillips DJ, Thiele BL, et al. Detection of carotid occlusive disease by ultrasound imaging and pulsed Doppler spectrum analysis. *Surgery*. 1979;86: 698–706.

2. Strandness DE. *Duplex Scanning in Vascular Disorders*. 2nd ed. New York: Raven Press; 1993:1–21.

3. Zierler RE, Philips DJ, Beach KW, et al. Noninvasive assessment of normal carotid bifurcation hemodynamics with color flow ultrasound imaging. *Ultrasound Med Biol*. 1987;13(8)471–476.

4. Nichols WW, O'Rourke MF. *McDonalds Blood Flow*. 3rd ed. Philadelphia: Lea & Febiger; 1990:143–146.

5. Persson AV, Gibbons G, Griffey S. Noninvasive evaluation of the aorto-iliac segment. *J Cardiovasc Surg*. 1981;22(6)539–542.

6. Johnston KW, Maruzzo BC, Cobbold RSC. Doppler methods for quantitative measurement and localization of peripheral arterial occlusive disease by analysis of the blood velocity waveform. *Ultrasound Med Biol*. 1978;4(3):209–223.

7. van Bremmelen PS, Beach K, Bedford G, et al. The mechanism of venous valve closure. *Arch Surg*. 1990;125(5):617–619.

8. Beebe HG, Salles-Cunha SX, Scissons RP, et al. Carotid arterial ultrasound scan imaging: a direct approach to stenosis measurement. *J Vasc Surg*. 1999;(29)5:838–844.

9. Roederer GO,Langlois YE, Jager KA, et al. A simple spectral parameter for accurate classification of severe carotid disease. *Bruit*. 1984;15(4):605–613.

10. Roederer GO, Langlois YE, Jager KA, et al. The natural history of carotid arterial disease in asymptomatic patients with cervical bruits. *Stroke*. 1984;15:605–613.

11. Linguish J Jr., Reavis SW, Preisser JS, et al. Duplex ultrasound scanning defines operative strategies for patients with limb-threatening ischemia. *J Vasc Surg*. 1998;28(3):482–490.

12. Bendick PJ, Jackson VP. Evaluation of the vertebral arteries with duplex sonography. *J Vasc Surg*. 1986;3(3): 523–530.

13. Bartles E, Flugel KA. Evaluation of extracranial vertebral artery dissection with duplex color flow imaging. *Stroke*. 1996;27(2):290–295.

14. Kaneko A, Ohno R, Hattori K, et al. Color-coded Doppler imaging of subclavian steal syndrome. *Intern Med.* 1998; 37(3):259–264.

15. Ries S, Steinke W, Devuyst G, et al. Power Doppler imaging and color Doppler flow imaging for the evaluation of normal and pathological vertebral arteries. *J Neuroimaging.* 1998;8(2):71–74.

16. Ackersaff RG, Jansen C, Moll FL, et al. The significance of microemboli detection by means of transcranial Doppler ultrasonography monitoring in carotid endarterectomy. *J Vasc Surg.* 1995;21(6):963–969.

17. Bass A, Krupski WC, Schneider PA, et al. Intraoperative transcranial Doppler: limitations of the method. *J Vasc Surg.* 1989;10(5):549–553.

18. Moneta GL, Yeager RA, Lee RW et al. Noninvasive localization of arterial occlusive disease: a comparison of segmental Doppler pressures and arterial duplex mapping. *J Vasc Surg.* 1993;17(3):578–582.

19. Sivanesan S, How TV, Bakran A. Characterizing flow distributions in AV fistulae for haemodialysis access. *Nephrol Dial Transplant.* 1998;13(12):3108–3110

20. Won T, Jang JW, Lee S, et al. Effects of intraoperative blood flow on the early patency of radiocephalic fistulas. *Ann Vasc Surg.* 2000;14(5):468–472

21. Beathard GA, Settle SM, Shields MW. Salvage of the nonfunctioning arteriovenous fistula. *Am J Kidney Dis.* 1999;33(5):910–916.

22. Nix ML, Troilett RD, Nelson CL, et al. Is bilateral duplex examination necessary for unilateral symptoms of deep venous thrombosis? *J Vasc Technol.* 1991;15:296–298.

23. Elias A, Le Corff G, Bouvier JL, et al. Value of real-time B-mode ultrasound imaging in the diagnosis of deep vein thrombosis of the lower limbs. *J Mal Vasc.* 1987;12(3):246–248.

24. Mattos MA, Melendres G, Summer DS, et al. Prevalence and distribution of calf vein thrombosis in patients with symptomatic deep venous thrombosis. A color flow duplex study. *J Vasc Surg.* 1996;24(5):738–744.

25. Eklöf B, Rutherord R, Bergan J, et al. Revision of the CEAP classification for chronic venous disorders: consensus statement. *J Vasc Surg.* 2004;40(6):1248–1252.

26. Markel A, Meissner MH, Manzo RA, et al. A comparison of the cuff deflation method with Valsalva's maneuver and limb compression in detecting venous valvular reflux. *Arch Surg.* 1994;29(7):701–705.

27. Miller SS, Foote AV. The ultrasonic detection of incompetent perforating veins. *Br J Surg.* 1974;61(8): 653–656.

28. Sarin S, Scurr JH, Colerdidge Smith PD. Medial calf perforators in venous diseases: the significance of outward flow. *J Vasc Surg.* 1992;16(1):40–46.

29. Pierk EG, Toonder IM, van Urk H, et al. Validation of duplex ultrasonography in detecting competent and incompetent perforating veins in patients with venous ulceration of the lower leg. *J Vasc Surg.* 1997;26(1):49–52.

30. Grant EG, Benson CB, Moneta GL, et al. Carotid artery stenosis: gray-scale and Doppler US Diagnosis-Society of Radiologists in Ultrasound Consensus Conference. *Radiology.* 2003;19(4):340–346.

31. Moneta GL, Edwards JM, Papanicolaou G, et al. Screening for asymptomatic internal carotid artery stenosis: duplex criteria for discriminating 60% to 99% stenosis. *J Vasc Surg.* 1995;21(6):989–994.

32. Faught WE, Mattos MA, van Bremmelen PS, et al. Color-flow duplex scanning of carotid arteries: new velocity criteria based upon receiver operator characteristic analysis for threshold stenoses used in the symptomatic and asymptomatic carotid trials. *J Vasc Surg.* 1994;19(5):818–827.

33. Executive Committee for the Asymptomatic Carotid Atherosclerosis Study. Endarterectomy for asymptomatic carotid artery stenosis. *JAMA.* 1995 May 10;273(18): 1421–1428.

34. North American Symptomatic Carotid Endarterectomy Trial Collaborators. Beneficial effect of carotid endarterectomy in symptomatic patients with high grade carotid stenosis. *N Engl J Med.* 1991;325(7):445–453.

35. Lal BK, Hobson RW 2nd, Tofighi B, et al. Duplex ultrasound velocity criteria for the stented carotid artery. *J Vasc Surg.* 2008;47(1):63–73.

36. Ringer AJ, German JW, Guterman LR, et al. Follow up of stented carotid arteries by Doppler ultrasound. *Neurosurgery.* 2002;51(3):639–643.

37. Newell DW, Aaslid R. Transcranial Doppler: clinical and experimental uses. *Cerebrovasc Brain Metab Rev.* 1992;4(2):122–143.

38. Martin RL, Nanra RS, Wlodarczyk J. Renal hilar Doppler analysis in the detection of renal artery stenosis. *J Vasc Technol.* 1991;15(4):173–180.

39. Jorgensen LG, Schroeder TV. Defective cerebrovascular autoregulation after carotid endarterectomy. *Eur J Vasc Surg.* 1993;7(4):370–379.

40. Kohler TR, Zierler RE, Martin RL, et al. Noninvasive diagnosis of renal artery stenosis by ultrasonic duplex scanning. *J Vasc Surg.* 1986;4(5):450–456.

41. Norris CS, Pfeiffer JS, Rittgers SE, et al. Noninvasive evaluation of renal artery stenosis and renovascular resistance. *J Vasc Surg.* 1984;1(1):192–201.

42. Hansen KJ, Tribble RW, Reavis SW, et al. Renal duplex sonography: evaluation of clinical utility. *J Vasc Surg.* 1990;12(3):227–236.

43. Olin JW, Piedmonte MR, Young JR, et al. The utility of duplex ultrasound scanning of the renal arteries for diagnosing significant renal artery stenosis. *Ann Intern Med.* 1995;122(11):833–837.

44. Eidt JF, Fry RE, Claggett GP, et al. Post-operative follow up of renal artery reconstruction with duplex ultrasound. *J Vasc Surg.* 1988;8(6):667–673.

45. Taylor DC, Houston GTM, Anderson C, et al. Follow up of renal and mesenteric artery revascularization with duplex ultrasonography. *Can J Surg.* 1996;39(1):17–20.

46. Moneta GL, Yeager RA, Dalman R, et al. Duplex ultrasound criteria for diagnosis of splanchnic artery stenosis or occlusion. *J Vasc Surg.* 1991;14(4):511–518.

47. Moneta GL, Lee RW, Yeager RA, et al. Mesenteric duplex scanning: a blinded prospective study. *J Vasc Surg.* 1993;17(1):79–86.

48. Bowersox JC, Zwolak RM, Walsh DB, et al. Duplex ultrasonography in the diagnosis of celiac and mesenteric artery occlusive disease. *J Vasc Surg.* 1991;14(6):780–786.

49. Zwolak RM, Fillinger MF, Walsh DB, et al. Mesenteric and celiac duplex scanning: a validation study. *J Vasc Surg.* 1998;27(6):1078–1087.

50. LaBombard FE, Musson A, Bowersox JC, et al. Hepatic artery duplex as an adjunct in the evaluation of chronic mesenteric ischemia. *J Vasc Technol.* 1992;16L:7–11.

51. Cossman DV, Ellison JE, Wagner WH, et al. Comparison of contrast arteriography to arterial mapping with color flow duplex imaging in the lower extremities. *J Vasc Surg.* 1989;10(5):522–528.

52. Legemate DA, Teeuwen C, Hoeneveld H, et al. Value of duplex scanning compared with angiography and pressure measurement in the assessment of aortoiliac arterial lesions. *Br J Surg.* 1991;78(8):1003–1008.

53. Leng GC, Whyman MR, Donnan PT et al. Accuracy and reproducibility of duplex ultrasonography in grading femoropopliteal stenosis. *J Vasc Surg.* 1993;17(3):510–517.

54. Liguish J Jr, Reavis SW, Preisser JS, et al. Duplex ultrasound scanning defines operative strategies for patients with limb threatening ischemia. *J Vasc Surg.* 1998;28(3):482–491.

55. Mazzariol F, Ascher E, Hingorani A, et al. Lower extremity revascularization without pre-operative contrast arteriography in 185 cases: lessons learned with duplex ultrasound arterial mapping. *Eur J Vasc Endovasc Surg.* 2000;19(5):509–515.

56. Carter KA, Nelms CR, Bloch PHS, et al. Doppler waveform assessment of endoleak following endovascular repair of abdominal aortic aneurysm: predictors of endoleak thrombosis. *J Vasc Technol.* 2000;24(2):119–122.

57. Bendick PJ, Bove PG, Long GW, et al. Efficacy of ultrasound scan contrast agents in the noninvasive follow up of aortic stent grafts. *J Vasc Surg.* 2003;37(2):381–385.

58. McWilliams RG, Martin J, White D, et al. Use of contrast-enhanced ultrasound in follow-up after endovascular aortic aneurysm repair. *J Vasc Interven Radiol.* 1999;10(8):1107–1114.

59. Grassbaugh JA, Nelson PR, Rzucidlo EM, et al. Blinded comparison of preoperative duplex ultrasound scanning and contrast arteriography for planning revascularization at the level of the tibia. *J Vasc Surg.* 2003;37(6):1186–1190.

60. Wilson YG, George JK, Wilkins DC, et al. Duplex assessment of run-off before femorocrural reconstruction. *Br J Surg.* 1997;84(10):1360–1363.

61. Sensier Y, Hartshorne T, Trush A, et al. The effect of adjacent segment disease on the accuracy of colour duplex scanning for the diagnosis of lower limb arterial disease. *Eur J Vasc Endovasc Surg.* 1996;12(2):238–242.

62. Idu MM, Blankenstein JD, de Gier P, et al. Impact of color flow duplex surveillance program on infrainguinal vein graft patency. A five year experience. *J Vasc Surg.* 1993;17(1):42–52.

63. Disselhoff B, Bluth J, Jakimowicz J. Early detection of stenosis of femoral distal grafts: a surveillance study using color-duplex scanning. *Eur J Vasc Surg.* 1989;3(1):43–48.

64. Bandyk DF, Cato RF, Towne JB. A low flow velocity predicts failure of femoropopliteal and femorotibial bypass grafts. *Surgery.* 1985;98(4):799–809.

65. Westerband A, Mills JL, Kistler S, et al. Prospective validation of threshold criteria for intervention in infrainguinal vein grafts under-going duplex surveillance. *Ann Vasc Surg.* 1997;11(1):44–48.

66. Gupta AK, Bandyk DF, Cheanvechai D, et al. Natural history of infrainguinal vein graft stenosis relative to bypass grafting technique. *J Vasc Surg.* 1997;25(2):211–220.

67. Chao A, Daley T, Gruenewald S, et al. Duplex ultrasound criteria for assessment of stenosis in radiocephalic hemodialysis fistulas. *J Vasc Technol.* 2001;6:203–208.

68. Lockhart ME, Robbin ML. Hemodialysis access ultrasound. *Ultrasound Q.* 2011;17:157–167.

69. Older RA, Gizienski TA, Wilkowski MJ, et al. Hemodialysis access stenosis: early detection with color Doppler US. *Radiology.* 1998;207(1):161–164.

70. Robbin ML, Oser RF, Allon M, et al. Hemodialysis access graft stenosis. US detection. *Radiology.* 1998;208(3):655–661.

71. Won T, Jang JW, Lee S, et al. Effects of intraoperative blood flow on the early patency of radiocephalic fistulas. *Ann Vasc Surg.* 2000;14(5):468–472.

72. Robbin ML, Chamberlain NE, Lockhart ME, et al. Hemodialysis arteriovenous fistula maturity: US evaluation. *Radiology.* 2002;225(1):59–64.

73. Talbot SR. B-mode evaluation of peripheral veins. *Semin Ultrasound.* CT MR 1988;9:295.

74. Killewich LA, Bedford GR, Beach KW, et al. Diagnosis of the deep venous thrombosis: a prospective study comparing duplex scanning to contrast venography. *Circulation.* 1989;79(4):810–814.

75. Burbidge SJ, Finlay DE, Letourneau JG, et al. Effects of central venous catheter placement on upper extremity duplex US findings. *J Vasc Interv Radiol.* 1993;4(3):399–404.

76. Gooding GAW, Hightower DR, Moore EH, et al. Obstruction of the superior vena cava or subclavian veins: sonographic diagnosis. *Radiology.* 1986;159(11):663–665.

77. Lensing AW, Prandoni P, Brandjes D, et al. Detection of deep vein thrombosis by real time B-mode ultrasonography. *N Engl J Med.* 1989;320(6):342–345.

78. Dauzat M, Laroche J-P, Deklunder G, et al. Diagnosis of acute lower limb deep venous thrombosis with ultrasound. Trends and controversies. *J Clinical Ultrasound.* 1997;25(7):343–358.

79. Greenfield LJ. Free floating thrombus and pulmonary embolism. *Arch Intern Med.* 1997;157(2):2661–2662.

80. Voet D, Afschrift M. Floating thrombi: diagnosis and follow up by duplex ultrasound. *Br J Radiol.* 1991;64(767):1010–1014.

81. Baldridge ED, Martin MA, Welling RE. Clinical significance of free floating thrombi. *J Vasc Surg.* 1990;11(1):62–67.

82. Murphy TP, Cronan JJ. Evolution of deep venous thrombosis: a prospective evaluation with US. *Radiology.* 1990;177(2):543–548.

83. Prandoni P, Cogo A, Bernardi E, et al. A simple ultrasound approach for detection of recurrent proximal vein thrombosis. *Circulation.* 1993;88(4 Pt1):1730–1735.

84. Ohgi S, Ito K, Tanaka K, et al. Echogenic types of venous thrombi in the common femoral vein by ultrasonic B-mode imaging. *Vasc Surg.* 1991;25(4):253–258.

85. Baxter GM, Duffy P, MacKechnie S. Colour Doppler ultrasound of the post phlebitis limb: sounding a cautionary note. *Clin Radiol.* 1991;43(5):301–304.

86. van Bemmelen PS, Bedford G, Beach K, et al. Quantitative segmental evaluation of venous valvular reflux with duplex ultrasound scanning. *J Vasc Surg.* 1989;10(4):425–431.

87. Araki CT, Back TL, Padberg FT, et al. Refinements in the ultrasonic detection of popliteal vein reflux. *J Vasc Surg.* 1993;18(5):742–748.

88. Szendro G, Nicolaides AN, Zukowski AJ, et al. Duplex scanning in the assessment of deep venous incompetence. *J Vasc Surg.* 1986;4(3):237–42.

89. Neglen R, Raju S. A comparison between descending phlebography and duplex Doppler investigation in the evaluation of reflux in chronic venous insufficiency: a challenge to phlebography as the "gold standard." *J Vasc Surg.* 1992;16(5):687–698.

90. Rodriquez AA, Whitehead CM, McLaughlin RL, et al. Duplex derived valve closure times fail to correlate with reflux flow volumes in patients with chronic venous insufficiency. *J Vasc Surg.* 1996;23(4):606–610.

91. Howard G, Baker WH, Chambless LE, et al. An approach for the use of Doppler ultrasound as a screening tool for hemodynamically significant stenosis (despite heterogeneity of Doppler performance). *Stroke.* 1996;27(11):1951–1957.

92. Lewis BD, James EM, Welch TJ, et al. Diagnosis of acute deep venous thrombosis of the lower extremities: prospective evaluation of color Doppler flow imaging versus venography. *Radiology.* 1994;192(3):651–655.

93. Vaccaro JP, Cronan JJ, Dorfman GS. Outcome analysis of patients with normal compression US exams. *Radiology.* 1990;175(3):645–649.

94. Baker WH, Koustas G, Burke K, et al. Intraoperative duplex scanning and late carotid artery stenosis. *J Vasc Surg.* 1994;19(5):829–833.

95. Bandyk DF, Mills JL, Ghatan V, et al. Intraoperative duplex scanning of arterial reconstructions. Fate of repaired and unrepaired defects. *J Vasc Surg.* 1994;20:426–433.

96. Johnson BL, Bandyk DF, Back MR, et al. Intraoperative duplex monitoring of infrainguinal vein bypass procedures. *J Vasc Surg.* 2000;31(4):678–690

97. Morrison SL, Obrand DA, Steinmetz OK, et al. Treatment of femoral artery pseudoaneurysms with percutaneous thrombin injection. *Ann Vasc Surg.* 14(6):634–639.

98. Cox GS, Young JR, Gray BR, et al. Ultrasound guided compression repair of postcatheterization pseudoaneurysm: results of treatment in one hundred cases. *J Vasc Surg.* 1994;19(4):683–686.

99. Kang SS, Labropoulos N, Mansour MA, et al. Percutaneous ultrasound guided thrombin injection: a new method for treating postcatheterization femoral pseudoaneurysms. *J Vasc Surg.* 1998;27(6):1032–1038.

100. Krugger K, Zahringer M, Sohngen FD, et al. Femoral pseudoaneurysms: management with percutaneous thrombin injections-success rates and effects on systemic coagulation. *Radiology.* 2003:226(2):452–458.

101. Padberg FT, Calligaro K, Sidawy AN, et al. Complications of arteriovenous hemodialysis access: recognition and management. *J Vasc Surg.* 2008;48:55S–80S.

102. Ascher EA, Hingori AP, Marks NA, et al. Duplex-guided balloon angioplasty of failing or nonmaturing arterio-venous fistulae for hemodialysis: a new office based procedure. *J Vasc Surg.* 2009;50(3):594–599.

103. Fox D, Amador F, Clarke D, et al. *Duplex Guided Dialysis Access Angioplasty can be Performed Safely in the Office Setting: Techniques, Advantages and Results.* 2010 SVS Vascular Annual Meeting, June 9–13, Boston, MA, USA.

104. Van den Bos R, Arends L, Kockaert M, et al. Endovenous therapy of lower extremity varicosities: a meta-analysis. *J Vasc Surg.* 2009;49(1):230–239.

105. Pichot O, Kabnick LS, Creton D, et al. Duplex ultrasound scan findings two years after great saphenous vein radiofrequency endovenous obliteration. *J Vasc Surg.* 2004;39(1):189–95.

106. Min RJ, Zimmet SE, Isaacs MN, et al. Endovenous laser treatment of the incompetent greater saphenous vein. *J Vasc Interven Radiol.* 2001;12(10):1167–1171.

107. Puggioni A, Kalra M, Carmo M, et al. Endovenous laser therapy and radiofrequency ablation of the great saphenous vein: analysis of early efficacy and complications. *J Vasc Surg.* 2005;42(3):488–493.

15

ULTRASOUND-GUIDED REGIONAL ANESTHESIA

ANIS DIZDAREVIC, STEVEN YAP, EUGENE GARVIN, & CAMERON MARSHALL

INTRODUCTION

The use of ultrasound guidance for peripheral nerve blocks in regional anesthesia and pain management offers several advantages over traditional methods including the paresthesia technique and neural stimulation technique. Studies in regional anesthesia and pain medicine seem to indicate that ultrasound guidance can decrease the time required to perform a nerve block and hasten the onset of block, thus potentially improving efficiency between operative cases. Patient discomfort may also be reduced as ultrasound decreases the number of attempted needle passes while performing a block. Direct visualization of neural and vascular structures, including the use of Doppler and visual confirmation of local anesthetic spread around the target nerves, could decrease the risk of intravascular injection, intraneural injection, injury to the lung, or other nearby vital structures.

In this chapter, we provide an overview of the most commonly performed ultrasound-guided peripheral nerve blocks in regional anesthesia and pain medicine, along with their clinical indications.

THORACIC PARAVERTEBRAL BLOCK

Thoracic paravertebral block provides a viable alternative to intercostal nerve blocks and thoracic epidural catheter placement. Continuous paravertebral blockade using a catheter can provide a similar reduction in postoperative pain scores as thoracic epidural blockade, but is associated with less profound sympathetic blockade, resulting in less hypotension and urinary retention (especially when unilateral block is performed). Thoracic paravertebral blocks are indicated for surgical anesthesia and analgesia for thoracic, upper abdominal, cardiac, and breast surgeries, as well as chronic pain management for post-thoracotomy pain syndrome, rib fractures, intercostal neuralgia, and other painful conditions requiring analgesia of the trunk.

▶ Normal Anatomy

The paravertebral space is a wedge-shaped region demarcated by the superior costo-transverse ligament (posterior border), parietal pleura (anterolateral border), and lateral surface of the transverse process (medial border). It should be noted that the medial aspect of the paravertebral space communicates with the epidural space. The paravertebral space contains the intercostal or spinal nerves, blood vessels, rami communicantes, dorsal rami, and the sympathetic chain.

▶ Scanning Technique and Ultrasound Appearance

The procedure is performed with the patient in sitting, lateral decubitus, or prone positions. The ultrasound transducer can be positioned in the longitudinal parasagittal plane or transverse (axial) plane. Insertion of the needle in-plane with the ultrasound transducer is highly recommended (if not mandatory) to allow for complete visualization of the entire needle at all times and avoid puncturing the pleura.

Transverse approach

Using a linear, high-frequency (10–12 MHz) transducer, the ultrasound probe is placed parallel to the appropriate intercostal level, just lateral to the spinous process. The image is optimized by adjusting for the appropriate depth of field (usually within 3–5 cm), focus, and gain. The spinous process and the corresponding transverse process are visualized as hyperechoic lines with acoustic shadows underneath. The hypoechoic wedge-shaped paravertebral space is identified by scanning lateral to the transverse process. Care should be taken to identify the underlying pleura (Figure 15-1A, A1).

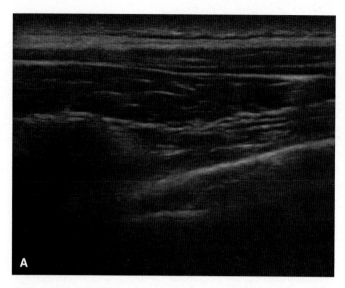

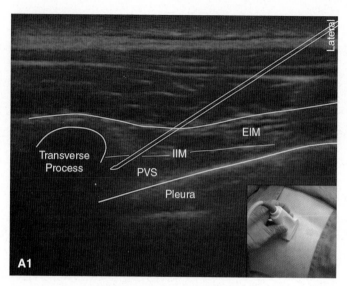

Figure 15-1. (A) Paravertebral space, ultrasound image. **(A1)** Paravertebral space anatomy, ultrasound probe orientation (inset). Transverse process, PVS = paravertebral space, pleura, IIM = internal intercostal membrane, EIM = external intercostal muscle.

NOTE: The pleura is distinguished as a hyperechoic line that moves with respiration and has underlying hyperechoic air artifacts. This is to be distinguished from the rib, which contains an underlying acoustic shadow.

The use of color Doppler may aid in the identification of intercostal vessels in the paravertebral space. Care must be taken to avoid intravascular injection or injury.

In-plane needle insertion approach

The patient's posterior midthoracic area and the ultrasound probe are prepared with standard sterile precautions. The underlying skin is infiltrated with local anesthetic. A 20- or 22-gauge needle is inserted at the lateral end of the ultrasound probe and advanced slowly into the paravertebral space under direct visualization in the lateral to medial direction. It is advisable to turn the bevel of the needle upward, toward the transducer, to reduce the risk of inadvertent puncture of blood vessels, nerves, or pleura. To facilitate better visualization of the needle tip, the hydrodissection technique may be utilized by intermittently injecting small volumes of normal saline to dissect tissue planes while under direct visualization. Once the needle tip penetrates the internal intercostal membrane and enters the paravertebral space, a test dose of local anesthetic (3 mL) can be administered after ensuring negative aspiration for blood or air.

▶ Clinical Pearls and Common Pitfalls

Injection of local anesthetic under direct visualization is highly recommended. If resistance to injection is encountered, the needle should be redirected either more laterally, or the bevel should be rotated into a different plane. Upon injection, the paravertebral space will distend and push the underlying pleura ventrally.

When performing the in-plane needle insertion approach, the needle tip should be visualized at all times in relation to the pleura to avoid the risk of pneumothorax. Frequent aspiration and incremental injection of local anesthetic are recommended to avoid inadvertent intravascular injection and systemic local anesthetic toxicity. Caution should be exercised in anticoagulated patients to avoid multiple needle passes and, thereby, decrease the risk of hematoma.

▶ Case Scenario

A 67-year-old woman with no significant past medical history presents with right-sided chest wall pain that started approximately six months ago. The pain is described as burning, pulling sensation, worse with movement. She describes no preceding rash or blister formation or trauma to the area. Chest x-ray imaging of the ribs and thoracic spine shows no abnormalities. On physical examination, the patient reports tenderness to palpation over the right T7 and T8 dermatomes, in the anterior and midaxillary line. Differential diagnosis includes intercostal neuralgia, and the patient is scheduled for a right T7 paravertebral block. The block is performed under direct ultrasound guidance using a mixture of local anesthetic and steroid. After the procedure, the patient reports greater than 75% decrease in pain intensity and an overall improvement in the activities of daily living. She is advised to return to the pain clinic for a repeat block in the future, if needed.

INTERSCALENE BLOCK

▶ Normal Anatomy and Indications

Motor, sensory, and sympathetic innervation to the upper extremity is supplied by the brachial plexus. The plexus is composed of five nerve roots (C5-T1 ventral rami), three trunks, six divisions, three cords, and five terminal nerves. The nerve roots travel through the interscalene groove, which is situated between the anterior and middle scalene muscles at the level of the cricoid cartilage (C6), superior to the subclavian artery. The vertebral artery lies anteriorly, and the phrenic nerve travels between the anterior scalene and sternocleidomastoid muscles.

The interscalene block was originally described by Winnie, and it targets the brachial plexus at the cervical root and trunk level. It is utilized mostly in regional anesthesia for operative procedures involving the shoulder and lateral clavicle to the elbow area. Continuous interscalene block with a catheter can also be used for postoperative analgesia.

▶ Normal Appearance on Ultrasound

In the interscalene groove, the roots/trunks of the brachial plexus appear hypoechoic with hyperechoic fascia sheaths, often described as a "honeycomb" appearance, in the short axis. Color Doppler should be used to identify and confirm the carotid, subclavian, and vertebral arteries.

▶ Scanning Technique

Images are obtained using a linear, high-frequency (10–15 MHz) transducer set to 2–3 cm depth with the patient supine and the head slightly turned to the contralateral side. The interscalene groove may be visualized by scanning from identifiable anatomical landmarks superiorly or inferiorly. Starting inferiorly, the probe is placed in the supraclavicular fossa, parallel to the clavicle, where the trunks of the brachial plexus are identified along with the subclavian artery. The neurovascular bundle is followed in short-axis view up to the interscalene groove, between the anterior and middle scalene muscles. The probe should be oriented perpendicular to the interscalene groove (Figure 15-2A, A1).

Alternatively, scanning superiorly, the probe may be placed in the interscalene groove at the level of the cricoid cartilage and swept laterally. Regardless of the approach, a systematic anatomical survey should always be performed with critical structures identified, including the carotid, vertebra,l and subclavian arteries, C6 transverse processes, and intervertebral foramina.

▶ Block Technique

After appropriate aseptic preparation of both the neck area and the ultrasound transducer, the injection site is infiltrated with local anesthetic, and a 22-gauge 5 cm needle is advanced either in-plane or out of plane to the ultrasound transducer. For the in-plane approach, the needle is inserted along the posterior-lateral border of the probe and is directly visualized as it advances lateral to medial through the medial scalene muscle into the interscalene groove. The out-of-plane approach may be performed on either the cranial or caudal side of the probe; this technique, however, is suboptimal as it does not allow for direct visual tracking of the needle through the tissue, and it is almost never used. Hydrodissection may be used to identify the tip of the needle, as visualization is more difficult with this approach. Injected solutions will appear hypoechoic.

▶ Common Findings/Abnormalities

Although frequently described as arising from C5-T1, the brachial plexus may be prefixed, with the ventral ramus of C4 contributing, or postfixed, with the ventral ramus of T2 contributing.

▶ Common Pitfalls

Complications may include nerve damage, intravascular injection, epidural and intrathecal injections, and hematoma. Pneumothorax can occur if the needle enters the cupola of the lung (block performed more distally). Local anesthetic central nervous system toxicity can occur if the

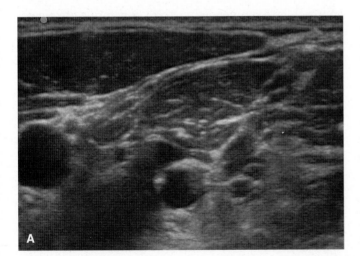
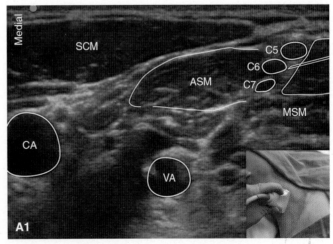

Figure 15-2. (A) Interscalene anatomy, ultrasound image. **(A1)** Interscalene anatomy, ultrasound probe orientation (inset). CA = carotid artery, SCM = sternocleidomastoid muscle, VA = vertebral artery, ASM = anterior scalene muscle, MSM = middle scalene muscle, C5, C6, C7 = cervical nerve roots.

needle enters the vertebral artery, and spinal or epidural anesthesia may occur if the needle enters the intervertebral foramina. Direct visualization of the needle tip should be maintained during advancement of the needle into tissue, as well as during injection of local anesthetic.

Injection too close to the transverse process may compress the roots against bony structures. The roots of C8 and T1 may be more difficult to visualize in the interscalene groove, and thus more difficult to anesthetize. If this occurs, "ulnar sparing" (or inadequate anesthesia of the medial forearm and hand) may occur with the absence of ulnar nerve blockade. If necessary, a selective ulnar nerve block may be performed, either at the infraclavicular level or at the elbow.

▶ Clinical Pearls

Common side effects that can occur, especially after a large-volume interscalene block, are Horner syndrome, as the sympathetic chain may be anesthetized, and phrenic nerve palsy, with resulting diaphragmatic hemiparesis. Thus, the interscalene block should be performed with caution in patients with respiratory insufficiency, as it may result in respiratory distress. In addition, due to the risk of phrenic nerve blockade and pneumothorax, the interscalene block should never be performed bilaterally.

▶ Case Scenario

A 72-year-old man presents for a right total shoulder replacement surgery. He has a history of obstructive sleep apnea and sensitivity to opioid medications, and is anxious about the postoperative pain control and recovery.

During preoperative anesthetic evaluation, risks and benefits of general anesthesia versus regional anesthesia using interscalene block are discussed. The benefits of regional anesthesia may include: decreased use of opioid medications and opioid-related side effects such as sedation, respiratory depression, mental status changes, nausea, decrease in anesthetic requirements during the surgery and faster recovery time, and avoidance of general anesthesia and its associated cardiopulmonary side effects.

Prior to surgery start, the patient undergoes an ultrasound-guided interscalene block with local anesthetic and catheter placement for postoperative pain control via infusion. He reports excellent pain relief after the surgery, requiring minimal amount of supplemental pain medications.

The interscalene catheter is removed on postoperative day 2, and the patient is discharged home soon after on an oral pain medication regimen.

SUPRACLAVICULAR BLOCK

▶ Normal Anatomy and Indications

As described previously, the trunks of the brachial plexus exit the interscalene groove and pass under the clavicle. In the supraclavicular fossa, the superior and middle trunks lie superior to the subclavian artery, and the inferior trunk lies posterior. The neurovascular bundle is immediately superior to the first rib and 1–2 cm superior to the pleura.

The supraclavicular block was originally described by Hirschel and Kulenkampff. It targets the trunks/divisions of the brachial plexus and is ideal for anesthesia and analgesia of the arm, forearm, and hand.

▶ Normal Appearance on Ultrasound

The subclavian artery can be visualized in the short axis as it passes under the clavicle. The subclavian vein is anterior and medial to the artery. The trunks, divisions, and cords appear hypoechoic, with hyperechoic surrounding fascia giving them the appearance of a "grapelike" structure. It should be noted that the number of fascicles visualized varies widely and can range from a few to as many as a dozen. Inferiorly, the first rib appears hyperechoic with an underlying acoustic shadow. Deep to it, the pleura appears as a hyperechoic line lacking an acoustic shadow. Deep to the pleura, the lung may be identified by its expansion during respiration and also by looking for the "comet tail artifact," which occurs when two highly reflective acoustic layers of different acoustic impedance cause the echo to bounce back and forth quickly, appearing as a narrow striped band.

▶ Scanning Technique

The scanning technique for a supraclavicular block is similar to that of an interscalene block. The patient is positioned supine, and the head is turned slightly to the contralateral side. A linear 10–15-MHz high-frequency probe is placed in the supraclavicular fossa parallel to the clavicle and rotated into a coronal oblique position. The probe is swept medially until the subclavian artery is identified. Once this landmark is obtained, a systematic anatomical survey should be performed with the artery, first rib, pleura, and lung identified (Figure 15-3A, A1).

The block may be performed with a 22-gauge 5-cm needle, with a scanning depth of 2–3 cm. The in-plane approach is recommended to avoid puncturing the pleura. For this approach, the needle is inserted lateral to the probe and slowly advanced in lateral to medial plane under direct visualization. Hydrodissection may help confirm the needle tip position. The tip of the needle should be lateral to the artery and superior to the pleura. A medial approach is also described in which the tip of the needle points away from the subclavian artery during injection; however, the subclavian artery can obscure the medial and inferior trunks with this approach.

▶ Common Findings and Clinical Pearls

On occasions, the clavicle may obstruct the view of the neurovascular bundle. A smaller ultrasound probe and slight angulation may be used to facilitate better visualization. If there is difficulty locating the subclavian artery, the carotid artery can be scanned first and traced down to the bifurcation. Hypoechoic vessels can sometimes be

general anesthesia. Prior to surgery, the patient undergoes an ultrasound-guided sciatic nerve block and femoral nerve block with a catheter placement for postoperative pain control. The surgery is performed under a spinal block and monitored anesthesia care.

HIP JOINT INJECTION

▶ Normal Anatomy and Indications

The hip joint, also known as the acetabulofemoral joint, is a ball-and-socket type synovial joint formed by articulation of the femoral head within the acetabulum of the pelvis. Three bones of the pelvis, the ilium, pubis, and ischium, join to form the acetabular socket. The femoral capsule surrounds the neck of the femur, thus securing the femoral head against the acetabulum.

The femoral neurovascular bundle overlies the hip joint anteriorly within the femoral triangle and should be avoided during injection of the hip joint. This triangle is bounded superiorly by the inguinal ligament, medially by the adductor longus muscle, and laterally by the sartorius muscle.

Palpation of the hip joint is limited mainly to the greater trochanter. As a result, blind injection of the hip can be difficult, may traumatize the femoral neurovascular bundle, and may result in injection outside the hip joint in 20% to 48% of the time. Flouroscopically guided injections facilitate accurate placement of the needle near the hip joint, but do not aid in avoidance of the femoral neurovascular bundle. Hip joint injection is indicated in chronic painful hip joint conditions, such as osteoarthritis of the hip.

▶ Normal Appearance on Ultrasound

In the longitudinal view, the femur appears as a hyperechoic line with an underlying acoustic echo. The concavity of the femoral neck lies between the femoral head and femoral shaft. The iliofemoral ligament overlies the femoral head and terminates proximal to the anterior synovial recess.

▶ Scanning Technique

The patient is positioned supine with the hip placed in a neutral position. After skin sterilization and draping, the femoral pulse is palpated, or alternatively, the femoral neurovascular bundle is visualized under ultrasound so as to avoid injury during the procedure. A 1–5 MHz curvilinear transducer is placed in a longitudinal plane parallel to the femoral neck and lateral to the femoral neurovascular structures. Color Doppler should be used to exclude any blood vessels along the path of injection. A 22-gauge, 9-cm spinal needle is inserted and advanced in-plane to the target site at the anterior synovial recess, maintaining visualization of the needle tip at all times. As the needle is advanced, resistance may be felt as the iliofemoral ligament is penetrated. The syringe is then aspirated prior to injection of steroid, local anesthetic, or hyaluronate (Figure 15-6A, A1).

▶ Common Findings and Abnormalities

Palpation of the hip joint is obscured by overlying muscular tissue and subcutaneous fat. As a result, the success rate of blind hip injections may be as low as 52%, and may pass within 4.5 mm of the overlying femoral nerve. While the hip joint may be adequately visualized with a 5- to 10-MHz linear transducer in thin patients, a 1- to 5-MHz curvilinear transducer may be required in most patients.

▶ Common Pitfalls

Paresthesia in the anterolateral aspect of the ipsilateral lower extremity upon insertion of the needle should alert the practitioner to possible puncture of the femoral nerve. Failure to inject local anesthetic into the hip joint, or injection of a large volume of local anesthetics may result in weakness or numbness of the muscles overlying the hip joint. Care should be taken to avoid intra-arterial injection of particulate steroids, especially near the femoral neck, as this may result in steroid particles lodging in the blood vessels and compromising the perfusion to the joint, possibly leading to avascular necrosis of the hip.

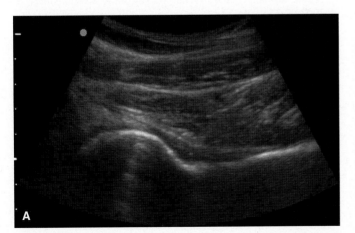

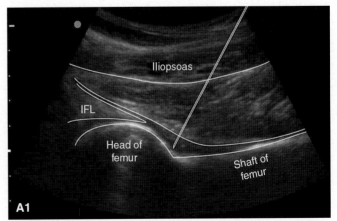

Figure 15-6. (**A**) Hip joint anatomy, ultrasound image. (**A1**) Hip joint anatomy, Iliopsoas muscle, IFL = iliofemoral ligament.

▶ Clinical Pearls

Intra-articular injection can be confirmed by injection of air into the anterior synovial recess under ultrasound visualization. Collection of hyperechoic air in a nondependent fashion along the joint capsule is indicative of an intra-articular injection, whereas collection of air locally around the needle tip suggests incorrect needle placement.

▶ Case Scenario

A 65-year-old woman presents to a pain clinic with several months' history of left anterior hip and groin pain. The pain is very limiting, worse with walking and physical activity and better with rest. She is unable to take non-steroidal-anti-inflammatory (NSAIDS) medications due to her chronic renal insufficiency and gastroesophageal reflux disease. Hip imaging reveals severe osteoarthritis without fracture or dislocation.

The patient undergoes an ultrasound-guided hip joint injection with local anesthetic and steroid, reporting greater than 50% pain relief afterward, lasting for several weeks.

The patient is advised to return to the clinic if her pain worsens in the future, as the steroid injection can be repeated every 3–4 months, if needed.

In summary, ultrasound has evolved as a significant and valuable tool and advance in the field of regional anesthesia and pain medicine. Over the past decade there has been growing evidence to suggest some potential benefits of ultrasound over its comparator techniques. Future studies, especially randomized controlled trials and well-designed meta-analyses, will be needed to further explore the clinical advantages of ultrasound guidance in regional anesthesia, such as whether or not its use reduces the procedure-related complication rate, improves patient safety, and reduces the need to convert to general anesthesia or alternative technique.

SUGGESTED READINGS

Bendtsen T, Nielsen, T, Rhode C, Kibak K, Linde F. Ultrasound guidance improves continuous popliteal sciatic nerve block when compared with nerve stimulation. *Reg Anesth Pain Med.* 2011;36:181–184.

Brull R, Macfarlane A, Parrington S, Koshkin A, Chan V. Is circumfrential injection advantageous for ultrasound-guided popliteal sciatic nerve block? *Reg Anesth Pain Med.* 2011;36:266–270.

Cheng P, Kim H, et al. Ultrasound-guided injections of the knee and hip. *Tech Reg Anesth Pain Manag.* 2009;13:191–197.

Davies R, Myles P, Grahamm J. A comparison of the analgesic efficacy and side-effects of paravertebral vs epidural blockade for thoracotomy—a systematic review and meta-analysis of randomized trials. *Brit J Anesth.* 2006;96(4): 418–426.

Kapral S, Greher M, Huber G, Willschke H, Kettner S, Kdolsky R, Marhofer P. Ultrasonographic guidance improves the success rate of interscalene brachial plexus blockade. *Reg Anesth Pain Med.* 2008 May–Jun;33(3): 253–258.

Liu SS, Ngeow JE, YaDeau JT. Ultrasound-guided regional anesthesia and analgesia. *Reg Anesth Pain Med.* 2009;34(1):47–59.

Marhofer P, Schrogendorfer K, Wallner T, Koinig H, Mayer N, Kapral S. Ultrasonographic guidance reduces the amount of local anesthetic for 3-1 block. *Reg Anesth Pain Med.* 1998;26:584–588.

Neal JM, Brull R, Chan VW, Grant SA, Horn JL, Liu SS, McCartney CJ, Narouze SN, Perlas A, Salinas FV, Sites BD, Tsui BC. The ASRA evidence-based medicine assessment of ultrasound-guided regional anesthesia and pain medicine: Executive summary. *Reg Anesth Pain Med.* 2010 Mar–Apr; 35(2 Suppl):S1–9.

O Riain SC, Donnell BO, Cuffe T, Harmon DC, Fraher JP, Shorten G. Thoracic paravertebral block using real-time ultrasound guidance. *Anesth Analg.* 2010 Jan 1;110(1): 248–251.

Prasad A, Perlas A, Ramlogan R, Brull R, Chan V. Ultrasound guided popliteal block distal to sciatic nerve bifurcation shortens onset time. *Reg Anesth Pain Med.* 2010;35: 267–271.

Shibata Y, Nishiwaki K. Ultrasound-guided intercostal approach to thoracic paravertebral block. *Anesth Analg.* 2009 Sep;109(3):996–997.

Smith J, Hurdle MF, Weingarten TN. Accuracy of sonographically guided intra-articular injections in the native adult hip. *J Ultrasound Med.* 2009;28:329–335.

Soong J, Schafhalter-Zoppoth I, Gray AT. The importance of transducer angle to Ultrasound visibility of the femoral nerve. *Reg Anesth Pain Med.* 2005;30:505.

Ultrasound for Regional Anesthesia. 2008. July 20, 2011 http://www.usra.ca

Vincent W S C, Anahi P, Regan R, Olusegun O. Ultrasound-guided supraclavicular brachial plexus block. *Anesth Analg.* 2003;97:1514–1517.

Xavier D, Pascal H, Nathalie B, Christian F, Jean-Paul F, Anne C. Sonographic mapping of the normal brachial plexus. *Am J Neuroradiol.* 2003;24:1303.

16

THERAPEUTIC ULTRASOUND

BETH SCHROPE

One of the chief reasons for using ultrasound as a diagnostic modality relates to its superior safety profile, where the principle of ALARA (as low as reasonably achievable) yields great information at low energy. Yet, when ultrasound energy is employed at higher powers, it offers a number of therapeutic possibilities. Not needing the high frequencies required for imaging resolution also permits greater depth of penetration if desired.

Therapeutic ultrasound interventions can be divided into two categories: low-power and high-power applications. The low-power group includes physiotherapy, sonophoresis and sonoporation (both methods of enhancing drug delivery), gene therapy, ultrasound-assisted thrombolysis, and bone healing. High-intensity focused ultrasound (HIFU), surgical energy devices, and lithotripsy are the more common applications in the high-power group.

The physics of therapeutic ultrasound encompasses both thermal and nonthermal effects of acoustic energy. At high intensity or energy, heating of surrounding tissue from absorption dominates, while at lower intensities, the nonthermal or mechanical effects of cavitation, acoustic streaming, and microstreaming are observed. The latter effects are thought to result from scattering of the ultrasound energy, leading to mechanical changes in the medium (tissue).

As described in detail in the physics chapter, as it travels through tissue the ultrasound wave is subject to absorption, scattering, reflection, rarefaction, etc. Absorption leads to the generation of heat within the tissue, the degree of which depends on the intensity of the incident wave. Intensity is simply defined as the power density within an area (spatial average), or at its peak (spatial peak). However, when considering pulsed ultrasound (which allows for delivery of greater power), one must take into account the duration of the pulse when describing intensity. One could, for example, describe the power delivered only over the duration of the pulse itself (pulse average), or averaged over a period to include the time between pulses (temporal average). From this discussion it can be seen then that intensity may be described in a number of ways, including I_{SATA} (spatial average, temporal average), I_{SPTA} (spatial peak, temporal average), or I_{SPPA} (spatial peak, pulse average). Generally, in therapeutic ultrasound applications where tissue heating is the goal, the term I_{SATA} is used as it gives the best sense of the net thermal effect of the ultrasound beam.

A focused rise in temperature such as that afforded by ultrasound offers therapeutic benefits for perhaps a number of reasons. For example, hyperemia occurs as tissue is warmed, and the increased blood supply in a certain area may enhance the therapeutic effects of certain drugs or radiation therapy. Hyperthermia treatments in the temperature range of 43–50°C cause cessation of cell reproduction. Delivery of the heat must be sustained for up to an hour. HIFU results in a concentration of heat to temperatures of around 56°C, which causes instantaneous cell death (and thus need only be sustained for a few seconds).

To summarize then the thermal effects of ultrasound can be manipulated for different therapeutic goals. Higher frequency results in greater absorption, and thus increased thermal energy; as in diagnostic ultrasound; however, higher frequency sacrifices depth of penetration. Intensity is manipulated by increasing the power delivery to the transducer, or by increasing the duty cycle. Finally, treatment time is adjusted for desired therapeutic effect.

The nonthermal effects are thought to arise from the scattering of the ultrasound beam as it traverses tissue. The perturbation of the tissue causes mechanical changes in the medium. Cavitation refers to the formation and behavior of microbubbles in tissue. If certain conditions are met, microbubbles may be formed from dissolved gas in the medium. Or, air cavities may be naturally occurring, such as in the lung alveoli, or bubbles may be iatrogenically introduced, as in ultrasound contrast agents. As the ultrasound wave compresses and rarefacts through the medium, it causes microbubbles in the tissue to contract and expand.

The potential for cavitation to occur and its relative magnitude is related to numerous factors, including frequency, amplitude, pulse duration, and pulse repetition frequency. Acoustic streaming is related to the concept of cavitation, except that it describes the behavior of the medium around the bubbles as a consequence of their vibration. These shear stresses have been shown to be capable of displacing ions and small molecules, potentially rendering cell membranes transiently more permeable, for example.

LOW-POWER APPLICATIONS

▶ Physical Therapy

Physical therapists utilize several energy-based therapies in their arsenal to treat specific injuries or illnesses, including ultrasound, laser, electrical nerve stimulation, or even hydrotherapy. These therapies including ultrasound are used to accelerate and enhance tissue repair and regeneration. As indicated above, there are two mechanisms of action of therapeutic ultrasound: thermal and nonthermal. Heat generated by the absorption of ultrasound energy in tissue dilates blood vessels, increasing the volume of a multitude of circulating factors for tissue repair. In addition, heat has an analgesic effect on nerves. Tissue composition also determines the magnitude of thermal effect; protein has a higher absorption coefficient than fat and water. Thus, fatty tissue and blood (high water and/or fat content) do not experience as much of a thermal effect as ligament and tendon (higher protein, lower water content). Although cartilage and bone have the highest protein content, acoustic impedance mismatching results in a higher proportion of ultrasound energy being reflected than absorbed. The best absorbing tissues in terms of clinical practice are those with high collagen content: ligament, tendon, fascia, joint capsule, and scar tissue. Nonthermal mechanisms, such as acoustic streaming and cavitation, effect changes in membrane permeability and hence the movement of essential ions and nutrients into and out of the cell. Thus, it can be said to achieve an upregulation of cellular activity triggered by ultrasound energy.

Although there is conflicting clinical evidence to support the use of ultrasound to facilitate the treatment of injured ligaments, tendons, and joints, and to alleviate symptoms associated with excessive scar tissue, it is widely used today for such purposes. Indeed, much of the conviction surrounding the efficacy of ultrasound in treating soft tissue injury and pain originates from in vitro studies, which have not been duplicated in vivo (Baker et al, 2001). Within the most recent decade more clinically oriented papers have attested to the utility of therapeutic ultrasound in conditions such as osteoarthritis, carpal tunnel syndrome, myofascial pain syndrome, among others. Despite its widespread application in clinical use, there remains little standardization in terms of duration of therapy, frequency and intensity range, and number of treatments. The most common frequency range found on physical therapy ultrasound units is 0.7 to 3.3 MHz.

▶ Bone Healing

There have been many published reports of the benefit of ultrasound on bone regeneration in all types of bone injury including fresh fractures, nonunion and delayed union fractures, and for enhanced ossification in distraction osteogenesis. Fracture healing is a complex process that can be divided into three phases: reactive, reparative, and remodeling. The reactive phase is characterized by hemostasis and inflammation; the reparative phase heralds the formation of a fracture callus, where primitive bone and collagen cells begin the process of rebuilding across the fracture, and in the remodeling phase, the final constitution of mature compact bone is gradually replaced along the fracture. The first phase is relatively brief, and the cells of the reparative phase are seen within days of bone injury; complete healing is only seen 3 to 5 years after injury. It is the hyperactive first two phases that are the most sensitive to ultrasound therapies. Low-intensity pulsed ultrasound or LIPUS was approved by the FDA in 1994 for stimulating bone growth in a number of applications including fracture healing and dental applications. It generally utilizes 1.5-MHz frequency pulses, with a pulse width of 200 μs, duty cycle of 1 kHz, at an intensity of 30 mW/cm^2, 20 min/day.

Observations of ultrasound stimulation of bone healing are based on in vitro and animal models, and include increased secretion of cytokines (IL-1β) and angiogenesis-inducing factors (IL-8, b-FGF, VEGF), leading to cell proliferation, collagen production, bone formation, and angiogenesis. The biophysical principle of this cellular recruitment by ultrasound, however, remains unproven. Hypotheses include: a thermal effect from the absorption of energy in tissues, which may increase collagenase activity; the strain effect from the acoustic energy that may stimulate periosteal bone formation; and cavitation that increases protein and collagen synthesis, but the exact mechanism is yet unknown.

LIPUS has the advantage of being a safe, low-energy, low-cost and efficacious method for encouraging more rapid healing of bony fractures. Although there is a lack of rigorous randomized controlled studies, this shortcoming is shared with all other treatments of fractures. Some may hail the necessary duration of treatment as lengthy, in the range of 3 to 6 months, although this likely represents an acceleration of the natural healing process.

▶ Sonophoresis

Transdermal drug delivery offers the advantage of improved patient comfort and thus compliance over needle injection, and avoids the first-pass metabolism observed with many oral drugs. The composition of human skin, however, limits the usefulness of this technique to a few low-molecular weight (<500 Da) lipophilic drugs, and in small doses. In particular, the stratum corneum, with its matrix of corneocytes embedded in lipid bilayers, is a highly impermeable membrane. Insonifying skin with acoustic waves in the frequency range 20 to 100 kHz has been shown to increase its permeability to macromolecules, a process known as sonophoresis. Initially devised for local delivery of drugs, it is now being investigated for systemic drug delivery.

Low-frequency sonophoresis can be divided into two types: simultaneous sonophoresis and pretreatment. As is implied, simultaneous sonophoresis involves administering the drug in synchrony with the application of ultrasound. This technique increases skin's permeability to the molecule by enhancing diffusion via structural alterations of the skin (defects in the stratum corneum), and by inducing convective solvent flow by cavitation. This effect can be quantified by measuring the skin's electrical resistivity or impedance, which decreases in the presence of ultrasound.

Clinically sonophoresis has been used to enhance the local delivery of topical local anesthestic, by decreasing dramatically the application time needed for effect. Animal studies are ongoing with respect to systemic delivery of macromolecules, including proteins such as insulin and heparin, or immunogens such as tetanus toxoid. Sonophoresis is generally a safe process, if maintained within certain parameters of frequency, intensity, duty cycle, and application time. Specifically, intensities greater than 4 W/cm^2 have been shown to result in epidermal detachment and dermal necrosis. Continuous monitoring of skin's impedance can be employed to ensure safety during use.

▶ Sonoporation and Gene Therapy

Sonoporation refers to enhancing the permeability of a cell membrane with ultrasound (as opposed to skin structure in sonophoresis). This effect is being studied to allow the introduction of large molecules, such as DNA, into the cytoplasm of a cell. The ability to focus ultrasound naturally offers a method for targeted therapy of only diseased tissue. The mechanism of action is presumed to be cavitation-induced deformation or disruption of the cell membrane; a balance must naturally be achieved in choosing therapeutic parameters to avoid cell death, if that is not the desired effect. Genetic material may be introduced in various ways, including local administration, whereby it is transfected as the cell membrane is rendered permeable by ultrasound, or bound to a microbubble membrane or contained within the confines of the bubble, where it will be released with the resultant cavitation response to ultrasound.

▶ Ultrasound-Assisted Thrombolysis

Several observations have been published indicating that ultrasound can enhance the dissolution of blood clots, either through an inherent acoustic property or with the delivery of microbubble-encapsulated thrombolytic agents. Although no definitive mechanism of ultrasound-alone sonothrombolysis has been proven, it is supposed that acoustic cavitation plays a role by inducing changes in the fibrin microstructure and disaggregation of the fibrin into smaller units. Most of the efforts at sonothrombolysis today focus on augmenting delivery of clot-dissolving

enzymes such as tPA or urokinase into the clot, perhaps by jettisoning the drug into the clot via acoustically generated channels. A widely quoted study (TRUMBI – transcranial low-frequency ultrasound-mediated thrombolysis in brain ischemia) showed definitive improvement in intracranial recanalization after ischemic stroke, 49% in the ultrasound group versus 30% in the tPA group alone. Unfortunately this trial was prematurely aborted due to a high intracranial hemorrhage rate.

HIGH-POWER APPLICATIONS

▶ Lithotripsy

Extracorporeal shockwave lithotripsy (ESWL) first came into clinical use in the early 1980s, and now is a standard first-line treatment for nephrolithiasis. This procedure involves the application of a focused, high-intensity acoustic pulse to genitourinary stones, breaking them into small pieces that can then be passed spontaneously via the urine stream. Guidance systems are generally fluoroscopic, but ultrasound guidance may also be used. Sometimes a ureteral stent is placed to facilitate passage of the stone fragments. ESWL is the least invasive of the treatment modalities for nephrolithiasis, which includes percutaneous nephrolithotomy and laser-assisted ureteroscopy, and, in select circumstances, has an equivalent success rate. ESWL has also been applied to other stone diseases, such as gallstones and pancreatic stones, with less success and adoption for various reasons.

A typical acoustically generated shock wave is a very short pulse of about 5-μs duration, with near instantaneous (nanosecond) escalation to peak positive pressure, from 30 to 110 MPa. The positive portion of the pulse (shock front) has duration of about 1 μs, which is followed by a drop to a negative pressure (compressive phase) of about –10 MPa. Finally there is a short tail or tensile phase, familiar in the context of this text as a rarefaction of the acoustic wave. The pulse does not have a dominant frequency; rather, its energy is spread over a large range, typically from 100 kHz to 1 MHz.

Three different types of shockwave generators have been applied in clinical lithotripsy applications: electrohydraulic, electromagnetic, and piezoelectric. In the electrohydraulic generator, a high-voltage spark between two electrodes at the tip of a probe creates a hydraulic shockwave that can be focused on a calculus by an ellipsoid reflector. The electromagnetic lithotripter uses an electrical coil to generate the electrical pulse, which in turn creates a force on a metal plate to generate an acoustic wave. A concave plate is used to focus the acoustic wave in a predictable manner. Lastly, piezoelectric generators produce shockwaves via ultrasonic vibrations, resulting from the application of high-frequency electrical pulses to piezoelectric elements.

Numerous mechanisms of stone fragmentation have been proposed. The shockwaves propagate through the body with minimal collateral damage, as there is little difference in density among the soft tissues. At the stone-tissue/fluid interface, however, the marked difference in density causes the generation of compressive forces in the denser medium. At proper settings this energy is greater than the tensile strength of the stone, and the stone fragments. Spallation occurs when the shockwave passes through the stone and reflects from the rear border. This interface then inverts the positive pressure pulse, creating a tensile stress (as opposed to the compressive stress on the way in). The alternating compression and tension further weakens or fatigues the stone. Cavitation in the urine around the stone is seen in response to the tensile tail of the acoustic impulse. Collapse of microbubbles generates a microjet that impacts the stone surface. In addition, secondary shockwaves are generated with similar effect as the focused shockwave. Delivery of repeated shockwaves eventually leads to pulverization of the stone, which then ideally passes via the urine stream.

▶ High-Intensity Focused Ultrasound (HIFU)

High-frequency diagnostic ultrasound has the advantage of precise definition of structures, albeit at the cost of increased attenuation of the signal and thus a limitation on imaging depth. When the acoustic energy is to be employed as therapy, and high incident intensities are desirable, this translates to a precise delivery of therapeutic ultrasound. In this case, the effect is predominantly thermal, with temperatures of approximately 60°C in the focal region when an exemplary intensity of 1,500 W/cm^2 is applied for 1–2 seconds. This leads to instantaneous cell death and coagulative necrosis, with a margin of 6–10 cells between the focal zone and unaffected tissue. Incorporation of dual diagnostic and therapeutic imaging modes builds a targeted therapy system for tissue destruction. HIFU has been used historically as one of many treatments for prostate cancer, and is gaining popularity in treatment of tumors of the liver, kidney, uterus, and breast, as well as treatment for atrial fibrillation.

The need for precise temperature monitoring as an indicator of therapy progress has led to the development of MRI as a concurrent diagnostic imaging mode, to monitor therapy online. Unfortunately this is limited by motion artifact, equipment, and cost issues. Diagnostic ultrasound presents limited ability to monitor tissue changes related to temperature, but advances in elastography, ultrasound-stimulated acoustic emission, and radiation force measurement are potentially opening the door for accurate ultrasound-based therapy monitoring.

Although the primary effect of HIFU is coagulative necrosis by thermal absorption, investigation into utilizing the cavitation effect for enhanced heat delivery and reduced treatment times is underway. Previously avoided as unpredictable, controlled promotion of cavitation with more sophisticated monitoring and the introduction of microbubble-based contrast agents reduce treatment times and deliver more accurate beam shapes.

Many treatment options exist for prostate cancer, including traditional surgery, radiation therapy, cryosurgery, brachytherapy, and hormone therapy. HIFU emerged in the late 1980s as a viable option in appropriate circumstances of early-stage cancers. It is typically delivered via a dual diagnostic-therapeutic endorectal probe, with the patient under spinal or general anesthesia. Three-dimensional imaging advances have increased the accuracy of treatment, and advances in tissue signature detection allow monitoring of the effectiveness of the ablation in real time. Several commercial systems are available, delivering therapy in the frequency range of 3 to 4 MHz with intensities of 1300 to 220 W/cm^2. These systems produce temperatures in the focal zone of around 60°C. Because of the ability to target therapy precisely, effect on adjacent structures such as the bladder neck or sphincter is greatly reduced, thus diminishing the risk of urinary dysfunction.

HIFU for treatment of symptomatic uterine fibroids was approved by the FDA in 2004. Again, HIFU confers an advantage over surgery in that it minimally invasively targets the diseased tissue only, sparing surrounding structures. HIFU treatment systems for uterine fibroids often employ magnetic resonance imaging for targeting and monitoring of tissue temperature as a gauge for therapy.

Given the success and widespread adoption of HIFU for treatment of cancer of the prostate, the technology has been applied to many other tumors including kidney, breast, brain, bone, liver, pancreas, rectum, and testes. The above-mentioned advantages apply to these cancers as well, avoiding radical surgery and surrounding tissue damage with precise treatment of the tumor, in some cases curative and in other cases palliative.

HIFU ablation for the minimally invasive treatment of atrial fibrillation offers an exciting alternative to the more invasive MAZE and energy (RF, microwave, and cryotherapy) ablative procedures. In addition, HIFU may be performed on a beating heart, thus obviating the need for coronary bypass. HIFU effectively destroys tissue in the focal region, thus disrupting transmission of abnormal electrical impulses. Several early case series reported successful ablation and return to normal rhythm at rates comparable to RF and cryotherapy, and better than microwave ablation, on the order of 70–80% in one year. There is controversy over disparate data, however, with concern that acoustic radiation force and acoustic cavitation in conjunction with inconsistent thermal deposition can increase the risk of lesion discontinuity and result in gap sizes that promote ablation failure.

▶ Ultrasound-Assisted Lipoplasty

In this technique, high-intensity focused ultrasound is used to liquefy subcutaneous fat before it is removed by suction. In contrast, conventional liposuction involves the operator (surgeon) dislodging the fat by moving a thin cannula in the subcutaneous space. UAL delivers acoustic energy in the frequency range of 22 to 36 kHz. The probe vibrates longitudinally, thus creating standing waves at the tip of the probe. Thermal, cavitation, and mechanical mechanisms have all been postulated to achieve the fat liquefaction effect. What is observed is a fragmentation of the adipose tissue and the formation of an emulsion, with the relative sparing of collagen structures, vessels, and nervous tissue. Advocates of UAL claim that this results in a smoother end result with less blood loss and less pain. However, certain complications, most importantly burns, heed careful use of the technology with proper training and instrumentation.

HEMOSTASIS

HIFU has been used as a tool for hemostasis for blood vessels as well as organ surfaces such as the spleen, liver, and lungs. At high intensities such as 1–10 kW/cm^2 the thermal effect is significant, where direct cauterization causes coagulation necrosis. In addition to this, however, there is a cellular biological response to ultrasound exposure as evidenced by enhanced deposition of collagen, elastin, and proteoglycans at the treated site. The cavitation effect has also been shown to induce platelet activation, aggregation, and adhesion, perhaps by disrupting platelets, which then releases β-thromboglobulin, ADP, and other factors. The presence of these circulating factors in turn induces recruitment of new platelets for accelerated clot formation.

SURGICAL ENERGY DEVICES

Ultrasonic dissectors were first applied in cataract surgery (phacoemulsification) in the late 1960s. Gradual adoption by other specialties has led to the widespread use and commercialization of the technology, which uses ultrasonic vibration for tissue dissection, division, and hemostasis. These are high power (10–300 W/cm^2), relatively low-frequency (20–60 kHz) systems. Unlike the remote applications described above, the vibratory energy is imparted at the instrument tip that is placed in contact with the tissue. Thus, it is direct tissue effects, ie, cutting, coaptation, cavitation, and coagulation, which are the treatment goals in this case. Numerous tip configurations including hooks, blades, balls, or clamps are available for various applications.

Vibration excursion is on the order of a few hundred microns, either parallel or transverse to the axis of the probe. Several mechanisms of action result from this vibration. Firstly, there is a direct mechanical effect on tissues, where the vibrating probe results in tissue damage. In addition, shear forces around the device tip result in tissue fragmentation. Secondly, cavitation occurs during the negative pressure excursion, where microbubbles expand and collapse and generate microjets or shockwaves. This force is theorized to be responsible for cellular destruction. Finally, thermal mechanisms play a major role in tissue effects, in terms of both direct desired effect and potential for collateral damage. Coagulation results from

denaturation of proteins, and a minimum temperature rise of 4°C is required. Heat production in an ultrasonic dissector is directly proportional to application time and power setting. In an animal study of the Harmonic scalpel (Ethicon, New Jersey, the United States), temperature rises of up to 40°C within 1 mm of the probe were recorded. On measuring at varying intervals away from the probe, it was found that by a 5 mm distance away tissue perfusion had restored the temperature to normal. Based on the results, they concluded that a safety margin of 3 mm is adequate to avoid unwanted thermal damage. The magnitude and significance of these effects vary across different tissue types. Tissues with higher collagen content are less susceptible to the direct mechanical effects of the vibration. Softer tissues are more compliant and more responsive to shear forces and cavitation.

SUGGESTED READINGS

Baker KG, Robertson VJ, Duck FA. A review of therapeutic ultrasound: biophysical effects. *Phys Ther.* 2001;81: 1351–1358.

Cimino A. Ultrasound-assisted lipoplasty: basic physics, tissue interactions, and related results/complications. In: Prendergast PM, Shiffman MA, eds. *Aesthetic Medicine.* Berlin, Heidelberg: Springer-Verlag; 2011:519–528.

Cleveland R, McAteer J. The physics of shock wave lithotripsy. In: Smith AD, Badlani GH, Preminger GM, Kavoussi LR, eds. *Smith's Textbook of Endourology.* Oxford, UK: Wiley-Blackwell; 2012:I&II:317–331.

Grasso M, Green D, Rukstalis D, Talavera F, Wolf JS, Schwartz B. *Extracorporeal Shockwave Lithiotripsy.* Medscape reference, www.emedicine.medscape.com, accessed online June 4, 2012; last update January 19, 2012.

Mitragotri S. Healing sound: the use of ultrasound in drug delivery and other therapeutic applications. *Nat Rev Drug Discov.* 2005;4(3):255–260.

Mitragotri S. Sonophoresis: a 50-year journey. *Drug Discov Today.* 2004 Sept;9(17):735–736.

Nakamura Y, Kiaii B, Chu M. Minimally invasive surgical therapies for atrial fibrillation. *ISRN Cardiol.* 2012; Volume 2012. Article ID 606324.

O'Dalya B, Morris E, Gavinc G, O'Byrne J, McGuinness G. High-power low-frequency ultrasound: a review of tissue dissection and ablation in medicine and surgery. *J Mater Process Technol.* 2008;200:38–58.

Oguram M, Paliwal S, Mitragotri S. Low-frequency sonophoresis: current status and future prospects. *Adv Drug Deliv Rev.* 2008 June;60(10):1218–1223.

Paliwal S, Mitragotri S. Therapeutic opportunities in biological responses of ultrasound. *Ultrasonics.* 2008 August;48(4): 271–278.

Robertson VJ, Baker KG. A review of therapeutic ultrasound: effectiveness studies. *Phys Ther.* 2001;81:1339–1350.

Romano CL, Romano D, Logoluso N. Low-intensity pulsed ultrasound for the treatment of bone delayed union or nonunion: a review. *Ultrasound Med Biol.* 2009 April;35(4): 529–536.

ter Haar G. Therapeutic applications of ultrasound. *Prog Biophys Mol Biol.* 2007 Jan–April;93(1–3):111–129.

17

DOCUMENTATION, CODING, BILLING, AND COMPLIANCE

BETH SCHROPE

No starry-eyed future doctor goes to medical school to learn how to document, code, bill, etc. Furthermore, most residency programs fall far short of instructing their residents on how to comply with CMS and commercial insurance regulations. Yet, this is the reality that each practitioner faces daily. In this chapter, I hope to provide guidelines on how to document your ultrasound examination and code appropriately for maximum reimbursement.

CURRENT PROCEDURAL TERMINOLOGY (CPT)

This discussion begins with a review of the notion of CPT, or current procedural terminology, coding. Designed and maintained by the American Medical Association as a universal language for identifying and reporting medical, surgical, and diagnostic services, CPT codes enable clear communication for utilization review and claims processing by government and commercial payers. The CPT code describes the service performed, regardless of the performing individual (surgeon, radiologist, gastroenterologist, etc.). Most ultrasound examinations and procedures have CPT descriptors, and can be listed in addition to evaluation and management (E & M) codes.

Many ultrasound examinations performed by interventionalists as an adjunct to a procedure are of the "limited" variety, where a focused examination is performed. For example, a complete ultrasound examination of the abdomen (76700) consists of real-time scans of the liver, gallbladder, common bile duct, pancreas, spleen, both kidneys, upper abdominal aorta, and inferior vena cava. Ultrasound assessment for hepatic lesion ablation, however, would fall under code 76705, "Ultrasound, abdominal, real time with image documentation, limited," where a limited study refers to a single quadrant, diagnostic problem, or even a follow-up study. The most recent definition for a limited examination by CPT is one in which less than the required elements for a complete examination are performed and documented.

Category III codes are a temporary set of codes for emerging technologies, services, and procedures. They are used predominantly to track the usage of these procedures, and may be in the FDA approval process, or for research purposes. Category III codes are archived after a period of 5 years, unless the original requestor petitions for either retention as a Category III or conversion to a Category I (if Category I criteria are met). These codes are identified as four-digit numeric followed by a T. There are several vascular ultrasound procedure codes that fall under this category.

Certain modifiers may be added to the primary CPT code to clarify or further the information provided by the code alone. The most common modifiers used with ultrasound procedure codes are:

▶ -26 Professional Component

Unmodified ultrasound CPT codes are "global" service codes, where the technical and professional components are combined. Technical component refers to the facility portion, and includes equipment cost and maintenance, technician services, and supplies. Professional component refers to the physician interpretation services accompanied by a separate, distinctly identifiable report. When a physician uses an ultrasound machine in the operating room, for example, the machine is typically owned and maintained by the hospital or facility, and the physician should only bill for the professional component of the procedure (even though the physician may be performing the actual examination). On the other hand, a physician in a private office who owns and maintains the equipment is justified in submitting the unmodified code for an ultrasound examination.

▶ -50 Bilateral Procedure
▶ -51 Multiple Procedures

These modifiers would seem self-explanatory. For example, ultrasound-guided ablation of multiple hepatic lesions would fall into this category, or ultrasound-guided drainage of bilateral breast cysts.

-52 Reduced Services

At times the ultrasound examination performed will not fulfill all of the requirements of the CPT code descriptor. An example of this may include using ultrasound guidance for assessment of a pleural effusion, where a complete examination including the mediastinum as described in code 76604 (ultrasound, chest, (includes mediastinum) real time with image documentation) would not be indicated. Note that there exist many separate CPT codes that indicate a "limited" examination, so a "complete" examination with modifier -52 would be inappropriate in this circumstance.

-53 Discontinued Procedure

This modifier should be appended when a procedure was started but abandoned due to extenuating circumstances. The portion of the procedure completed as well as a description of the circumstances leading to discontinuance should be documented.

-59 Distinct Procedural Service

Circumstances may arise where a service performed was distinct from a similar or same service performed on that same day. These may include separate sessions on the same day, or a different site, organ, or lesion. As always, adequate documentation of the need for additional procedures is required. To distinguish this from modifier 51, multiple procedures, multiple submissions of the same CPT code with modifier 59 may be submitted, whereas modifier 51 is used with a singly submitted procedure code. An example for this may be ultrasound-guided removals of foreign bodies in two separate anatomic regions.

-76 Repeat Procedure by Same Physician

Repeat examinations on the same day by the same physician may be submitted as long as documentation for the necessity of the examination is provided. An easily understandable scenario is that of a FAST examination, repeated for hemodynamic changes. The second examination contains the modifier, not the first.

-77 Repeat Procedure by Another Physician

A physician with a different TIN who performs a repeat procedure as above would append modifier 77 to the procedure code.

A reference-coding guide is included at the end of this chapter in an appendix, categorized by the specialties contained in this text.

DOCUMENTATION AND ARCHIVING

In order to fulfill billing compliance regulations the following documentation is required: (1) medical necessity; (2) image interpretation; and (3) image archive. Addressing each element specifically, the medical necessity for the utilization of ultrasound must be clearly recorded. According to the American College of Radiology guidelines, this requirement is fulfilled with documentation of relevant history (including known diagnoses) and signs and symptoms. Relevant diagnosis codes (ICD-9, or, after October 2013, ICD-10) are often used by payers to determine the necessity for a given procedure; indeed, private carriers often use lists of specific ICD codes that support certain CPT codes. Medicare carriers are required to make such lists available to providers.

Next, a written report of findings and interpretations must be maintained in the patient's medical record, with key identifiers (name, date of birth, and medical record number). Additionally, the report should reflect the examiner and interpreting physician (if different), as well as the date, time, and location of the examination. Key positive and negative findings are typically provided, with specific measurements or quality descriptors (for example, anechoic) as appropriate. When ultrasound guidance is used in conjunction with another procedure, the report of the ultrasound may be included in the procedure note.

Although a relatively recent mandate, it is now compulsory to permanently store relevant images and have these available for future review. As an example to underscore this last requirement, the unambiguous descriptor for the code 76700 is "Ultrasound, abdominal, real time *with image documentation*, complete." There are no specific rules from CPT or CMS for image documentation, such as number of views, measurements, or modality of image storage. To meet this ambiguous requirement a minimum of one image should be produced and stored. Good clinical practice dictates the necessity for additional, relevant images as needed. Or, practitioners may look to local policies, such as those in place in the facility where they practice. Of course when performing a complex procedure it may not be possible to acquire and archive images throughout, but representative images obtained before and after the procedure may be considered the relevant images and should suffice. Finally, images and reports are governed by HIPAA policies, and should be stored as secure data.

CREDENTIALING AND BILLING COMPLIANCE

The next chapter of this book is devoted to a detailed and specialty-specific discussion of physician privileging and credentialing in performing and interpreting ultrasound examinations and procedures. With regard to billing compliance, the Center for Medicare and Medicaid Services offers regulatory guidance for the technical component of ultrasound procedures, ie, technologist, equipment, and facility, but no specific requirements for nonradiologist physician credentialing. Similarly, private or commercial insurance (for example, CareCore National) often makes available equipment standards but puts forth no official document on physician credentials. Therefore, nonradiologist physicians integrating ultrasound into their practice should look to fulfilling local privileging and credentialing, whether that be through a facility or professional society, as discussed in greater detail in the credentialing chapter.

SUGGESTED READINGS

ACR-SPR-SRU Practice Guideline for Performing and Interpreting Diagnostic Ultrasound Examinations, Resolution 7, revised 2011, accessed online www.acr.org/guidelines.

CPT Professional Edition 2012, *American Medical Association*, Chicago, 2011.

CODING GUIDE

CPT CODE	CPT Description	Notes
Head and Neck		
76942	Ultrasonic guidance for needle placement (eg, biopsy, aspiration, injection, and localization device), imaging, supervision, and interpretation	
10021	Fine needle aspiration, with imaging guidance	Code with 76942
60100	Biopsy thyroid, percutaneous core needle	Code with 76942 for imaging guidance
76998	Ultrasound guidance, intraoperative	
Breast		
76645	Ultrasound, breast(s) (unilateral or bilateral) real time with image documentation	
76942	Ultrasonic guidance for needle placement (eg, biopsy, aspiration, injection, and localization device), imaging, supervision, and interpretation	
76998	Ultrasound guidance, intraoperative	
10021	Fine needle aspiration, with imaging guidance	
19000	Puncture aspiration of cyst of breast	Use with 76942
19001	Puncture aspiration of cyst of breast, each additional cyst (list separately in addition to code for primary procedure)	Use with 76942
19102	Biopsy of breast; percutaneous, needle core, and using imaging guidance	Use with 76942
19103	Biopsy of breast; percutaneous, automated vacuum assisted or rotating biopsy device, and using imaging guidance	Use with 76942
19295	Image-guided placement, metallic localization clip, percutaneous, during breast biopsy (list separately in addition to code for primary procedure)	
Chest/Critical Care		
76942	Ultrasonic guidance for needle placement (eg, biopsy, aspiration, injection, and localization device), imaging, supervision, and interpretation	
76998	Ultrasound guidance, intraoperative	
75989	Radiological guidance (eg, fluoroscopy, ultrasound or computed tomography) for percutaneous drainage (eg, abscess, specimen collection) with placement of catheter, radiological supervision, and interpretation	Use with
76930	Ultrasonic guidance for pericardiocentesis, imaging supervision, and interpretation	Use with 33010 (initial) or 33011 (subsequent)
76937	Ultrasound guidance for vascular access requiring ultrasound evaluation of potential access sites, documentation of selected vessel patency, concurrent real-time ultrasound visualization of vascular needle entry, with permanent recording and reporting (list separately in addition to code for primary procedure)	Add-on code (reported in conjunction with the primary procedure and may not be reported as a stand-alone code)
76942	Ultrasonic guidance for needle placement (eg, biopsy, aspiration, injection, and localization device), imaging, supervision, and interpretation	
93304	Transthoracic echocardiography for congenital cardiac anomalies; follow-up or limited study	
93306	Echocardiography, transthoracic, real time with image documentation (2D), includes M-mode recording, when performed, complete, with spectral Doppler echocardiography, and with color flow Doppler echocardiography	

(continued)

CODING GUIDE (continued)

CPT CODE	CPT Description	Notes
93307	Echocardiography, transthoracic, real time with image documentation (2D), includes M-mode recording, when performed, complete, without spectral or color flow Doppler echocardiography	
93308	Echocardiography, transthoracic, real time with image documentation (2D), includes M-mode recording, when performed; follow-up or limited study	
93312	Echocardiography, transesophageal, real time with image documentation (2D) (with or without M-mode recording); including probe placement, image acquisition, interpretation, and report	
93313	Echocardiography, transesophageal, real time with image documentation (2D) (with or without M-mode recording); and placement of transesophageal probe only	
93314	Echocardiography, transesophageal, real time with image documentation (2D) (with or without M-mode recording); image acquisition, interpretation, and report only	
93318	Echocardiography, transesophageal (TEE) for monitoring purposes, including probe placement, real-time 2-dimensional image acquisition and interpretation leading to ongoing (continuous) assessment of (dynamically changing) cardiac pumping function, and to therapeutic measures on an immediate time basis	
+93320	Doppler echocardiography, pulsed wave and/or continuous wave with spectral display (list separately in addition to codes for echocardiographic imaging), complete	Add-on code (reported in conjunction with the primary procedure and may not be reported as a stand-alone code)
+93321	Doppler echocardiography, pulsed wave and/or continuous wave with spectral display; follow-up or limited study (list separately in addition to codes for echocardiographic imaging)	Add-on code (reported in conjunction with the primary procedure and may not be reported as a stand-alone code)
+93325	Doppler echocardiography color flow velocity mapping (list separately in addition to codes for echocardiography)	Add-on code (reported in conjunction with the primary procedure and may not be reported as a stand-alone code)
93971	Duplex scan of extremity veins including responses to compression and other maneuvers; unilateral or limited study	

Ultrasound-Guided Regional Anesthesia

76942	Ultrasonic guidance for needle placement (eg, biopsy, aspiration, injection, and localization device), imaging, supervision, and interpretation	
+76937	Ultrasound guidance for vascular access requiring ultrasound evaluation of potential access sites, documentation of selected vessel patency, concurrent real-time ultrasound visualization of vascular needle entry, with permanent recording and reporting (list separately in addition to code for primary procedure)	Add-on code (reported in conjunction with the primary procedure and may not be reported as a stand-alone code)

Vascular

93880	Duplex scan of extracranial arteries; complete bilateral study	
93882	Duplex scan of extracranial arteries; unilateral or limited study	
93925	Duplex scan of lower extremity arteries or arterial bypass grafts; complete bilateral study	
93926	Duplex scan of lower extremity arteries or arterial bypass grafts; unilateral or limited study	
93965	Noninvasive physiologic studies of extremity veins, complete bilateral study (eg, Doppler waveform analysis with responses to compression and other maneuvers, phleborheography, and impedance plethysmography)	

(continued)

CODING GUIDE *(continued)*

CPT CODE	CPT Description	Notes
93970	Duplex scan of extremity veins including responses to compression and other maneuvers; complete bilateral study	
93971	Duplex scan of extremity veins including responses to compression and other maneuvers; unilateral or limited study	
93975	Duplex scan of arterial inflow and venous outflow of abdominal, pelvic, scrotal contents, and/or retroperitoneal organs; complete study	
93976	Duplex scan of arterial inflow and venous outflow of abdominal, pelvic, scrotal contents, and/or retroperitoneal organs; limited study	
93978	Duplex scan of aorta, inferior vena cava, iliac vasculature, or bypass grafts; complete study	
93979	Duplex scan of aorta, inferior vena cava, iliac vasculature, or bypass grafts; unilateral or limited study	
93980	Duplex scan of arterial inflow and venous outflow of penile vessels; complete study	
93981	Duplex scan of arterial inflow and venous outflow of penile vessels; follow-up or limited study	
93990	Duplex scan of hemodialysis access (including arterial inflow, body of access and venous outflow)	
G0365	Vessel mapping of vessels for hemodialysis access (services for preoperative vessel mapping prior to creation of hemodialysis access using an autogenous hemodialysis conduit, including arterial inflow and venous outflow)	
G0389	Ultrasound B-scan and/or real time with image documentation; for abdominal aortic aneurysm (AAA) screening	
36475	Endovenous ablation therapy of incompetent vein, extremity, inclusive of all imaging guidance and monitoring, percutaneous radiofrequency, and first vein treated	Code inclusive of imaging guidance; therefore ultrasound guidance not separately reported
+36476	second and subsequent veins treated in a single extremity, each through separate access sites (list separately in addition to code for primary procedure)	Code inclusive of imaging guidance; therefore ultrasound guidance not separately reported;add-on code (reported in conjunction with the primary procedure and may not be reported as a stand-alone code)
36478	Endovenous ablation therapy of incompetent vein, extremity, inclusive of all imaging guidance and monitoring, percutaneous laser, and first vein treated	Code inclusive of imaging guidance; therefore ultrasound guidance not separately reported
+36479	second and subsequent veins treated in a single extremity, each through separate access sites (list separately in addition to code for primary procedure)	Code inclusive of imaging guidance; therefore ultrasound guidance not separately reported;add-on code (reported in conjunction with the primary procedure and may not be reported as a stand-alone code)
76936	Ultrasound guided compression repair of arterial pseudoaneurysm or arteriovenous fistulae (includes diagnostic ultrasound evaluation, compression of lesion, and imaging)	
+76937	Ultrasound guidance for vascular access requiring ultrasound evaluation of potential access sites, documentation of selected vessel patency, concurrent real-time ultrasound visualization of vascular needle entry, with permanent recording and reporting (list separately in addition to code for primary procedure)	Add-on code (reported in conjunction with the primary procedure and may not be reported as a stand-alone code)
76942	Ultrasonic guidance for needle placement (eg, biopsy, aspiration, injection, and localization device), imaging, supervision, and interpretation	

(continued)

CODING GUIDE (continued)

CPT CODE	CPT Description	Notes
Abdomen and Retroperitoneum		
76705	Ultrasound, abdominal, real time with image documentation, and limited (eg, single organ, quadrant, and follow-up)	Use with 93308 for FAST examination
76770	Ultrasound, retroperitoneal (eg, renal, aorta, and nodes), real time with image documentation, complete	A complete ultrasound examination of the retroperitoneum consists of real-time scans of the kidneys, abdominal aorta, common iliac artery origins, and inferior vena cava, including any demonstrated retroperitoneal abnormality.
76775	Ultrasound, retroperitoneal (eg, renal, aorta, and nodes), real time with image documentation, limited	
76776	Ultrasound, transplanted kidney, real time and duplex Doppler with image documentation	
76940	Ultrasound guidance for, and monitoring of, parenchymal tissue ablation	Do not report with 50250, 50542, 76942, and 76998
76942	Ultrasonic guidance for needle placement (eg, biopsy, aspiration, injection, and localization device), imaging, supervision, and interpretation	
76998	Ultrasound guidance, intraoperative	
93308	Echocardiography, transthoracic, real time with image documentation (2D), includes M-mode recording, when performed; follow-up or limited study	Use with 76705 for FAST examination
Genitourinary		
93976	Duplex scan of arterial inflow and venous outflow of abdominal, pelvic, scrotal contents, and/or retroperitoneal organs; limited study	
93980	Duplex scan of arterial inflow and venous outflow of penile vessels; complete study	
93981	Duplex scan of arterial inflow and venous outflow of penile vessels; follow-up or limited study	
51798	Measurement of postvoiding residual urine and/or bladder capacity by ultrasound; nonimaging	"Nonimaging" refers to the intent of the procedure, which is to obtain only postvoid residual, not to obtain an image
76700	Ultrasound, abdominal, real time with image documentation, complete	A complete ultrasound examination of the abdomen consists of real-time scans of the liver, gallbladder, common bile duct, pancreas, spleen, kidneys, and the upper abdominal aorta and inferior vena cava, including any demonstrated abdominal abnormality.
76705	Ultrasound, abdominal, real time with image documentation, and limited (eg, single organ, quadrant, and follow-up)	Use with 93308 for FAST examination
76770	Ultrasound, retroperitoneal (eg, renal, aorta, and nodes) real time with image documentation, and complete	A complete ultrasound examination of the retroperitoneum consists of real-time scans of the kidneys, abdominal aorta, common iliac artery origins, and inferior vena cava, including any demonstrated retroperitoneal abnormality.
76775	Ultrasound, retroperitoneal (eg, renal, aorta, and nodes) real time with image documentation, and limited	
76776	Ultrasound, transplanted kidney, real time and duplex Doppler with image documentation	

(continued)

CODING GUIDE (*continued*)

CPT CODE	CPT Description	Notes
76856	Ultrasound, pelvic (nonobstetric), B-scan and/or real time with image documentation, complete	
76857	Ultrasound, pelvic (nonobstetric), B-scan and/or time time with image documentation, limited (eg, for follicles)	
76870	Ultrasound, scrotum, and contents	
55700	Biopsy, prostate, needle or punch, single or multiple, and any approach	Use with 76872
76872	Ultrasound, transrectal	
76873	Ultrasound, transrectal, and prostate volume study for brachytherapy treatment planning (separate procedure)	
55859	Transperineal placement of needles or catheters into prostate for interstitial radioelement application, with or without cystoscopy	Use with 76965
76965	Ultrasound guidance for interstitial radioelement application	
76376	3D rendering with interpretation and reporting of computed tomography, magnetic resonance imaging, ultrasound, or other tomographic modality; not requiring postprocessing on an independent workstation	
76377	3D rendering with interpretation and reporting of computed tomography, magnetic resonance imaging, ultrasound, or other tomographic modality; requiring postprocessing on an independent workstation	
76942	Ultrasonic guidance for needle placement (eg, biopsy, aspiration, injection, and localization device), imaging, supervision, and interpretation	
76998	Ultrasound guidance, intraoperative	

Endoscopic

43232	Esophagoscopy, rigid or flexible, diagnostic, with or without the collection of specimen(s) by brushing or washing (separate procedure) with transendoscopic-guided intramural or transmural fine needle aspiration/biopsy(s)	Do not report with 76975
43237	Upper gastrointestinal endoscopy including esophagus, stomach, and either the duodenum and/or jejunum as appropriate; diagnostic, with or without collection of specimen(s) by brushing or washing (separate procedure) with endoscopic ultrasound examination limited to the esophagus	Do not report with 76942, 76975
43238	Upper gastrointestinal endoscopy including esophagus, stomach, and either the duodenum and/or jejunum as appropriate; diagnostic, with or without collection of specimen(s) by brushing or washing (separate procedure) with transendoscopic-guided intramural or transmural fine needle aspiration/biopsy(s), esophagus (includes endoscopic ultrasound examination limited to the esophagus)	Do not report with 76942, 76975
43242	Upper gastrointestinal endoscopy including esophagus, stomach, and either the duodenum and/or jejunum as appropriate; diagnostic, with or without collection of specimen(s) by brushing or washing (separate procedure) with transendoscopic-guided intramural or transmural fine needle aspiration/biopsy(s) (includes endoscopic ultrasound examination of the esophagus, stomach, and either the duodenum and/or jejunum as appropriate)	Use for EUS-guided FNA of pancreas, bile duct, lymph node, and liver do not report with 76942, 76975

(*continued*)

CODING GUIDE *(continued)*

CPT CODE	CPT Description	Notes
43259	Upper gastrointestinal endoscopy including esophagus, stomach, and either the duodenum and/or jejunum as appropriate; diagnostic, with or without collection of specimen(s) by brushing or washing (separate procedure) with endoscopic ultrasound examination, including the esophagus, stomach, and either the duodenum and/or jejunum as appropriate)	Do not report with 76975
45341	Sigmoidoscopy, flexible, diagnostic, with or without collection of specimen(s) by brushing or washing (separate procedure), with endoscopic ultrasound examination	Do not report with 76942, 76975
45342	Sigmoidoscopy, flexible, diagnostic, with or without collection of specimen(s) by brushing or washing (separate procedure), with transendoscopic ultrasound-guided intramural or transmural fine needle aspiration/biopsy(s)	Do not report with 76942, 76975
76872	Ultrasound, transrectal	
0249T	Ligation, hemorrhoidal vascular bundle(s), including ultrasound guidance	Do not report with 46020, 46221, 46250-46262, 46600, 46945, 46946, 76872, 76942, and 76998
45391	Colonoscopy, flexible, proximal to splenic flexure, diagnostic, with or without collection of specimen(s) by brushing or washing, with or without colon decompression (separate procedure), with transendoscopic ultrasound guided intramural or transmural fine needle aspiration/biopsy(s)	Do not report with 45330, 45341, 45342, 45378, 76872
45392	Colonoscopy, flexible, proximal to splenic flexure, diagnostic, with or without collection of specimen(s) by brushing or washing, with or without colon decompression (separate procedure), with endoscopic ultrasound examination	Do not report with 45330, 45341, 45342, 45378, 76872
76942	Ultrasonic guidance for needle placement (eg, biopsy, aspiration, injection, and localization device), imaging, supervision, and interpretation	
76975	Gastrointestinal endoscopic ultrasound, supervision, and interpretation	
64680	Destruction by neurolytic agent, celiac plexus, with or without radiologic monitoring	Report with 76975

V

18

CREDENTIALING

BETH SCHROPE

INTRODUCTION

Since the first surgeon-performed ultrasound examinations in the 1980s, the field has matured and expanded to include many surgical, and indeed other medical, specialties. In fact, in 1999 the American Medical Association passed a resolution (Res. 802, I-99; Reaffirmed: Sub. Res. 108, A-00) acknowledging the extensive application of the technology in medical practice and its use was within the scope of practice of "appropriately trained physicians." The resolution states that hospitals should be responsible for granting privileges to individuals within their scope of ultrasound practice. Furthermore, the AMA resolution recommends that specialties using ultrasound develop specialty-specific recommendations for its use. As the ranks of physicians comfortable with the performance and interpretation of ultrasound grow, guidelines for verification of competency and standardization of practice are essential. This chapter provides a historical context for current standards, justification for those standards, and a practical guide for those seeking credentialing in ultrasound in many interventional specialties.

PRECEDENT

Clearly the field of medicine, like many other advanced and highly technical disciplines, has and will continue to experience an exponential growth in the adoption of new technologies. With this evolution comes the need for practitioner training, credentialing, and continuing education. There are several notable precedents, or at least contemporaries, to the use of ultrasound by nonradiologists. Perhaps the most apparent is laparoscopy. Dismissed by many in the early years as too difficult, too expensive, and too time-consuming, it has now become the standard approach for many surgical procedures, relegating "open" approaches in

many cases to the barbaric. Although ultrasound cannot be compared directly to laparoscopy, as it represents an adjunct to current techniques, rather than a whole new approach, the history of training and credentialing can be paralleled.

In the late 1980s and early 1990s practicing surgeons struggled to find venues in which to learn the emerging technique of laparoscopy. Courses using simulators, cadavers, and animal models were created to introduce the instrumentation and methods of the procedures. Proctors were dispatched from the ranks of early adopters to assist in the acquisition of laparoscopic skills and to ensure safe practices. Junior partners graduating from large academic programs were recruited in some cases to propel a group practice forward into the era of laparoscopy. Hospitals and surgical departments were called upon to credential their staff on these new privileges, based on tangible criteria, tradition, or even wisdom from the more seasoned staff. Gradually, training programs together with the ACGME (Accreditation Council of Graduate Medical Education) and the American Board of Surgery developed minimum training standards and objective criteria as a condition for successful completion of a residency in general surgery that includes laparoscopic skills. In other words, completion of a residency in general surgery now qualifies a graduate as competent in laparoscopy, pending successful examination by the ABS.

Thus, the lesson learned from laparoscopy may be simplified as follows. An emerging technique is identified and verified independently by the surgical innovators. Through peer-reviewed communications at conferences and journals, the technique, including its appropriate use, is refined and agreed upon. Forums for disseminating the technique are developed and offered to a qualified audience. These forums often take the guise of courses in which some form of examination or, at minimum, verification of attendance is recorded. New practitioners of the technique can be expected to keep track of their experience, by logging cases, and perhaps verifying (in the case of ultrasound) results with independent findings. As awareness of the technique grows, hospital credentialing bodies assume the role of regulator of privileges. Eventually, professional organizations, including educational training councils as well as specialty societies, adopt the role as governors of the credentialing.

The application of this scheme to ultrasound is at various stages of maturation across the numerous subspecialties discussed in this book. What follows is a summary of the particulars for each area of expertise.

GENERAL SURGERY

As any physician who has completed a residency, possibly fellowship, and passed their written and oral board certifications knows, there is ample opportunity for proof of acquisition of didactic knowledge. Perhaps most shockingly in the case of interventionalists, however, there is no standardized mechanism for proof of adequate acquisition of skills. One assumes that during formal training this is continuously evaluated, and inadequate skills will be remediated prior to successful completion of the training program. As a physician practices, though, over time new technologies and skills will need to be incorporated into the proceduralists' armamentarium. In general the acquisition of new skills should follow a standard rubric, namely: (1) didactic instruction by experts in the field; (2) hands-on training; (3) proctoring for an agreed amount of cases with eventual demonstration of satisfactory skill; and (4) continuing education, both practical (meeting a minimum number of cases per year, for example) and quality assurance. Particulars for each of the steps above should be determined by governing societies forming committees of experts in the field.

▶ The American Institute for Ultrasound in Medicine

One might look to either a surgery-based or a radiology-based organization to offer guidelines for credentialing for ultrasound for surgeons. The largest ultrasound-specific society in the United States is the American Institute for Ultrasound in Medicine. In its official statement entitled "Training Guidelines for Physicians Who Evaluate and Interpret Diagnostic Ultrasound Examinations" approved on November 6, 2010, the AIUM outlines stringent criteria for training (full document may be found in Appendix 1). Outside of specialty certifications in breast, neck, trauma, obstetrics and gynecology, and musculoskeletal ultrasound, the association dictates the performance, evaluation, and interpretation of at least 300 sonograms, in addition to 100 hours of didactic lesson. This implies that a surgeon with a practice concentration in the abdominal arena will not be considered competent by the AIUM until they have been using ultrasound for likely a period of years. Contrast this to the "learning curve" for a laparoscopic cholecystectomy during the time of its adoption, where numbers oft-quoted were in the range of 25 to 50 cases. Dr. Grace Rozycki, a pioneer in surgical ultrasound and steadfast proponent of

surgeon-performed procedures, argues that this does not apply to surgeons for the following reasons: (1) a surgeon has the benefit of direct responsibility for the patient, and thus is more familiar with the patient's anatomy, symptomatology, and disease process than a technician or impartial proceduralist;(2) knowledge of three-dimensional anatomy is enhanced by the surgeon's operative experience; and (3) surgeon-performed ultrasounds are generally more focused, with the "ask question, get answer" approach. Although it may be instinctive to look to an ultrasound specialty society for guidance on credentialing ultrasound, in this author's opinion, the naiveté to a surgeon's practice, in fact, hinders proper judgment and is even dangerous if looked to for guidance by payers, litigation specialists, and the like.

▶ The American College of Surgery

For reasons that become obvious it is more appropriate for surgeons (and other interventionalists) to govern the adoption of ultrasound for themselves, knowing the full scope of the application of the technique as well as the applicability to the physician's practice. Looking now to the model described earlier for adoption of emerging technologies, the full and exemplary history of the American College of Surgery as a proponent and governor of surgeon-performed ultrasound is described.

The first ultrasound session at the national meeting of the ACS occurred in 1995 at the 80th Clinical Congress in New Orleans, with a general session entitled "The Surgeon and Ultrasound". The day-long meeting included discussions on ultrasound physics, breast, colorectal, hepatobiliary, vascular, laparoscopic, and trauma ultrasound. In addition, even at that earliest meeting, recognition of the importance of certification was apparent with a lecture entitled "Credentialing, Liability, and Turf Wars." Following rapidly was the first meeting of a core group of early adopters, the ACS Ultrasound Users Group. The goals and objectives of this meeting were enumerated: develop course of instruction for ACS, develop educational format for US, interface with manufacturers, interface with ACS hierarchy, and interface with ABS (American Board of Surgery) and APDS (Association of Program Directors in Surgery). The first postgraduate course was held at the 24th Spring Meeting in April 1996 in New York. A National Ultrasound Faculty was approved by the ACS Board of Regents in 1998. Key to this organization's responsibility was the development of an Ultrasound "Blue Book," or ultrasound educational program for surgeons and surgical residents. Quoting from the preface, "A voluntary verification process for surgeons performing ultrasound has been created and is intended to ensure that surgeons who use ultrasound are qualified and that the ultrasound facilities and equipment they use are appropriate for the medical application and met and maintain quality standards." Quickly a Verification Program was endorsed for surgeons and surgical residents, and included three components: Level 1, verification of attendance; Level 2, verification of satisfactory completion of course objectives; and Level 3, instructor. This program was constructed with modules, including both a curriculum in basic ultrasound and numerous advanced, specialty curricula.

The official statement developed by the College's Committee on Emerging Surgical Technology and Education (CESTE) was approved by the Board of Regents in the February 1998 meeting and may be found in Appendix 2. Briefly, it insures the surgeon either received adequate training in basic ultrasonography during residency, or acquired this knowledge through a basic approved educational program. This statement then describes the qualifications for use of specialty ultrasound, including knowledge of the specialty itself as well as documentation of expertise in the application of ultrasound to this specialty area (ie, by evidence of formal training or by examination). Recommendations for maintenance of skills by individuals as well as facility guidelines complete this document.

▶ The Society for American Gastrointestinal Endoscopic Surgeons

SAGES can perhaps be considered a surgical specialty society for the adoption of advanced surgical technologies, particularly in the field of "general" surgery. As such, in January 2011, SAGES released their own privileging guidelines for institutions granting ultrasonography privileges to surgeons. The full document is found in Appendix 3, but will be summarized here.

Interestingly and uniquely, this document specifically addresses hospital credentialing committees. It also specifies that ultrasonography privileges should be granted separately for each major category of practice, ie, trauma, abdominal, vascular, thoracic, urology, and gynecology. This document outlines explicit, minimum requirements for granting privileges in ultrasound. First is successful completion of an ACGME-accredited surgical residency program. If this program incorporated a structured experience in ultrasonography, documentation of this is to be provided. If the residency program did not include such training, a separate, structured training program is required. They indicate curriculum requirements such as didactic training and hands-on scanning with animate or inanimate models, and suggest courses such as those offered by the ACS or SAGES. Lastly, an applicant's experience should be adequate and documented as an appropriate number of cases, including proctored cases. The particular number of cases is left to the discretion of the institution. Further discussion is directed to maintenance of privileges, with guidelines for granting of provisional privileges, monitoring of performance, renewal of privileges, and denial of privileges with mechanisms for appeal.

NECK ULTRASOUND

The utility of ultrasound in the neck for diagnosis and treatment of various endocrine disorders is well established. The American Association of Clinical Endocrinologists (AACE) is a specialty society for physicians (largely medical specialists in endocrinology) who provide expertise in thyroid and parathyroid disorders. This group has established a certification in neck ultrasound, and provides a comprehensive handbook for the achievement and maintenance of this certification. Unlike the above general guidelines, the AACE is the sponsor of a formal course for neck ultrasound certification (ECNU, Endocrine Certification in Neck Ultrasound). Although neither required nor recognized by CMS or major insurers, this rigorous curriculum certainly identifies the necessary credentials and skills for neck ultrasound. This is a three-step program, including a written certifying examination that has a mandatory prerequisite of a thyroid ultrasound course (minimum 15 AMA PRA Category I credits), a validation of technical competency, and finally granting of certification. Certification entitles the recipient to a designation of "ECNU" after his or her name, and is valid for 10 years.

The validation of technical competency requirement is uniquely specific. Fifteen cases are required, 5 being thyroid nodules, 2, parathyroid adenomas, 2, malignant lymph nodes, 1, Hashimoto's thyroid case, and 5, FNAs. In addition, specific instructions for reporting are outlined, including indications for imaging, various measurements, exact images of the thyroid (A-P and transverse images of each lobe and the isthmus, and longitudinal images of each lobe), a description of the parenchyma of the thyroid, characterization of abnormal findings, diagnostic impression, and recommendations for additional studies, if indicated. FNA cases must also be accompanied by cytology reports and recommendations based on these and the ultrasound findings.

Although the AACE is predominantly an association for medical specialists, endocrine surgery fellows in this author's surgical program also participate in the ECNU course. There is currently no such rigorous curriculum designed specifically for surgeons, resulting in special certification, although the ACS offers a postgraduate course on thyroid and parathyroid ultrasound, based on their three-level requirements outlined previously.

BREAST ULTRASOUND

As with ultrasound of the thyroid and parathyroid, the clinical utility of ultrasound of the breast is well recognized. Certification is similarly rigorous, and is governed by the American Society of Breast Surgeons. Guidelines published in 2002 are based on the opinions of a panel of members of the society who are expert in breast ultrasound, as well as reviews of evidence-based literature. The specific guidelines are included in Appendix 4, and will be summarized here.

There are two components to the breast ultrasound certification process: a clinical application and a written examination. Prerequisites for the clinical application include: board certification by the American Board of Surgery or the American Osteopathic Board of Surgery, or international equivalent; appropriate level of training and a minimum of 1-year experience in the performance and interpretation of breast ultrasound; documented performance of at least 100 ultrasound examinations with review of 100 mammography examinations; and formal education in breast ultrasound with a minimum of 15 AMA credits. In addition, maintenance of skills is specified with demonstration of at least 50 breast ultrasounds a year, at least 12 ultrasound-guided invasive procedures per year, and at least 3 hours of AMA category 1 CME credits in breast ultrasound every 3 years.

Particular attention to ultrasound-guided procedures is found in these guidelines; with the requirement that the surgeon sonographer be proctored on at least two interventional procedures. The proctor's qualifications are also specified and include current certification in breast ultrasound by the ASBS, AIUM, or the American College of Radiology, and documentation of 5 years' clinical experience in breast ultrasound. The surgeon sonographer candidate is required to demonstrate certain maneuvers and skills during these proctoring sessions (found in Appendix 3), including adherence to written documentation stipulations. Guidelines for availability of proper equipment, performance verification, and quality control complete the document.

ENDOSCOPIC ULTRASOUND

Logically we look to the American Society for Gastrointestinal Endoscopy for guidance in credentialing endoscopic ultrasound. In 2001 the AGSE published their guidelines for credentialing and granting privileges for endoscopic ultrasound, found in Appendix 5 and summarized here. In this case, the society provides these guidelines to institutions or organizations for granting privileges to their staff, not as a certification in and of itself. This treatise is based on expert opinion and review of literature with regard to learning curves for specific procedures.

The ASGE specifies that endoscopic ultrasound is a distinct skill and should not be bundled with general endoscopy privileges. As with the other ultrasound credentialing already reviewed, demonstration of competence of EUS involves both didactic knowledge and practical skills. Candidates must demonstrate adequate training either in residency or in fellowship, or if this training was not available to the candidate, demonstration of an adequate number of supervised cases (special mention is made that self-teaching is not adequate). A minimum number of EUS procedures that should be documented before competency can be assessed is provided in this document. Detailed EUS training guidelines are referenced in the ASGE document "Guidelines for Training in Endoscopic Ultrasound" (*Gastroint Endosc.* 1999;49:829–833).

As with the other credentialing documents already reviewed, very specific measures are provided in all general aspects of EUS including imaging of mucosal tumors, submucosal tumors (both upper and lower GI tract), pancreaticobiliary imaging, and EUS-guided fine needle aspiration. Recognition is provided to the fact that once competence is achieved in one aspect of EUS, the minimum numbers required to achieve competence in another aspect of EUS may be decreased. Finally, the document reviews recredentialing and assurance of continued competence.

It should be mentioned that, analogous to the practice of thyroid and parathyroid ultrasound, no such specific guidelines for EUS are provided by surgical societies, such as the American Society for Colon and Rectal Surgeons, other than the more generic guidelines from the ACS and SAGES. Indeed, the ASCRS points to the ASGE document as guidance for education and credentialing in endoscopic ultrasound (Wexner et al. 2002).

UROLOGIC ULTRASOUND

Urologists were early adopters of ultrasound into their practice. As such, the education of ultrasound in residency training is well-developed, and clinical competency of this skill is inherent to the successful completion of an accredited urology residency training program. Formal guidelines for this particular aspect of urologic practice were first published in 1987 and are outlined in the "AIUM Practice Guideline for the Performance of an Ultrasound Examination in the Practice of Urology", available for review in Appendix 6. This document was created in a joint effort between the American Urologic Association and the American Institute for Ultrasound in Medicine.

Briefly, the AIUM provides general guidance for equipment, documentation instructions, patient safety and specific clinical applications including transrectal imaging of the prostate, renal ultrasound, scrotal ultrasound, penile and urethral ultrasound, and Doppler studies in urology. Provided under each of these clinical applications are equipment specifications for that particular application, indications for the exam as well as technique and documentation targets.

VASCULAR ULTRASOUND

Ultrasound is invaluable to the practice of vascular surgery, so much so that beginning in 2014 the Vascular Surgery Board of the American Board of Surgery will require all physicians applying for the Vascular Surgery Qualifying Examination to have attained the RPVI (Registered Physician in Vascular Interpretation) credential. This certification is administered by the American Registry for Diagnostic Medical Sonographers, and is offered to all physicians who diagnose and treat vascular disease. Prior to the creation of this credential, many vascular physicians (surgeons and nonsurgeons alike) sought certification as Registered Vascular Technologists, a credential that reflects competency in the *performance* of the vascular ultrasound examination and maintenance and quality assurance of a vascular lab. Alternatively, or even in addition to the RVT distinction, many vascular surgeons and other physicians treating peripheral vascular disease establish their own diagnostic vascular laboratories, and obtain certification through the Intersocietal Commission for the Accreditation of Vascular

Laboratories (ICAVL). In contrast, the RPVI, given exclusively to physicians, distinguishes the holder as expert in the *interpretation* of the vascular laboratory examinations.

The ARDMS administers the PVI examination and indicates six different prerequisites under which to apply (Appendix 7). The prerequisites, or categories of qualified physicians, are distinguished among those with U.S. or Canadian training versus international training. Further distinction is then made to those physicians who already hold the RVT credential or who hold ICAVL or American College of Radiology (ACR) vascular ultrasound accreditation, versus those who do not. The latter category is further subdivided into those with formal versus informal training in vascular ultrasound. Applicants must provide evidence of at least 12 credit hours of ARDMS-accepted CME as well as a record of interpretation experience with a minimum of 500 vascular laboratory studies. Fulfillment of one of these prerequisites and passage of a written examination thus entitles a physician to hold the RVPI credential.

ULTRASOUND-GUIDED REGIONAL ANESTHESIA

Governance for ultrasound-guided regional anesthesia (UGRA) has emerged from a joint meeting of the American Society of Regional Anesthesia and Pain Medicine and the European Society of Regional Anesthesia and Pain Therapy, with the full recommendations published in 2009 in the journal *Regional Anesthesia and Pain Medicine*. A detailed outline of their recommendations is appended to the manuscript and is included here in Appendix 8. The Joint Committee cautions the use of the document not as a mandate for those seeking credentialing in ultrasound-guided regional anesthesia, but rather as a basis for institutions that credential physicians, to fit within their practice scope and patterns.

The document outlines the indications for ultrasound-guided regional anesthesia and lists commonly performed ultrasound-guided nerve blocks. It segments training qualifications into two distinct pathways: a residency-based pathway and a practice pathway. The former applies to individuals who graduated from an ACGME-accredited residency program where the curriculum incorporates the 6 core competencies for training in UGRA. The practice pathway, which will eventually become obsolete as ultrasound becomes the standard for UGRA, exists for the anesthesiologist who was not exposed to sufficient training in residency or fellowship. This pathway recommends the usual didactic training, imaging practice on phantoms and humans, and ultimate proctored incorporation into one's practice. A fundamental skill set is outlined for both pathways, and includes obtaining the proper views using anatomical landmarks, optimization of scanning technique, fine-tuning device settings, and needle insertion and injection. Finally, an institutional program for quality improvement is recommended, including a formal analysis of results as well as biomedical engineering support for instrumentation maintenance.

TRAUMA ULTRASOUND

The use of ultrasound, primarily the FAST examination, has become a component of the physical examination in the rapid evaluation of a trauma patient. Although the FAST examination is not the basis for an image-guided intervention, it can critically guide the management of trauma patients. In addition, the skills acquired in becoming facile with the FAST examination can form the basis of other image-guided procedures (ie, paracentesis, pericardiocentesis). Other techniques used in the "trauma" setting include thoracic ultrasound for the detection of hemothorax, or the image-guided bedside drainage of an acutely decompensating patient with any hemodynamically significant pleural fluid. Obese or otherwise anatomically suboptimal patients clearly benefit from the use of ultrasound in the placement of venous and arterial catheters for rapid resuscitation and monitoring.

In 2007 the AIUM published practice guidelines for the FAST examination. Similar to the other practice guidelines reviewed, this document outlines indications for the procedure, training and credentialing physicians, detailed guidance on scanning techniques, views and documentation, equipment specifications, and quality assurance. This is not a credential administered by the AIUM, but rather falls into the category of guidelines for institutions that credential their physicians. This publication refers physicians to their specialty society such as the ACEP or AIUM for published standards.

With regard to training a practitioner in the performance of trauma ultrasound, one can look again to the American College of Surgery and their modular program for verification of ultrasound competency. After completion of the Basic Course in Ultrasound (ACS or equivalent), a candidate can then take the "FAST Ultrasound Skills Course," after successful completion of which the practitioner can verify knowledge and skills of trauma ultrasound. What remains is verification of preceptorial experience and verification of satisfactory patient outcomes.

REMARKS

Credentialing is a key issue in any profession. Specific to the fields of medicine are reimbursement requirements and medicolegal issues. Unfortunately in our current society, healthcare environment, and economy, proper credentialing is paramount, yet not unconditionally protective. In the case of ultrasound, we as practitioners are fortunate to have the leadership of many professional organizations that have put forth well-organized, robust guidelines to support our endeavors.

SUGGESTED READINGS

American College of Endocrinology. *ECNU Candidate Handbook*. 2011. Available at https://www.aace.com/files/CandidateHandbook.pdf.

American College of Surgeons.[ST-31] Ultrasound examination by surgeons. *Bull Acad Natl Med*. 1998;83:6.

American Institute for Ultrasound in Medicine. AIUM practice guideline for the performance of the focused assessment with sonography for trauma (FAST) examination. 2010. Available at: http://www.aium.org/publications/Statements.aspx.

American Institute for Ultrasound in Medicine. Standards and guidelines for the accreditation of ultrasound practices. 2010. Available at: http://www.aium.org/publications/Statements.aspx.

American Institute for Ultrasound in Medicine. Training guidelines for physicians who evaluate and interpret diagnostic ultrasound examinations. 2010. Available at: http://www.aium.org/publications/Statements.aspx.

American Medical Association policy H-230.960. Privileging for ultrasound imaging. Available at: http://www.ama-assn.org.

American Registry for Diagnostic Medical Sonography. Prerequisites for the physicians vascular interpretation examination. 2011. Available at: http://www.ardms.org/files/downloads/PVIprereq.pdf.

American Society for Gastrointestinal Endoscopy. Guidelines for credentialing and granting privileges for endoscopic ultrasound. *Gastrointest Endosc*. 2001;54(6):811–814.

American Society for Gastrointestinal Endoscopy. Guidelines for training in endoscopic ultrasound. *Gastrointest Endosc*. 1999;49:829–833.

American Society of Breast Surgeons. Performance and practice guidelines for breast ultrasound. 2010. Available at: http://www.breastsurgeons.org/statements/PDF_Statements/Perf_Guidelines_Breast_US.pdf.

American Urological Association. Consensus statement on urologic ultrasound utilization. 2007. Available at: http://www.auanet.org/content/guidelines-and-quality-care/policy-statements/c/consensus-statement-on-urologic-ultrasound-utilization.cfm.

Damewood S, Jeanmonod D, Cadigan B. Comparison of a multimedia simulator to a human model for teaching fast exam image interpretation and image acquisition. *Acad Emerg Med*. 2011;18:413–419. doi: 10.1111/j.1553-2712.2011.01037.

Knudson MM, Sisley AC. Training residents using simulation technology: experience with ultrasound for trauma. *J Trauma*. 2000;48:659–665.

Knudson M, Jamshidi R. Bedside procedures for general surgeons. ACS surgery: principles and practice. 2009. Available at: http://74.205.62.209/bcdecker/pdfs/acs/part00_ch11.pdf.

Rose S. Ultrasound in abdominal trauma. *Emerg Med Clin N Am*. 2004;22:581–599.

Rozycki G. Surgeon-performed ultrasound privileges, competency and practice. Available at: http://www.slideshare.net/u.surgery/surgeon-performed-ultrasound-privileges-competency-and-practice.

Sites B, Chan V, Neal J, Weller R, Grau T, Koscielniak-Nielsen Z, Ivani G. American Society of Regional Anesthesia and Pain Medicine and the European Society of Regional Anesthesia and Pain Therapy Joint Committee Recommendations for Education and Training in Ultrasound-Guided Regional Anesthesia. *Reg Anesth Pain Med*. 2010;35(1):64–101.

Society of American Gastrointestinal Endoscopic Surgeons. Guidelines for institutions granting ultrasonography privileges to surgeons. 2011. Available at: http://www.sages.org/publication/id/20/.

Sturm LP, Windsor JA, Cosman PH, et al. A systematic review of skills transfer after surgical simulation training. *Ann Surg*. 2008;248:166–179.

Wexner S, Eisen G, Simmang C. Principles of privileging and credentialing for endoscopy and colonoscopy. *Dis Colon Rectum*. 45(2):161–164.

APPENDIX 1

AIUM TRAINING GUIDELINES FOR PHYSICIANS WHO EVALUATE AND INTERPRET DIAGNOSTIC ULTRASOUND EXAMINATIONS

Approved November 6, 2010

Physicians who evaluate and interpret diagnostic ultrasound examinations should be licensed medical practitioners who have a thorough understanding of the indication and guidelines for ultrasound examinations as well as familiarity with the basic physical principles and limitations of the technology of ultrasound imaging. They should be familiar with alternative and complementary imaging and diagnostic procedures and should be capable of correlating the results of these other procedures with the ultrasound examination findings. They should have an understanding of ultrasound technology and instrumentation, ultrasound power output, equipment calibration, and safety. Physicians responsible for ultrasound examinations should be able to demonstrate familiarity with the anatomy, physiology, and pathophysiology of those organs or anatomic areas that are being examined. These physicians should provide evidence of training and requisite competence needed to successfully perform and interpret diagnostic ultrasound examinations in the area(s) they practice. The training should include methods of documentation and reporting of ultrasound studies.

Physicians performing diagnostic ultrasound examinations should meet at least 1 of the following:

1. Completion of an approved residency program, fellowship, or postgraduate training that includes the equivalent of at least 3 months of diagnostic ultrasound training in the area(s) they practice, under the supervision of a qualified physician(s),* during which the trainees will have evidence of being involved with the performance, evaluation, and interpretation of at least 300** sonograms.

2. Certification in breast ultrasound by the American Society of Breast Surgeons is accepted as proof of sufficient training in breast ultrasound.

3. Successful completion of the Endocrine Certification in Neck Ultrasound (ECNU) Program by the American Association of Clinical Endocrinologists (AACE) is accepted as proof of sufficient training in thyroid/parathyroid ultrasound.

4. Completion of training in "Focused Assessment with Sonography for Trauma (FAST)" as recommended by the American College of Emergency Physicians (ACEP) is accepted as proof of sufficient training for the performance of the FAST Examination.

5. Demonstration of at least 1 of the criteria listed in the AIUM's official statement "Training Guidelines for the Performance of the Musculoskeletal Ultrasound Examination" is accepted as proof of sufficient training in musculoskeletal ultrasound.

6. Proof of completion of an ABOG- or ACOOG-approved fellowship in Maternal-Fetal Medicine, with a brief written description of experience in performance of fetal echocardiography, including both normal and abnormal cases, is accepted as proof of sufficient training in fetal echocardiography. Physicians must be Active Candidates or Diplomates of ABOG or ACOOG. Others, including Pediatric Cardiologists and Radiologists, who have not completed formal MFM fellowship but who can demonstrate education and skills in performing fetal echocardiography should submit documentation of their educational and clinical experience.

7. In the absence of formal fellowship or postgraduate training or residency training, documentation of clinical experience could be acceptable, provided the following could be demonstrated:

   a. Evidence of *100 AMA PRA Category 1 Credits*™ dedicated to diagnostic ultrasound in the area(s) the physicians practice.

   b. Evidence of being involved in the performance, evaluation, and interpretation of the images of at least 300** sonograms within a 3-year period. It is expected that in most circumstances, examinations will be under the supervision of a qualified physician(s).* These sonograms should be in the specialty area(s) in which the physicians are practicing.

---

*A qualified physician is one who, at minimum, meets the criteria defined above in this document.
**Three hundred cases were selected as a minimum number needed to gain experience and proficiency with sonography as a diagnostic modality. This is necessary to develop technical skills, to appreciate the practical applications of basic physics as it affects image quality and artifact formation, and to acquire an experience base for understanding the range of normal and recognizing deviations from normal.

The number of required cases will be greater for physicians utilizing ultrasound for multiple subspecialty applications or anatomic areas (at least 500 cases). It is recognized, however, that the experience gained in the initial 300 cases provides an important foundation of knowledge and skill, which may reduce the number of additional cases needed to master other diagnostic ultrasound uses.

Cases presented as preselected, limited image sets, such as in lectures, case conferences, and teaching files, are excluded. The ability to analyze a full image set, determining its completeness and the adequacy of image quality, and performing the diagnostic process, distinguishing normal from abnormal, is considered a primary goal of the training experience.

APPENDIX 2

[ST-31] ULTRASOUND EXAMINATIONS BY SURGEONS*

By the American College of Surgeons

INTRODUCTION

Ultrasonography is a technology applicable in a wide variety of surgical practices and surgical specialties, and has become a routine tool for noninvasive evaluation of many organ systems and targeting areas for intervention. Examples include ultrasonic evaluation of the eye, the neck, reproductive organs, and the vascular, nervous, and musculoskeletal systems. Clinical applications of ultrasound require unique knowledge and skill.

To ensure that surgeons who use ultrasound are qualified and that the ultrasound facilities and equipment they use are appropriate for the medical application and meet and maintain quality standards, a voluntary verification process has been made available to Fellows. There are several components to this process: first, the surgeon must meet the requirements for education and/or experience; second, the facilities and equipment should meet recommended standards; third, the surgeon should maintain qualifications through continued experience and formal continuing medical education in the technique and its applications; and fourth, surgeon's outcomes using ultrasound should be assessed through a program of continuous quality improvement.

AMERICAN COLLEGE OF SURGEONS' VOLUNTARY VERIFICATION PROGRAM FOR SURGEONS IN THE USE OF ULTRASOUND

Surgeons performing ultrasound examinations and ultrasound-guided procedures must be familiar with the principles of ultrasound physics, and the indications, advantages, limitations, performance, and interpretation of the ultrasound examinations. The facilities used by the surgeon should be adequate and the equipment should be appropriate to the application. Technologists working under the supervision of the surgeon must be appropriately trained and certified and their performance regularly evaluated within the framework of the quality improvement process.

▶ Surgeon Eligibility and Verification in Basic Ultrasonography

The surgeon should provide evidence of training by meeting the following criteria:

1. Satisfactory completion of an accredited residency program in a surgical specialty, for example, through documentation of current certification by an ABMS Board or its equivalent.

2. When residency and/or fellowship did include documented training in the principles of ultrasound physics, the indications, advantages, and limitations of ultrasound, and personal experience with performance and interpretation of the ultrasound examination and ultrasound-guided interventional procedures, including knowledge of the indication for these procedures, complications that might be incurred, and techniques for successful completion of these procedures, the surgeon will be eligible for verification of qualifications in the basic use of ultrasound on review of their documentation.

3. When residency or fellowship training did not include education and personal experience in the use of ultrasound, completion (Level 2) of a basic approved educational program** in ultrasound physics and instrumentation, including didactic and practical components, is required for verification of qualifications in the basic use of ultrasound.

The basic level of ultrasound expertise includes the ability to acquire and interpret images of normal ultrasound anatomy.

▶ Verification of Surgeons Who Independently Perform Specific Ultrasound Examinations and Procedures

Examples of specific ultrasound applications are: FAST examination in trauma; breast examination and biopsy; evaluation of the thyroid and parathyroid; transrectal examination of the prostate and rectal tumors; endoscopic examination of the upper gastrointestinal (GI) tract and hepatobiliary system; intraoperative and laparoscopic examination of intra-abdominal and thoracic organ systems; and vascular, obstetric, gynecologic, ophthalmologic, and transcranial examinations. The surgeon using specific applications of ultrasound in an independent mode must have basic and specific expertise.

---

*Reprinted from **Bulletin of the American College of Surgeons,** Vol. 83, No. 06, June 1998.
**Courses must meet the criteria for Approval of Courses in New Skills, American College of Surgeons, 1998.

Specific applications require: (a) verification of qualifications in the basic use of ultrasound and (b) fundamental knowledge of and current competence in the management of the relevant clinical condition together with additional clinical expertise and training in diagnostic ultrasound. The ability to distinguish abnormal findings and perform ultrasound-guided procedures in the relevant clinical condition is also necessary.

These qualifications can be demonstrated by: (a) completion (Level 2) of an approved educational program in the specific application of ultrasound pertaining to the specific clinical area of interest (trauma, and so forth), or (b) documented experience and satisfactory outcomes in the use of specific application of ultrasound in the specific clinical area of interest and meeting the specified learning objectives of the specific module (for example, successful completion of the written examination).

[Criteria (a) and (b) may be fulfilled in a residency or fellowship that specifically includes sufficient education and experience under the supervision of a qualified physician.]

▶ Recommendations for Maintenance of Qualifications

To maintain proficiency in ultrasound applications, surgeons are encouraged to perform and interpret ultrasound examinations and have regular ultrasound-related Category 1 CME. These surgeons must document that a continuous quality improvement process is established and proper records are maintained.

▶ Ultrasound Facility Guidelines

Medical staff/medical director

A licensed physician is specified and responsible for determination and documentation of the quality and appropriateness of testing. This individual should oversee the development of a written policy for the granting of privileges for the medical staff. Such a policy should specify the scope of the privileges, specialty background, and education and experience in ultrasonography.

Scope of practice

The scope of practice (listing of all types of examinations and procedures) should be explicitly stated and documented.

Electrical safety

Testing of electrical safety of the ultrasound equipment must be performed on a regular basis and the results documented.

Equipment

For the proposed examinations and/or procedures the equipment and transducer selection should be the most appropriate to obtain optimal images of high resolution.

Quality control

The ultrasound equipment should be calibrated at installation and at least annually thereafter. The following tests are recommended for inclusion in the quality control program on, at least, an annual basis:

1. Maximum depth of visualization and hard copy recording with a tissue mimicking phantom
2. Distance accuracy: vertical distance accuracy and horizontal distance accuracy
3. Uniformity
4. Anechoic void perception
5. Ring down and dead space determination
6. Lateral resolution
7. Axial resolution
8. Data logs on system performance and examples of results

The process for testing and the standards for performance should be referenced. Technologists should be evaluated on a quarterly basis, and the results of that evaluation documented.

Minimum performance evaluation should include the following:

1. Adherence to universal infection control precautions
2. Distance calibration–quarterly
3. Gray scale photography–quarterly
4. Clinical images: Photographic images or films of normal and abnormal examinations should be available for review. In those facilities performing procedures, pre- and postprocedure films or photographs should be clearly labeled.
5. Equipment quality control: Each facility should have documented policies and procedures for monitoring and evaluating the effective management and proper performance of imaging equipment. Quality control programs should be designed to maximize the quality of the diagnostic information. Equipment performance should be monitored regularly in conformity with standards for ultrasound imaging and phantom testing for resolution. Such monitoring may be accomplished as part of a routine preventive maintenance program.
6. Quality improvement: Quality improvement procedures should be systematically monitored for appropriateness of examination, for technical accuracy, and for the accuracy of interpretation. The total number of examinations and procedures should be documented on a quarterly basis. Incidences of complications and adverse events incurred during ultrasound-guided interventional procedures should be recorded and regularly reviewed to identify opportunities to improve patient care.

APPENDIX 3

GUIDELINES FOR GRANTING OF ULTRASONOGRAPHY PRIVILEGES FOR SURGEONS
PRIVILEGING GUIDELINES published on: 01/2011

By the Society of American Gastrointestinal and Endoscopic Surgeons (SAGES)

PRINCIPLES OF CREDENTIALING

▶ Preamble

The Society of American Gastrointestinal Endoscopic Surgeons (SAGES) recommends the following guidelines for privileging qualified surgeons in the performance of ultrasound (transabdominal, laparoscopic, endoscopic, thoracoscopic surgery, and endovascular). The basic premise is that the surgeon(s) must have the judgment and training to perform ultrasonography safely and interpret the findings accurately.

▶ Disclaimer

Guidelines for clinical practice are intended to indicate preferable approaches to medical problems as established by experts in the field. These recommendations will be based on existing data or a consensus of expert opinion, when little or no data are available. Guidelines are applicable to all physicians who address the clinical problem(s) without regard to specialty training or interests, and are intended to indicate the preferable, but not necessarily the only, acceptable approaches due to the complexity of the healthcare environment. Guidelines are intended to be flexible. Given the wide range of specifics in any health care problem, the surgeon must always choose the course best suited to the individual patient and the variables in existence at the moment of decision.

Guidelines are developed under the auspices of the Society of American Gastrointestinal Endoscopic Surgeons and its various committees, and approved by the Board of Governors. Each clinical practice guideline has been systematically researched, reviewed, and revised by the guidelines committee, and also reviewed by an appropriate multidisciplinary team. The recommendations are therefore considered valid at the time of its production based on the data available. Each guideline is scheduled for periodic review to allow incorporation of pertinent new developments in medical research knowledge and practice.

▶ Purpose

The purpose of this statement is to assist hospital credentialing committees in their task of granting privileges to surgeons for the performance of ultrasonography (transabdominal, laparoscopic, endoscopic, intraoperative, thoracoscopic, and endovascular) for diagnostic and therapeutic purposes. In conjunction with the standard JCAHO guidelines for granting hospital privileges, implementation of these methods should help to insure that ultrasonography performed by surgeons is performed only by individuals with appropriate competency, thus assuring optimal patient care and procedure utilization.

Ultrasound is being increasingly used as a diagnostic tool in real time and as an aid to therapeutic decisions during surgery. A wide array of uses have been well described, spanning the various surgical subspecialties. Several publications have confirmed high degree of specificity and sensitivity of ultrasound examinations, equivalent to radiologist performed ultrasound when performed by surgeons with adequate training.[5,6]

▶ Uniformity of Standards

Uniform standards should be developed that are applicable to all surgeons requesting privileges to perform ultrasonography. Criteria must be established that are medically sound and take into account the skills that a surgeon already possesses as part of his/her surgical training.

▶ Specificity of Privileging for Ultrasonography

Privileges should be granted for each major category of ultrasonography separately. The ability to perform one ultrasonographic procedure does not automatically imply adequate competency to perform another. Associated skills generally considered to be an integral part of an ultrasonographic category may be required before privileges for that category can be granted. Major categories include Focused Assessment with Sonography for Trauma (FAST), abdominal (staging—laparoscopic and open), vascular, thoracic, urology, and gynecology.

▶ Responsibility for Credentialing

The credentialing structure and process are the responsibility of each hospital. It should be the responsibility of the Department of Surgery, through its Chief, to recommend individual surgeons for privileges in ultrasonography as for all other procedures performed by members of his/her department.

MINIMUM REQUIREMENTS FOR GRANTING PRIVILEGES

Part II A is mandatory, and must be accompanied by either part II B, II C, or at least one component of part II D.

▶ Formal Fellowship or Surgical Residency Training

Prerequisite training must include satisfactory completion of an accredited surgical residency program, with subsequent certification by the American Board of Surgery as required by the institution. The residency program must be accredited by the Accreditation Council for Graduate Medical Education or the equivalent body if the program is based outside the United States or Canada.

▶ Formal Training in Ultrasonography

For surgeons who successfully completed a residency and/or fellowship program that incorporated a structured experience in ultrasonography, the applicant's program director and, if desired, other faculty members should supply the appropriate documentation of training.

▶ No Formal Residency Training in Ultrasonography

For those surgeons without residency and/or fellowship training, which included structured experience in ultrasonography, or without documented prior experience in these areas, a structured training curriculum is required. The curriculum should be defined by the institution, and may include a formal course. The curriculum should include an appropriate number of opportunities for the applicant to observe, assist, and serve as the primary operator for the procedure for which privileges are being sought. The curriculum should include didactic sessions and hands-on experience with inanimate and/or animate models. Other teaching aids may include video review and interactive computer programs. Several fellowships and courses by relevant professional societies including SAGES and American College of Surgeons are available throughout the year and can be used to gain ultrasonographic skills pertaining to a particular topic.

▶ Practical Experience

Applicant's experience

Documented experience that includes an appropriate volume of cases equivalent to the procedure in question in terms of complexity. The chief of surgery should determine the appropriateness of this experience.

Experience with preceptor and/or proctor

The specific role and qualifications of the preceptor and/or proctor, if required, must be determined by the institution. Criteria of competency for each procedure should be established in advance, and should include evaluation of familiarity with instrumentation and equipment, competence in their use, appropriateness of patient selection, safety, and successful completion of the procedure. The criteria should be established by the Chief of Surgery in conjunction with the specific specialty chief where appropriate. It is essential that proctoring be provided in an unbiased, confidential, and objective manner.

MAINTENANCE OF PRIVILEGES

▶ Provisional Privileges

Once competence has been determined, a period of provisional privileges may be appropriate. The time frame and/or the number of cases required during this period should be determined by the Chief of Surgery and/or the appropriate institutional committee, board, or governing body.

▶ Monitoring of Ultrasonographic Performance

To assist the hospital credentialing body in the ongoing renewal of privileges, there should be a mechanism for monitoring each surgeon's performance. This should be done through existing quality assurance mechanisms or an appropriate hospital committee. Monitoring may include ultrasound utilization, image quality, diagnostic and therapeutic benefits to patients, complications, and tissue review in accordance with previously developed criteria.

▶ Renewal of Privileges

For renewal of privileges an appropriate level of continuing clinical activity should be required, in addition to satisfactory performance as assessed by monitoring of procedural activity through existing quality assurance mechanisms. Continuing education related to ultrasonography should be part of the periodic renewal of privileges.

▶ Denial of Privileges

Institutions denying, withdrawing, or restricting privileges should have an appropriate mechanism for appeal in place. The procedural details of this should be developed by the institution, and must satisfy the institution's bylaws and JCAHO recommendations.

Sumeet K. Mittal, MD
William S. Richardson, MD (Co-Chair)
Ziad T. Awad, MD
Simon Bergman, MD
Ronald H. Clements, MD
David B. Earle, MD
David S. Edelman, MD
Liane S. Feldman, MD
Erika K. Fellinger, MD
Shannon A. Fraser, MD
Stephen P. Haggerty, MD
William W. Hope, MD
Ifeoma J. Igboeli, MD
Geoffrey P. Kohn, MD
Henry J. Lujan, MD

Lisa R. Martin Hawver, MD
Erica A. Moran, MD
David W. Overby, MD
Jonathan P. Pearl, MD
Raymond R. Price, MD
Kurt E. Roberts, MD
John S. Roth, MD
Alan A. Saber, MD
Dimitrios Stefanidis, MD
Andrew S. Wright, MD
Jin S. Yoo, MD
Joerg Zehetner, MD
Marc Zerey, MD
Robert D. Fanelli, MD, FACS (Chair)

REFERENCES

1. Society of American Gastrointestinal Endoscopic Surgeons: Granting of Privileges for Gastrointestinal Endoscopy by Surgeons. Los Angeles, CA, 1992.
2. Society of American Gastrointestinal Endoscopic Surgeons: Framework for Post-Residency Surgical Education & Training – A SAGES Guideline. *Surg Endosc.* 1994;8(9):1137–1142.
3. Richardson W, Stefanidis D, Mittal S, Fanelli RD. Society of American Gastrointestinal Endoscopic surgeons: SAGES guidelines for the use of laparoscopic ultrasound. *Surg Endosc.* 2010 Apr;24(4):745–756.
4. Position statement ST 31 by American College of Surgeons Committee on Emerging Surgical Technology and Education (CESTE). February 1998.
5. Boneti C, McVay MR, Kokoska ER, Jackson RJ, Smith SD. Ultrasound as a diagnostic tool used by surgeons in pyloric stenosis. *J Pediatr Surg.* 2008 Jan;43(1):87–91; discussion 91.
6. Soon PS, Delbridge LW, Sywak MS, Barraclough BM, Edhouse P, Sidhu SB. Surgeon performed ultrasound facilitates minimally invasive parathyroidectomy by the focused lateral mini-incision approach. *World J Surg.* 2008 May;32(5):766–771.

This statement was reviewed and approved by the Board of Governors of the Society of American Gastrointestinal and Endoscopic Surgeons (SAGES) on Jan 2011.

This is a revision of SAGES publication #20 printed Oct 2003, revised Jan 2011.

APPENDIX 4

THE AMERICAN SOCIETY OF BREAST SURGEONS

PERFORMANCE AND PRACTICE GUIDELINES FOR BREAST ULTRASOUND

The American Society of Breast Surgeons (the Society) was formed to encourage the study of breast surgery, promote research and development of advanced surgical techniques, improve standards of practice for breast surgery in the United States, and serve as a forum for the exchange of ideas.

ARTICLE I. INTRODUCTION

This publication, *The American Society of Breast Surgeons Performance and Practice Guidelines for Breast Ultrasound*, is intended to provide the surgeon sonographer with guidelines for performing and recording high-quality ultrasound examinations of the breast in order to attain optimal breast ultrasound practices. The following guidelines reflect what the Society considers to be the basic criteria for the complete diagnostic examination of the breast, as well as for ultrasound-guided invasive breast procedures. However, use of these guidelines may require modification to adapt to a specific clinical situation.

These guidelines are based on the opinions of a panel of Society members who are experts in breast ultrasound. Panel members have served on the faculty of breast ultrasound courses sponsored by the Society and the American College of Surgeons, as well as many stand-alone courses for more than a decade. Multiple published sources were also reviewed in establishing these guidelines.[1-6]

ARTICLE II. INDICATIONS FOR BREAST ULTRASOUND

Breast ultrasound is useful and appropriate in multiple clinical situations, including but not limited to the following:

1. Identification and characterization of palpable abnormalities noted on clinical breast examination

2. Identification and characterization of localized breast symptoms, such as breast pain, fullness, and nipple discharge

3. Identification and characterization of nonpalpable abnormalities detected on other breast imaging modalities

4. Guidance for percutaneous and surgical procedures

5. Evaluation and assessment of the breast after surgical or medical therapy

6. Preoperative evaluation of breast and axilla in diagnosed breast cancer (ie, ultrasound mapping, BIRADS 6)

7. Identification and characterization of abnormalities associated with implants

8. Evaluation and assessment for radiation therapy planning

9. Intraoperative assessment of lumpectomy margins

ARTICLE III. QUALIFICATIONS OF THE SURGEON SONOGRAPHER

To be qualified as a surgeon sonographer, a surgeon should: (a) have successfully completed an American Board of Medical Specialties (ABMS)-approved residency program, and must have attained board certification by the appropriate certifying board upon completion of training, or be admissible for certification; (b) have at least 15 hours AMA-PRA Category I CME credits in breast ultrasound, including at least one full-day course including diagnostic and interventional components; and (c) demonstrate maintenance of skills by performing at least 50 breast ultrasound examinations and at least 12 ultrasound-guided invasive procedures per year, and must earn at least 3 hours of AMA category 1 CME credit in breast ultrasound every 3 years.

To perform ultrasound-guided interventional procedures, the surgeon should be proctored on at least two ultrasound-guided interventional procedures. The proctor must be a physician that can satisfy at least one of the following:

1. Current certification/accreditation in breast ultrasound by the Society, the American Institute of Ultrasound in Medicine, or the American College of Radiology

2. Documentation of 5 years' clinical experience in breast ultrasound with at least 15 hours of American Medical Association (AMA) category 1 continuing medical education (CME) credit in breast ultrasound earned in the preceding 5 years

ARTICLE IV. ULTRASOUND EXAMINATION REQUIREMENTS

▶ Diagnostic

For characterization of palpable or nonpalpable abnormalities: (a) the patient should be properly positioned to minimize thickness of the portion of the breast examined;

(b) minimally acceptable ultrasound device settings should include proper depth, proper gain, and appropriate focal zones; (c) described lesions should be imaged in two orthogonal projections; (d) at least two sets of lesion images should be obtained, one set with calipers and one without, except for follow-up examination or lesions large enough that calipers would not significantly obscure the margins; (e) all described lesions should be measured in three dimensions including height, width, and depth, unless shadowing obscures the accurate measurement of height; (f) each image should have complete labeling, including: date and time of the examination, a unique patient identifier; right or left breast, transducer orientation, and lesion location described by either written or pictorial methods. The location of the lesion should be recorded by either clock notation or the quadrant of the breast with distance of the lesion from the nipple noted in centimeters or by zone; (g) the imaged lesion should be correlated with the physical examination of the breast and appropriate imaging studies; and (h) each identified lesion should have complete documentation in a written report.

▶ Interventional

Indications

1. Guidance for office procedures, including cyst aspiration, fine needle aspiration cytology, core needle biopsy, rotational cutter or vacuum-assisted needle biopsy, placement of marking clips or guide wires, placement of brachytherapy devices, targeted breast tissue ablation, and similar procedures

2. Intraoperative use, including guidance for surgical excision with or without placement of a hook wire or needle localization device, assessment of adequacy of surgical excision for both palpable and nonpalpable lesions, and the use of other intraoperative devices (eg, ablative procedure)

Technical aspects

1. Guidance technique should align the biopsy (needle) device as perpendicular to the acoustic beam as possible (parallel to the chest wall) in order to optimize visualization of the device and to minimize the risk of injury to surrounding structures.

2. Simple core tissue sampling should use a minimum of a 14-gauge needle, with or without a coaxial system.

3. Multiple images of the guidance procedure should be obtained, including an image just prior to intervention as well as an image showing the device in the proper location after deployment.

ARTICLE V. WRITTEN DOCUMENTATION

1. Each ultrasound study should have a permanent written record along with the accompanying set of images in retrievable image storage format. The images and report should become a part of the patient's permanent medical record.

2. Each individual image should include the facility name, date of examination, patient's first and last name, and identification number, if applicable. A notation of left or right breast and the location of the lesion should be shown on all images. Diagnostic images should also indicate transducer orientation within the breast. *All of the above notations should be made using the icon or the annotation script capability of the instrument.*

   The distance of the lesion from the nipple should be noted either in centimeters or by zone *using the instrument's script. Handwritten notes on the images should be used only to correct errors on previously printed images.*

3. Standard form reports may be used as long as they are comprehensive in nature.

4. Reports of diagnostic procedures should include the indication for the study (including correlation with physical and/or imaging studies), description of technique, findings (including size, shape, echogenicity, and physics artifacts), impression (with provisional diagnosis, if possible), and recommendation.

5. Reports of ultrasound-guided interventional procedures should include the location of the lesion; the approach (lateral to medial, etc); the type of prep and local anesthesia; skin incision, if any; the type of device used; the number of cores taken; and the type of clip placed, if any. If specimen radiographs or sonograms are done, the information should be recorded in the report.

6. Final reports should be completed and sent to the referring clinician in a timely manner, if indicated.

7. A written note should be made documenting concordance (or discordance) of imaging findings with pathology, complications (if any), and a disposition based upon correlation of physical, imaging, and pathology findings.

8. Optional classification of breast ultrasound lesions may be used employing the American College of Radiology Breast Imaging Reporting and Data System, or BIRADS (see Appendix 4A).

ARTICLE VI. EQUIPMENT SPECIFICATIONS AND QUALITY CONTROL

1. High-resolution linear array transducers of at least 7.5 MHz frequency should be utilized for breast ultrasound diagnostic examinations and for ultrasound-guided interventional procedures.

2. Each facility should have written policies and procedures for monitoring and evaluating the effective management and proper performance of imaging equipment.

3. Quality control programs should be designed to maximize the quality of the diagnostic information. (See Article VII.)

4. Equipment performance should be monitored at least annually in conformity with standards for ultrasound imaging and phantom testing for resolution. Such monitoring may be accomplished as part of a routine preventive maintenance program unless such routine maintenance is not recommended by the manufacturer.

ARTICLE VII. QUALITY ASSESSMENT/ IMPROVEMENT

1. Policies and procedures related to quality, personnel and patient safety, and infection control should be developed in accordance with the appropriate American College of Surgeons policies.

2. Quality assessment procedures should exist and should be systematically monitored for appropriateness of examinations, technical accuracy, and accuracy of interpretations. The Society encourages participation in quality monitoring programs that may exist on a national level.

3. The volume of examinations and procedures should be documented and assessed on a continuous basis.

4. Complications and adverse events incurred during ultrasound-guided interventional procedures should be recorded and regularly reviewed to identify opportunities to improve patient care.

5. Results of ultrasound-guided interventional procedures should be recorded, monitoring the false-negative rates, inadequate tissue samples, and follow-up recommendations. Concordance/discordance of imaging findings and pathology reports should be addressed by policies developed for resolution of discordant findings.

ACKNOWLEDGMENTS

These guidelines were developed by the members of The American Society of Breast Surgeons Breast Ultrasound Certification Committee and have been approved by the Board of Directors of The American Society of Breast Surgeons.

Sara Fredrickson, MD, Chair
Stephen Auda, MD
Aaron D. Bleznak, MD
Beth Boyd, RN
Kambiz Dowlat, MD
Richard A. Fine, MD
Mark A. Gittleman, MD
Linsey Gold, DO
Ronda Henry-Tillman, MD
Scott Karlan, MD

Dan Kopen, MD
Alison L. Laidley, MD
Arthur G. Lerner, MD
Howard C. Snider, MD
Angela Soto-Hamlin, MD
Carrie Thoms, MD
Gary Unzeitig, MD
Dariush Vaziri, MD
Eric Whitacre, MD
Victor Zannis, MD

REFERENCES

1. American College of Radiology. ACR practice guideline for the performance of a breast ultrasound examination. 1994 (revised 1998, 2002; amended 2006, revised 2007). Available at: http://www.acr.org/guidelines.

2. American College of Radiology. ACR practice guidelines for the performance of ultrasound guided percutaneous breast interventional procedures. 1996 (revised 2000, 2005, amended 2006, revised 2009). Available at: http://www.acr.org/guidelines.

3. American Institute of Ultrasound in Medicine. AIUM standard for the performance of breast ultrasound examination. 2002. Available at: http://www.aium.org/publications/clinical/breast.pdf.

4. Canadian Association of Radiologists. Standard for the performance of breast ultrasound examination. 2003. Available at: http://www.car.ca/EN/About_the_CAR/Standards_and_Guidelines/library/breast_interventional.pdf.

5. Canadian Association of Radiologists. Standards for the performance of ultrasound-guided percutaneous breast interventional procedures. 2003. Available at: http://www.car.ca/EN/About_the_CAR/Standards_and_Guidelines/library/breast_interventional.pdf.

6. American College of Surgeons. [ST-31] Ultrasound examinations by surgeons. 1998. Available at: http://www.facs.org/fellows_info/statements/st-31.html.

Developed October 2006
Revised February 2007
Revised October 2008
Revised April 2010

APPENDIX 4A

AMERICAN COLLEGE OF RADIOLOGY BREAST IMAGING REPORTING AND DATA SYSTEM—ULTRASOUND ASSESSMENT CATEGORIES*

▶ A. Assessment Is Incomplete

Category 0: Need additional imaging evaluation

In many instances, the ultrasound (US) examination completes the evaluation of the patient. If US is the initial study, other examinations may be indicated. An example would be the need for mammography if US were the initial study for a patient in her late 20's evaluated with US for a palpable mass that had suspicious sonographic features.

Another example might be where mammography and US are nonspecific, such as differentiating between scarring and recurrence in a patient with breast cancer treated with lumpectomy and radiation therapy. Here, MRI might be the recommendation. A need for previous studies to determine appropriate management might also defer a final assessment.

▶ B. Assessment Is Complete— Final Categories

Category 1: Negative

This category is for sonograms with no abnormality, such as a mass, architectural distortion, thickening of the skin, or microcalcifications. For greater confidence in rendering a negative interpretation, an attempt should be made to correlate the ultrasound and mammographic patterns of breast tissue in the area of concern.

Category 2: Benign finding(s)

Essentially a report that is negative for malignancy. Simple cysts would be placed in this category, along with intramammary lymph nodes (also possible to include in Category 1), breast implants, stable postsurgical changes, and probable fibroadenomas noted to be unchanged on successive US studies.

Category 3: Probably benign finding— short interval follow-up suggested

With accumulating clinical experience and by extension from mammography, a solid mass with circumscribed margins, oval shape, and horizontal orientation, most likely a fibroadenoma, should have a less than 2% risk of malignancy.

Although additional multicenter data may confirm safety of follow-up rather than biopsy based on US findings, short-interval follow-up is currently increasing as a management strategy. Nonpalpable complicated cysts and clustered microcysts might also be placed in this category for short-interval follow-up.

Category 4: Suspicious abnormality— biopsy should be considered

Lesions in this category would have an intermediate probability of cancer, ranging from 3% to 90%. An option would be to stratify these lesions, giving them a low, intermediate, or moderate likelihood of malignancy. In general, Category 4 lesions require tissue sampling. Needle biopsy can provide acytologic or a histologic diagnosis. Included in this group are sonographic findings of a solid mass without all of the criteria for a fibroadenoma.

Category 5: Highly suggestive of malignancy—appropriate action should be taken (almost certainly malignant)

The abnormality identified sonographically and placed in this category should have at least a 90% or higher risk of malignancy so that definitive treatment might be considered at the outset. With the increasing use of sentinel node imaging as a way of assessing nodal metastases and also with the increasing use of neoadjuvant chemotherapy for large malignant masses or those that are poorly differentiated, percutaneous sampling, most often with imaging-guided core needle biopsy, can provide the histopathological diagnosis.

Category 6: Known biopsy-proven malignancy—appropriate action should be taken

This category is reserved for lesions with biopsy proof of malignancy prior to institution of therapy, including neoadjuvant chemotherapy, surgical excision, or mastectomy.

---

*American College of Radiology (ACR). ACR BI-RADS®—Ultrasound. First Edition. ACR Breast Imaging Reporting crd Data System, Breast Imaging Atlas; BI-RADS—US Assessment Categories. Reston, VA. American College ofRadiology; 2003. (Reprinted with permission of the American College of Radiology). No other representation of this material is authorized without expressed, written permission from the American College of Radiology.

APPENDIX 5

AMERICAN SOCIETY FOR GASTROINTESTINAL ENDOSCOPY

GUIDELINES FOR CREDENTIALING AND GRANTING PRIVILEGES FOR ENDOSCOPIC ULTRASOUND

VOLUME 54, NO. 6, 2001 GASTROINTESTINAL ENDOSCOPY 811

This is one of a series of statements discussing the utilization of gastrointestinal endoscopy in common clinical situations. In preparing this guideline, a MEDLINE literature search was performed, and additional references were obtained from the bibliographies of the identified articles and from recommendations of expert consultants. When little or no data exist from well-designed prospective trials, emphasis is given to results from large series and reports from recognized experts.

Guidelines for the appropriate use of endoscopy are based on a critical review of the available data and expert consensus. Controlled clinical studies are needed to clarify aspects of this statement and revision may be necessary as new data appear. Clinical considerations may justify a course of action at variance from these recommendations.

This document is intended to provide the principles by which credentialing organizations may create policy and practical guidelines for granting endoscopic ultrasound (EUS) privileges. For information on credentialing for other endoscopic procedures, please refer to "Guidelines for Credentialing and Granting Privileges for Gastrointestinal Endoscopy" (*Gastrointest Endosc.* 1998;48:679–682).

DEFINITIONS OF TERMS

Clinical Privileges: Authorization by a local institution to perform a particular procedure or clinical service.

Competence: The minimum level of skill, knowledge, and/or expertise derived through training and experience, required to safely and proficiently perform a task or procedure.

Credentialing Process: The process of assessing and validating the qualifications of a licensed independent practitioner to provide patient care. The determination is based on an evaluation of the individual's current license, knowledge base, training or experience, current competence, and ability to perform the procedure or patient care requested.

Credentials: Documents provided after successful completion of a period of education or training as an indication of clinical competence.

Endoscopic ultrasound (EUS): A group of related techniques whereby an endoscope is used to place an ultrasound transducer within the gastrointestinal lumen to perform ultrasonography of the wall, wall-associated lesions, and structures surrounding the gastrointestinal tract.

Echoendoscope: A device used to perform EUS, consisting of a flexible fiberoptic or video endoscope incorporating an ultrasound transducer in its design.

Catheter ultrasound probe: A through-the-scope ultrasound device that allows the insertion of a transducer through the working channel of standard endoscopic instruments to perform endoluminal ultrasonography.

EUS-guided fine needle aspiration (FNA): Use of EUS for real-time guidance of an aspiration needle into a lesion within or adjacent to the GI tract for diagnostic sampling.

PRINCIPLES OF INITIAL CREDENTIALING IN EUS

1. Credentials for EUS should be determined independently from other endoscopic procedures such as colonoscopy, sigmoidoscopy, esophagogastroduodenoscopy (EGD), endoscopic retrograde cholangiopancreatography (ERCP), or any other endoscopic procedure.[1]

2. Competence in EUS requires both cognitive and technical components.[2,3]

3. Appropriate documentation should be required in the determination of competence in EUS. This may include the completion of a formal training program (residency or fellowship) or documentation of equivalent training in other settings.

   Documentation of continued competence should be required for the renewal of EUS privileges.[1,4]

4. After the successful completion of EUS training (as detailed in—Guidelines for training in endoscopic ultrasound. *Gastrointest Endosc.* 1999;49:829–833) the trainee:

   a. Must be able to integrate EUS into the overall clinical evaluation of the patient.

   b. Should have sound general medical or surgical training.

   c. Must have completed at least 24 months of a standard GI fellowship (or equivalent) and have documented competence in routine endoscopic procedures.

   d. Must have a thorough understanding of the indications, contraindications, individual risk factors, and benefit-risk considerations for the individual patient.

   e. Must be able to clearly describe the EUS procedure and obtain informed consent.

TABLE 18-1

Minimum Number of EUS Procedures Before Competency Can Be Assessed

Site/Lesion	No. of Cases Required
Mucosal tumors (cancers of esophagus, stomach, rectum)	75
Submucosal abnormalities	40
Pancreaticobiliary	75
EUS-guided FNA	
Nonpancreatic*	25
Pancreatic†	25

For competence in imaging both mucosal and submucosal abnormalities, a minimum of 125 supervised cases is recommended.
For comprehensive competence in all aspects of EUS, a minimum of 150 supervised cases, of which 75 should be pancreaticobiliary and 50 EUS-guided FNA, is recommended.
*Intramural lesions or lymph nodes. Must be competent to perform mucosal EUS.
†Must be competent to perform pancreaticobiliary EUS.

f. Must have knowledge of the gastrointestinal and surrounding anatomy as imaged by EUS, and of the technical features of the equipment, work station, and accessories.

g. Must be able to safely intubate the esophagus, pylorus, and duodenum, and obtain imaging of the desired organ or lesion.

h. Must be able to accurately identify and interpret EUS images and recognize normal and abnormal findings.

i. Must be able to perform imaging such as tumor staging in agreement with surgical findings or findings of EUS trainer.

j. Must be able to document EUS findings and communicate with referring physicians.

k. Must competently perform those EUS procedures that were taught.

5. A clinician can obtain training in formal settings such as fellowship or residency programs. Less formal settings may be an option if an adequate number of supervised cases can be provided.

Short courses, use of animal models, and computer-based learning are useful adjuncts but should not be used in lieu of direct supervised training.[3]

Self-teaching through trial and error is not appropriate.

6. New EUS procedures or significant advances in existing procedures may occur. Endosonographers may wish to acquire privileges to perform these procedures. The degree of training, direct supervision, and proctoring will vary with the experience of the endoscopist.[5] When possible, objective criteria of competence should be developed and met.[6]

EUS is performed in several anatomic locations for various indications.[7] These include the evaluation and staging of mucosally based malignancies (esophagus, stomach, colon, and rectum), evaluation of submucosal abnormalities, assessment of pathology involving the pancreas and bile ducts, and performance of EUS-guided FNA. It is recognized that a practitioner may be competent in one or more of these areas. Privileging should consider each of

these areas separately and training must be adequate for the major category for which privileges are sought. Performance of an arbitrary number of procedures does not guarantee competency. The number of supervised procedures necessary to obtain competency will vary between trainees. Whenever possible, competence should be determined by objective criteria and direct observation.[3]

Threshold numbers of procedures that should be done before competency can be assessed are presented in Table 18-1. These numbers represent a minimum standard and should not be taken to indicate that competency has been achieved. These numbers are derived from studies on training in EUS, published expert opinion, and the consensus of the Ad Hoc EUS and Standards of Practice committees of the ASGE.

MUCOSAL TUMORS

The evaluation of esophageal, gastric, and duodenal tumors requires safe intubation of the esophagus, pylorus, and duodenum, accurate imaging of the lesion, and identification of lymphadenopathy with special attention to the celiac axis region. In a prospective study, competent intubation of the above sites was achieved in 1 to 23 procedures (median 1–2), with visualization of the gastric or esophageal wall in 1 to 47 procedures (median 10–15).

Evaluation of the celiac axis required 8 to 36 procedures (median 25).[8] Two articles have addressed the issue of the learning curve in the staging of esophageal cancer. Fockens et al.[9] found that adequate staging accuracy was achieved only after 100 examinations, and Schlick et al.[10] found 75 cases to be the minimum to attain 89.5% T stage accuracy.

Both of these articles involved largely self-taught practitioners and it is possible that competency maybe achieved with fewer cases in the setting of a formalized training program. A survey of the American Endosonography Club suggested an average 44.3 cases for competent gastric imaging, 42.9 for the esophagus, and 37.1 for the rectum.[11] It is recognized that once competence is achieved in one anatomic location (eg, esophageal cancer), the number of cases required in other sites (eg, stomach cancer) may be reduced. For this reason it is recommended that for the evaluation of mucosal tumors and malignancies, a minimum of 75 supervised cases, at least 2/3 in the upper GI tract, should be performed before competency can be assessed.

SUBMUCOSAL ABNORMALITIES

EUS is indicated for the evaluation of submucosal abnormalities such as neoplasms, varices, and enlarged gastric folds, and to determine intramural versus extrinsic location of an abnormality.[12] With the availability of inexpensive catheter-based EUS systems, practitioners may wish to become competent in the evaluation of these abnormalities separately from other indications for EUS. Although the number of cases required to accurately assess submucosal abnormalities has not been studied, the Standards of Training Committee of the ASGE recommends 40 to 50.[13]

PANCREATICOBILIARY IMAGING

Consensus opinion recognizes that accurate imaging and interpretation of images of the pancreas, bile duct, gallbladder, and ampulla is more technically demanding than that of intramural lesions.[2,11] The number of pancreaticobiliary cases needed to achieve competency may be higher than that for other anatomic sites. In a prospective study, adequate imaging of the pancreas required 15 to 74 cases (median 34), imaging of the bile and pancreatic ducts required 13 to 135 cases (median 55), and imaging of the ampulla required 13 to 134 cases (median 54).[8] A survey of the American Endosonography Club found that although technical competence in pancreaticobiliary imaging could be achieved in 94 cases, interpretive competence required 121,[11] whereas other expert opinion suggested 150 cases were needed for interpretative competence.[2]

EUS-GUIDED FNA

The addition of EUS-guided FNA to standard EUS imaging adds both complexity and risk to the procedure.[3] FNA is performed in three general sites: intramural lesions, perigastrointestinal lymphadenopathy, and pancreatic lesions.[14] Of these sites, the most technically difficult and the one that carries the highest risk of complications is biopsy of pancreatic lesions and cysts.[14,15] Therefore, pancreatic and nonpancreatic FNA are considered separately. Successful and safe FNA first requires competence in standard EUS imaging.[2] The number of FNA cases needed to achieve competence has not been studied. EUS has similarities to ERCP in that each uses side-viewing instruments and combined endoscopic/radiologic imaging. For therapeutic ERCP it has been recommended that a minimum of 25 supervised cases be performed in addition to 75 diagnostic.[13] For nonpancreatic FNA (intramural lesions, lymph nodes) it is recommended that the trainee be competent to perform mucosal tumor EUS and have done at least 25 supervised FNA of nonpancreatic lesions. For pancreatic FNA it is recommended that the trainees be competent to perform pancreaticobiliary EUS and have done at least 25 supervised FNA of pancreatic lesions.

COMPREHENSIVE EUS COMPETENCE

It is recognized that once clinical competence in one area of EUS practice has been achieved (eg, staging mucosal tumors), the number of cases required to achieve competence in other areas (eg, submucosal tumors) may be decreased. For practitioners interested in achieving competence in more than one area, training must include an adequate variety of clinical pathology. It is suggested that for those interested in mucosal and submucosal lesions but not pancreaticobiliary imaging, a minimum of 100 supervised cases be completed. For comprehensive competence in all aspects of EUS, at least 150 supervised cases should be performed, with 50 EUS-guided FNA, and at least 75 pancreaticobiliary cases.

PRINCIPLES OF RECREDENTIALING AND RENEWAL OF EUS PRIVILEGES

The goal of recredentialing is to assure continued clinical competence, promote continuous quality improvement, and maintain patient safety (see—Renewal of endoscopic privileges. *Gastrointest Endosc.* 1999;49:823–825).

ASSURING CONTINUED COMPETENCE IN EUS REQUIRES

1. Documentation of an adequate case load to maintain skills. Documentation can include procedure log books or patient records and should include objective measures of the number of cases, procedure success, and complications.

2. Review of above statistics in a continuous quality improvement setting.

3. Documentation of continued cognitive training through participation in educational activities.

The purpose of this review and documentation should be restricted to use in continuous quality improvement and endoscopic credentialing.

REFERENCES

1. ASGE. Guidelines for credentialing and granting privileges for gastrointestinal endoscopy. *Gastrointest Endosc.* 1998;48:679–682.
2. Boyce HW. Training in endoscopic ultrasonography. *Gastrointest Endosc.* 1996;43:S12–S15.

3. ASGE. Guidelines for training in endoscopic ultrasound. *Gastrointest Endosc.* 1999;49:829–833.

4. ASGE. Renewal of endoscopic privileges. *Gastrointest Endosc.* 1999;49:823–825.

5. Fleischer DE. Advanced training in endoscopy. *Gastrointest Endosc Clin North Am.* 1995;5:311–322.

6. ASGE. Methods for privileging for new technology in gastrointestinal endoscopy. *Gastrointest Endosc.* 1999;50:899–900.

7. Chak A, Cooper GS. Procedure-specific outcomes assessment for endoscopic ultrasonography. *Gastrointest Endosc Clin North Am.* 1999;9:649–656.

8. Hoffman B, Wallace MB, Eloubeidi MA, Sahai AV, Chak A, van Velse A, et al. How many supervised procedures does it take to become competent in EUS? Results of a multicenter three year study. *Gastrointest Endosc.* 2000;51:AB139.

9. Fockens P, Van den Brande JHM, van Dullemen HM, van Lanschot JJB, Tytgat GNJ. Endosonographic T-staging of esophageal carcinoma: a learning curve. *Gastrointest Endosc.* 1996;44:58–62.

10. Schlick T, Heintz A, Junginger T. The examiner's learning effect and its influence on the quality of endoscopic ultrasonography in carcinoma of the esophagus and gastric cardia. *Surg Endosc.* 1999;13:894–898.

11. Hoffman BJ, Hawes RH. Endoscopic ultrasound and clinical competence. *Gastrointest Endosc Clin North Am.* 1995;5:879–884.

12. Lightdale CJ. Indications, contraindications, and complications of endoscopic ultrasonography. *Gastrointest Endosc.* 1996;43:S15–S18.

13. ASGE. Principles of training in gastrointestinal endoscopy. *Gastrointest Endosc.* 1999;49:845–850.

14. ASGE. Tissue sampling during endosonography. *Gastrointest Endosc.* 1998;47:576–578.

15. Gress FG, Hawes RH, Savides TJ, Ikenberry SO, Lehman GA. Endoscopic ultrasound-guided fine-needle aspiration biopsy using linear array and radial scanning endosonography. *Gastrointest Endosc.* 1997;45:243–250.

PREPARED BY

▶ Standards of Practice Committee

Glenn M. Eisen, MD, Chair
Jason A. Dominitz, MD
Douglas O. Faigel, MD
Jay A. Goldstein, MD
Bret T. Petersen, MD
Hareth M. Raddawi, MD
Michael E. Ryan, MD
John J. Vargo II, MD
Harvey S. Young, MD
Jo Wheeler-Harbaugh, BS, RN, CGRN, MD

▶ Ad Hoc EUS Committee

Robert H. Hawes, MD, Chair
William R. Brugge, MD
John G. Carrougher, MD
Amitabh Chak, MD
Douglas O. Faigel, MD
Michael L. Kochman, MD
Thomas J. Savides, MD
Michael B. Wallace, MD, MPH
Maurits J. Wiersema, MD
Richard A. Erickson, MD

APPENDIX 6

CONSENSUS STATEMENT ON UROLOGIC ULTRASOUND UTILIZATION

Ultrasound is an integral part of standard urological practice. The American Urological Association, Inc.® (AUA) has developed guidelines and recommendations for these applications. These include: (1) Policy statement; (2) Equipment, documentation and indications for specific urologic examinations; (3) Education; and (4) Patient safety.

AUA POLICY STATEMENT ON IMAGING SERVICES

▶ Urologists' Use of Imaging Services

The American Urological Association, Inc.® (AUA) affirms that urologists are the physicians best qualified to diagnose, manage, and treat diseases and conditions of the genitourinary tract in patients of all ages. Urologists are trained in the performance and interpretation of diagnostic and interventional imaging studies including ultrasonography, radiography, axial scanning (CT and MRI), and other imaging techniques.

Urologists combine technical skill in the use of imaging equipment with the cognitive skills of the underlying disease processes. It is the urologist's role, using appropriate clinical indications, to select the study, or sequence of studies, needed to aid in the optimal diagnosis and management of urologic patients.

The acquisition and maintenance of skills and knowledge associated with imaging technology is assured by the Accreditation Council for Graduate Medical Education (ACGME) residency review committee for urology, continuing medical education provided by the AUA, and the certification, recertification, and maintenance of certification process of the American Board of Urology.

Urologists integrate an understanding of the risks and benefits of imaging technologies with the clinical care of the patient. Patient care is optimized when urologists coordinate the use of appropriate imaging techniques and equipment in the setting most beneficial to their patients.

Board of Directors, May 1993
Board of Directors, September 1995 (Revised)
Board of Directors, January 2001 (Reaffirmed)
Board of Directors, October 2006 (Revised)
Board of Directors, February 2007 (Revised)

EQUIPMENT, DOCUMENTATION, AND INDICATIONS

▶ Equipment

Ultrasound studies should be conducted with equipment capable of producing real-time images. Transducers should have a frequency range that will optimize tissue penetration and resolution. Appropriate transducer frequencies are 3.0 to 5.0 MHz for abdominal scanning, 6.0 to 9 MHz for transrectal, and 7.0 to 12.0 MHz for genital ultrasound. Intraoperative and laparoscopic renal ultrasound is performed with a 6- to 10-MHz linear array transducer. Transducers of higher frequency may be used for specialized examinations. The equipment should display mechanical and thermal indices and provide for adjusting power output. Equipment should have software-controlled options that allow the user to obtain the highest-quality image and documentation.

▶ Documentation

Appropriate images should be generated according to the type of study being performed. Images should be recorded on a permanent medium (digital format preferred) and stored in the patient's medical record. The ultrasound images should be labeled with patient identification, date of study, name of urologist, and type of probe.

TRANSRECTAL IMAGING OF THE PROSTATE AND SURROUNDING STRUCTURES

▶ Equipment

A biplane or end-fire transrectal ultrasound probe should be used to evaluate the prostate and surrounding structures. Prostate size and morphology may also be evaluated using a transabdominal approach with a curved linear array probe. The transrectal probe should be able to accommodate a needle guide for transrectal ultrasound-guided biopsy. The needle guide may be a single-use device or a reusable device. The probe should have an appropriate frequency range (usually 6.0 to 9.0 MHz).

▶ Documentation/Technique

The patient may be prepared by administering a cleansing enema prior to the procedure. An antibiotic may be administered if biopsy is anticipated. The prostate should be carefully scanned from base to apex in the transverse plane and from side to side in the sagittal plane. Specific abnormalities of the prostate should be documented. Surrounding structures including the bladder, seminal vesicles, ejaculatory ducts, and vascular structures should be evaluated. Prostate volume should be documented and may be calculated based on measurements of the length, width, and height of the prostate. The number of images obtained should be sufficient to document a complete examination and demonstrate all significant abnormalities.

APPENDIX 7

ARDMS RVPI CREDENTIAL – PREREQUISITE INFORMATION

PREREQUISITE A1

MD or DO with RVT (Active Status)

Physicians who currently hold the RVT credential with active status may apply directly for the PVI credential examination.

▶ **Documentation**

1. Copy of a current, valid medical license is the only documentation required.

2. Photocopy of a nonexpired government issued photo identification with signature; the name on the identification must exactly match the name under which you are applying for ARDMS examination.

PREREQUISITE A2

MD or DO, Current ICAVL or ACR Lab Accreditation

MD or DO degree with current, valid license to practice in the United States or Canada, and current Intersocietal Commission for the Accreditation of Vascular Laboratories (ICAVL) or American College of Radiology (ACR) vascular ultrasound accreditation.

▶ **Documentation**

1. Copy of MD or DO current, valid license to practice in the United States or Canada.

2. Letter from ICAVL or ACR identifying applicant as a current member of the medical staff of an accredited vascular ultrasound laboratory unit.
   The letter must be received directly from the accrediting organization and can be requested by contacting them.

3. Photocopy of a nonexpired government issued photo identification with signature; the name on the identification must exactly match the name under which you are applying for ARDMS examination.

PREREQUISITE B1

Formal Training (the United States and Canada) Education
MD or DO degree earned in the United States or Canada

▶ **Training**

Attendance of an Accreditation Council for Graduate Medical Education (ACGME) or Royal College of Physicians and Surgeons of Canada (RCPSC) accredited residency or fellowship that includes didactic and clinical vascular laboratory/ultrasound interpretation experience as an integral part of the program.

▶ **Interpretation Experience**

The applicant must be able to document interpretation experience with a minimum of 500 vascular laboratory studies as shown on page 3.
  These studies should be distributed over the following testing areas:

1. Carotid duplex ultrasound

2. Transcranial Doppler

3. Peripheral arterial physiologic testing

4. Peripheral arterial duplex ultrasound

5. Venous duplex ultrasound

6. Visceral vascular duplex ultrasound

▶ **Continuing Medical Education (CME)**

If the period of formal training ended more than 3 years prior to the candidate's application date, then the candidate must be able to document a minimum of 12 credit-hours of ARDMS-accepted CME, specifically related to vascular ultrasound earned within 3 years prior to the date of application for examination.

▶ **Documentation**

1. Copy of medical school diploma.

2. Original letter from residency/fellowship program director verifying dates of attendance and completion of a minimum of 500 vascular laboratory interpretation studies as shown on page 3.

3. If applicable, certificates or other original documentation for a minimum of 12 credit-hours of ARDMS-accepted CME, specifically related to vascular ultrasound.

4. Applicants should maintain a patient log or other record of interpretation experience with a minimum of 500 vascular laboratory studies. This log does not need to be submitted with the application, but may be requested as part of a random audit. This documentation should be maintained by the applicant for at least 3 years following the date of application for examination.

5. Photocopy of a nonexpired government-issued photo identification with signature; the name on the

identification must exactly match the name under which you are applying for ARDMS examination.

PREREQUISITE B2

Informal Training (the United States and Canada)
Education
MD or DO degree earned in the United States or Canada

▶ Interpretation Experience

The applicant must be able to document interpretation experience with a minimum of 500 vascular laboratory studies. These studies should be distributed over the following testing areas:

1. Carotid duplex ultrasound
2. Transcranial Doppler
3. Peripheral arterial physiologic testing
4. Peripheral arterial duplex ultrasound
5. Venous duplex ultrasound
6. Visceral vascular duplex ultrasound

▶ Continuing Medical Education (CME)

The applicant must document 12 credit-hours of ARDMS-accepted CME, specifically related to vascular ultrasound earned within 3 years prior to the date of application for examination.

▶ Documentation

1. Copy of medical school diploma.
2. Original letter from medical director of vascular laboratory or other physician describing the applicant's experience with vascular laboratory interpretation as shown on page 3; the applicant may write this letter if no other physician is available.
3. Certificates or other original documentation for 12 credit-hours of ARDMS-accepted CME, specifically related to vascular ultrasound.
4. Applicants should maintain a patient log or other record of interpretation experience with a minimum of 500 vascular laboratory studies. This log does not need to be submitted with the application, but may be requested as part of a random audit. This documentation should be maintained by the applicant for at least 3 years following the date of application for examination.
5. Photocopy of a nonexpired government issued photo identification with signature; the name on the identification must exactly match the name under which you are applying for ARDMS examination.

PREREQUISITE C1

Formal Training (outside the United States and Canada)

Education MD or DO degrees equivalent to those of the United States or Canada

▶ Training

Formal Training—Completion of a residency or fellowship that includes appropriate didactic and clinical ultrasound/vascular experience as an integral part of the program.

▶ Interpretation Experience

The applicant must be able to document interpretation experience with a minimum of 500 vascular laboratory studies. These studies should be distributed over the following testing areas:

1. Carotid duplex ultrasound
2. Transcranial Doppler
3. Peripheral arterial physiologic testing
4. Peripheral arterial duplex ultrasound
5. Venous duplex ultrasound
6. Visceral vascular duplex ultrasound

▶ Continuing Medical Education (CME)

If the period of formal training ended more than three (3) years prior to the candidate's application date, then the candidate must be able to document a minimum of 12 credit-hours of ARDMS-accepted CME, specifically related to vascular ultrasound earned within 3 years prior to the date of application for examination.

▶ Documentation

1. Original credential report or official notarized copy of the evaluation converting the foreign medical degree in the United States or Canada; a listing of organizations that produce individualized, written reports describing each certificate, diploma, or degree earned and specifying its U.S. or Canadian equivalent, can be found on page 17. If the applicant has taken and passed all three parts of, and earned, the Educational Commission for Foreign Medical Graduates (ECFMG®) certification, a copy of the ECFMG® certificate may be submitted with a copy of current, valid MD or DO license from the United States or Canada in lieu of the evaluation.
2. Original letter from residency/fellowship program director, verifying successful completion of the program, and describing the applicant's experience with vascular laboratory interpretation during the training period as shown on page 3.
3. Certificates or other documentation for a minimum of 12 credit-hours of ARDMS-accepted CME, specifically related to vascular ultrasound.
4. Applicants should maintain a patient log or other record of interpretation experience with a minimum of 500 vascular laboratory studies. This log does not need to be

submitted with the application, but may be requested as part of a random audit. This documentation should be maintained by the applicant for at least 3 years following the date of application for examination.

5. Photocopy of a nonexpired government issued photo identification with signature; the name on the identification must exactly match the name under which you are applying for ARDMS examination.

PREREQUISITE C2

Informal Training (outside the United States and Canada)

Education

MD or DO degrees equivalent to those of the United States or Canada

▶ Interpretation Experience

The applicant must be able to document interpretation experience with a minimum of 500 vascular laboratory studies. These studies should be distributed over the following testing areas:

1. Carotid duplex ultrasound
2. Transcranial Doppler
3. Peripheral arterial physiologic testing
4. Peripheral arterial duplex ultrasound
5. Venous duplex ultrasound
6. Visceral vascular duplex ultrasound+

▶ Continuing Medical Education (CME)

The applicant must document 12 credit-hours of ARDMS-accepted CME, specifically related to vascular ultrasound earned within 3 years prior to the date of application for examination.

▶ Documentation

1. Original credential report or official notarized copy of the evaluation converting the foreign medical degree in the U.S. or Canada; a listing of organizations that produce individualized, written reports describing each certificate, diploma, or degree earned and specifying its U.S. or Canadian equivalent, can be found on page 17. If the applicant has taken and passed all three parts of, and earned, the Educational Commission for Foreign Medical Graduates (ECFMG®) certification, a copy of the ECFMG® certificate may be submitted with a copy of a current, valid MD or DO license from the U.S. or Canada in lieu of the evaluation.

2. Original letter from the medical director of vascular laboratory or other physician, describing the applicant's experience with vascular laboratory interpretation as shown on page 3.

3. Certificates or other original documentation for 12 credit-hours of ARDMS-accepted CME, specifically related to vascular ultrasound.

4. Applicants should maintain a patient log or other record of interpretation experience with a minimum of 500 vascular laboratory studies. This log does not need to be submitted with the application, but may be requested as part of a random audit. This documentation should be maintained by the applicant for at least 3 years following the date of application for examination.

5. Photocopy of a nonexpired government issued photo identification with signature; the name on the identification must exactly match the name under which you are applying for ARDMS examination.

Note: Prerequisite requirements are subject to change from time to time and at any time. Applicants must meet current prerequisite requirements in effect at the time of application.

APPENDIX 8

AMERICAN SOCIETY OF REGIONAL ANESTHESIA AND PAIN MEDICINE AND THE EUROPEAN SOCIETY OF REGIONAL ANESTHESIA AND PAIN THERAPY JOINT COMMITTEE RECOMMENDATIONS FOR EDUCATION AND TRAINING IN ULTRASOUND-GUIDED REGIONAL ANESTHESIA

▶ ### Appendix I: The Ultrasound-Guided Regional Anesthesia Coordinator

Each department of anesthesiology at which UGRA is being performed or is sought to be performed may choose to identify a staff member, an UGRA coordinator, who will help facilitate the safe and skilled implementation of UGRA. The UGRA coordinator should be the designee of the anesthesiology department and will support the education and supervision of anesthesiologists practicing UGRA. The UGRA coordinator in a training institution would likely be responsible for developing and coordinating the educational process for residents learning and achieving core competencies in UGRA.

The Joint Committee suggests that the UGRA coordinator designation be granted to an individual following a review by the departmental leadership.

The Joint Committee recommends that the candidate obtain the following:

1. letter of recommendation from department leadership;

2. a written description of clinical experience including case volume, length of experience, and safety; and

3. participation in at least one accredited ultrasound workshop (as described in the Training section).

▶ ### Appendix II: Core Competencies for Residency Training in UGRA

The following list overlaps with the skills defined in the proficiency section of the Practice Pathway:

Patient care

1. Perform gentle ultrasound examinations, providing appropriate sedation

2. Demonstrate proper patient selection

3. Use appropriate monitoring during UGRA

4. Demonstrate proper nerve localization techniques

5. Perform effective and safe nerve blocks

Ultrasound knowledge

1. Understand the general principles of ultrasound physics

2. Understand benefits and limitations of UGRA techniques

3. Understand differences between in-plane vs out-of-plane techniques and their indications

4. Understand key artifacts and pitfall errors associated with UGRA

5. Develop an intimate knowledge of two-dimensional ultrasound anatomy of the major neurovascular structures of the upper and lower extremities

6. Appreciate common non-neural pathological states that are diagnosed by ultrasound: atherosclerotic disease and venous thrombosis

7. Establish familiarity with the major scientific literature related to UGRA

8. Learn techniques for UGRA (see list of applications in Table 18-1)

9. Understand the applications of color Doppler interrogation

10. Understand equipment specifications

11. Infection control and equipment cleaning

Interpersonal/communication skills

1. Communicate sensitively and effectively with patients and their families regarding ultrasound findings

2. Explain any complexities of UGRA in terms that the patient can understand

3. Demonstrate team leadership/management skills for the management of an effective regional anesthesia service

Professionalism

1. Be open to constructive criticism regarding ultrasound skills

System-based practice

1. Recognize costs associated with UGRA practice

2. Collaborate with other members of the health care team to ensure quality patient care

3. Use evidence-based, cost-conscious strategies in caring for all patients

Practice-based learning and improvement

1. Identify and acknowledge gaps in personal knowledge and skills in the care of patients presenting for UGRA

2. Use textbook and online and computer-based resources to broaden knowledge base regarding UGRA techniques

3. Perform electronic searches of the medical literature to identify articles that address the medical issues surrounding UGRA

4. Understand and critically evaluate outcome studies related to the influence of UGRA on perioperative outcome

5. Attend the department's required teaching conferences

6. Develop time management skills to perform the required tasks in a reasonable amount of time with satisfactory quality

▶ Appendix III: Recommended Ultrasound Curriculum

Equipment specifications

Minimal specifications include a machine with a linear transducer that has a frequency of 8 MHz or higher, color Doppler technology, and image storage capabilities.

Curriculum content: scanning techniques

1. The role of physics for UGRA; understand terminology (eg, piezoelectric effect, frequency, resolution, attenuation, echogenicity, and color Doppler)

2. The role of instrumentation in image acquisition (eg, image mode, gain, time gain compensation, and transducer types)

3. Equipment requirements: types of transducers (linear, curved, and phased array for different indications and scanning at different depths), footprint length, and frequency (range, 2–15 MHz)

4. Ultrasound acoustic artifacts and imaging artifacts (pitfalls). These include reverberation artifacts, acoustic enhancement, acoustic shadowing, gain-related artifacts, resolution-related artifacts, and mistaking tendon or muscle for nerve (11–12)

5. Techniques to perform effective ultrasound examinations; appreciate the Joint Committee recommended "PART" maneuvers for generating optimal imaging: Pressure, Alignment, Rotation, and Tilting (see Appendix IV)

Curriculum content: UGRA procedures

1. Define indications and contraindications

2. Practice procedural technique on available organic and inorganic simulators

3. Define relevant anatomy in each region, including the ability to identify muscle, pleura, nerve, tendon, and bone

4. Define needle insertion technique using the Joint Committee-recommended terminology (in-plane vs out-of-plane: see Appendix V)

5. Understand potential difficulties and pitfalls

6. Describe ultrasound appearance of common anatomical variations seen during upper and lower extremity block

7. Recognize correct and incorrect distributions of local anesthetic

8. Appreciate Joint Committee-recommended standardization of patient-screen relationships (see Appendix VI)

▶ Appendix IV: Recommended Technique for Ultrasound Scanning

1. Find landmark vascular structure (possibly assisted by color Doppler), bone, or muscle

2. Find nerve or plexus on short-axis imaging (transverse scan)

3. Place machine focus on target structures

4. Place depth setting at 1 cm deep to target structures

5. Adjust gain, time gain compensation, and frequency as necessary

6. Initiate the "PART" maneuvers to optimize image quality:

    a. **Pressure:** varying degrees of transducer pressure on skin

    b. **Alignment:** sliding movement of the transducer to define the lengthwise course of the nerve

    c. **Rotation:** the transducer is turned in either a clockwise or counterclockwise direction to optimize the image

    d. **Tilting:** the transducer is tilted in both directions to maximize the angle of incidence of the ultrasound beam with the target nerve. Scan anticipated needle trajectory with color Doppler to identify any unsuspected vascularity

▶ Appendix V: Recommended Terminology to Distinguish In-Plane Technique from Out-of-Plane Technique

Most peripheral nerves described in the anesthesia literature have been imaged in short axis (transverse or cross section) (Figure 18-1, top images). Alternatively, if the transducer is rotated 90 degrees from the short-axis view, the long-axis view (longitudinal scan) is generated (Figure 18-1, bottom images). The short-axis view is generally preferred because it allows the operator to assess the lateral-medial perspective of the target nerve, which is lost in the long-axis view. In the literature, two techniques have emerged regarding the orientation of the needle with respect to the ultrasound beam. The in-plane approach generates a long-axis view of the needle, allowing full visualization of the shaft and tip of the needle (Figure 18-2A, 18-2B). The out-of-plane view generates a short-axis view of the needle (Figure 18-2C, 18-2D). The in-plane approach has the disadvantage that, because the ultrasound beam is very thin, it can be challenging to maintain continuous needle imaging. The out-of-plane view has the limitation that a small block needle imaged in short axis can be hard to visualize. Furthermore, with the out-of-plane view, distinguishing the needle tip from

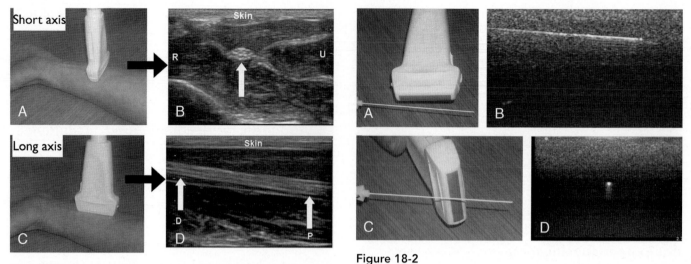

Figure 18-1

Figure 18-2

the shaft may be challenging. Regardless of the technique chosen, the goal is to steer the needle away from neighboring structures such as vessels and pleura and to confirm the spread of local anesthetic within correct fascial compartments and around the target nerves.

▶ Appendix VI: Recommended Procedure for Correlating Ultrasound Screen with Patient Sidedness for Patients in Prone, Supine, and Lateral Decubitus Positions

Before needle insertion, each neural structure should be referenced to key landmark structures in the anterior-posterior and lateral-medial planes. However, because of the bilateral nature of the peripheral nervous system, variations in patient positioning, differing presets of various ultrasound systems, and the nuances of individual techniques, it would be difficult to standardize the correlation of sidedness of the screen with an anatomical location. This is in contrast to transesophageal echocardiography where, in the transgastric short-axis view of the left ventricle (for example), the anterior aspect of the left

ventricle can be standardized to be on the bottom of the ultrasound screen.

Therefore, the Joint Committee recommends this simple procedure for correlation of the ultrasound screen with patient sidedness in any patient position.

1. After the application of the transducer onto the patient's skin, the landmark structure or peripheral nerve is identified. The primary operator states that the top of the ultrasound screen correlates with the patient's skin. To confirm this, pressure is applied with a finger onto the skin. This area should be visualized being compressed on the ultrasound screen.

2. For patients in any position, the operator states that screen left represents a defined anatomical aspect of the patient (eg, cephalad). To confirm this, the primary operator again applies pressure with a finger at this defined site. A corresponding indentation should be visualized on the left aspect of the ultrasound screen. If indentation occurs on screen right, then the operator must turn the transducer 180 degrees. After such a correction, the operator should return to step 1 until correct imaging has been obtained and confirmed.

APPENDIX 9

AIUM PRACTICE GUIDELINE FOR THE PERFORMANCE OF THE FOCUSED ASSESSMENT WITH SONOGRAPHY FOR TRAUMA (FAST) EXAMINATION

▶ **Introduction**

The clinical aspects of this guideline (Indications/Contraindications, Specifications for Individual Examinations, and Equipment Specifications) as well as Responsibilities of the Physician were developed collaboratively by the American Institute of Ultrasound in Medicine (AIUM) and the American College of Emergency Physicians (ACEP). Recommendations for physician qualifications, procedure documentation, and quality control vary among these organizations and are addressed by each separately.

This guideline has been developed to provide assistance to practitioners performing focused assessment with sonography for trauma (FAST) ultrasound examinations.

The FAST ultrasound examination is a proven and useful procedure for the evaluation of peritoneal spaces for bleeding after traumatic injury, particularly blunt trauma but including penetrating injury. Prior to its development, more invasive, including surgical, procedures were required to evaluate these patients. Over the last three decades, particularly with its wide advocation during the early 1990s, the FAST examination has evolved into one that now includes assessments of the peritoneal cavity for evidence of hemorrhage as well as analysis of the pericardium and pleural spaces for hemorrhage, particularly in cases of chest trauma. While it is not possible to detect every abnormality using the FAST examination for the analysis of the traumatized patient, adherence to the following guideline will maximize the probability of detecting free fluid and allowing rapid analysis for intraperitoneal hemorrhage and other abnormal fluids, such as urine and bile. In its extended form, the FAST examination allows analysis for possible hemopericardium, hemothorax, pneumothorax, solid organ damage, and retroperitoneal injury. The ready portability of ultrasound equipment allows the FAST examination to be used at the patient's bedside or in the rapid triaging of multiple individuals in mass casualty situations, including assessments in the field.

▶ **Indications/Contraindications**

Indications for the FAST examination of the torso include but are not limited to traumatic injury. FAST examinations should be performed when there is a valid medical reason. There are no absolute contraindications.

There are limitations to FAST assessments, including limitations in their ability to detect free fluid in some injured children, patients with mesenteric injury, and patients with isolated penetrating injury to the peritoneum.

Limitations to the diagnosis of free traumatic fluid in the peritoneum may be due to fluid present in patients for physiologic reasons, including ovarian cyst rupture, as well as pathologic reasons, such as patients with ascites. One must be wary of free fluid typically found intraperitoneally in patients with ventriculoperitoneal shunts and in those who undergo peritoneal dialysis. Free fluid may also be due to recent peritoneal lavage. Limitations to pericardial assessment for hemopericardium include pericardial cysts and pre-existing pericardial fluid. Limitations to pleural assessment for hemothorax include pre-existing pleural fluid from pre-existing pleural disease as well as extension into the pleural space of fluid from the pericardium or peritoneum.

▶ **Qualifications of the Physician**

See the training guidelines of the physician provider's respective specialty society, eg, the ACEP or the AIUM.

Training, as defined by the AIUM or the ACEP, is accepted as qualifying a physician for performance and/or interpretation of the FAST examination. Credentialing should be based on published standards of the physician's specialty society, such as the ACEP or the AIUM.

▶ **Responsibilities of the Physician**

Trauma ultrasound, or the FAST examination, provides information that is the basis for immediate decisions about further evaluation, clinical management, and therapeutic interventions. Rapid provision and interpretation of such examinations are critical to proper patient care.

The clinical care of patients in life-threatening situations should always take precedence over these guidelines.

Physicians/sonologists of a variety of medical specialties may perform the FAST examination. If appropriately trained, physician extenders, emergency medical personnel, and sonographers can obtain the ultrasound images.

Image interpretation should be performed by a supervising physician. Training of physicians in the diagnostic interpretation of FAST examinations should be in accordance with specialty-specific guidelines. Physicians who supervise nonphysician sonographers should render a diagnostic interpretation in a time frame consistent with the management of acute trauma, as outlined above.

▶ **Specifications for Individual Examinations**

The objective of the abdominal portion of the examination is to analyze the torso for free fluid. This requires examination of the abdomen's 4 quadrants and pelvis.

This is achieved by obtaining images of both upper quadrants as well as the pelvis. The ability to denote free fluid in the pelvis is aided by the presence of a fluid-filled bladder. As with all ultrasound examinations, orthogonal images (transverse, longitudinal, and coronal planes) help elucidate areas of concern seen in any single plane. Subtle changes in transducer angle and position can help improve analysis of a given area. Images may be obtained through anterior, coronal, or other approaches to denote free fluid in the evaluated areas.

As with most imaging and ultrasound examinations, techniques evolve over time and with increased clinical and imaging experience. The current primary FAST examination includes transverse and longitudinal images obtained through the heart to denote intrapericardial fluid. The images may be obtained by placing the transducer in the upper abdomen and pointing superiorly or placing the transducer directly above the heart in various echocardiographic planes, particularly a parasternal longitudinal plane. Pleural effusion can be analyzed by a midline transverse plane image in the upper abdomen, concentrating on the area posterior and therefore superior to the echogenic diaphragms. This may be the same image as that used to evaluate the (inferior) pericardium for fluid.

More specifically, primary ultrasound windows for the FAST examination include the following:

The right upper quadrant view (also known as the perihepatic, Morison pouch, or right flank view)

This uses the liver as an ultrasound window to interrogate the liver as well as the hepatorenal space (Morison pouch) for free fluid. Slight superior angulation of the transducer allows imaging of the right pleural space for free fluid. Inferior angulation allows visualization of the inferior pole of the right kidney as well as the right paracolic gutter for free fluid assessment.

The left upper quadrant view (also known as the perisplenic or left flank view)

This uses the spleen as a window to interrogate the spleen and the perisplenic space above the spleen, below the diaphragm, and above the left kidney. Angulation superiorly allows visualization of the left pleural space. Inferior angulation allows visualization of fluid above the left kidney or in the left paracolic gutter.

The pelvic view (also known as the retrovesical, retrouterine, or pouch of Douglas view)

This allows assessment of the most dependent space in the peritoneum for free fluid. Analysis through a fluid-filled bladder (which can be filled, if necessary, by fluid placed through a Foley catheter when possible) may help analysis for pelvic fluid. When free fluid is present, it is noted most often superior and posterior to the bladder and uterus.

The pericardial view (also known as the subcostal or subxiphoid view)

This uses the left lobe of the liver as a window for the analysis of the heart, particularly its right side. Both sagittal and transverse four-chamber planes may be used. The potential space of the pericardium is analyzed for the presence of any free fluid in an anterior or posterior location. Slight angulation posteriorly or inferiorly in this view allows visualization of the inferior vena cava and hepatic veins, including their normal respiratory variability.

Additional views may include the following:

The right and left paracolic gutter views

Longitudinal and transverse views through peritoneal windows inferior to the level of the ipsilateral kidney and next to the ipsilateral iliac crest may reveal free fluid surrounding bowel. These windows may be of limited use because of the absence of an ultrasound window, such as a fluid-filled bladder or a solid organ. Air-filled bowel may also limit these views. They rely on there being sufficient free fluid present to be imaged.

The pleural space views

Each pleural space may be investigated via angulation and superior movement of the transducer along the ipsilateral flank. Abnormal fluid collections in the pleural space are visualized as anechoic collections above the echogenic diaphragm.

The anterior pleural space view

The anterior visceral and parietal pleura may be analyzed through this view for free fluid. The pleura normally appose each other and slide on each other easily. Absence of this sliding and the potential separation of the pleura by a pneumothorax may be imaged typically in the second or third intercostal space with a higher-frequency near-field transducer, although lower-frequency transducers may also be used.

The parasternal view

The parasternal window allows visualization of the heart in sagittal or transverse planes. This view is used in cases in which a patient's subcostal view is suboptimal.

The apical view

The apical view may allow visualization of pericardial fluid in the difficult patient by placing the transducer at the nipple line at the left fifth intercostal space and aiming it toward the spine or the right shoulder.

Other considerations for the FAST examination are as follows:

Trendelenburg or sitting positions may increase the sensitivity of the ultrasound examination for visualizing abnormal fluid.

A FAST ultrasound examination may be repeated during the patient's stay for reassessment of the patient's condition either routinely or because of sudden clinical decompensation.

As a caveat, one must remember that a trauma ultrasound examination provides a picture of a patient's condition at one point in time. It never eliminates the possibility of injuries or fluid collections that are below the detectable threshold of a well-performed ultrasound examination.

Further information may be obtained by referring to the *ACEP Ultrasound Imaging Criteria–Trauma*.

▶ **Documentation**

Focused sonograms, as all sonograms, require documentation. Whenever feasible, images should be created and stored as part of the medical record, and a full description of the findings is required. The analysis of findings on FAST examinations is limited to those areas assessed and imaged. In particular, a FAST analysis may not allow the diagnostic evaluation of all abnormalities in the chest, abdomen, or pelvis.

▶ **Equipment Specifications**

FAST examinations should be conducted with real-time scanners, preferably using sector or linear (curved or straight) transducers. The equipment should be adjusted to operate at the highest clinically appropriate frequency, realizing that there is a trade-off between resolution and beam penetration. For most preadolescent pediatric patients, mean frequencies of 5 MHz or greater are preferred, and in neonates and small infants, a higher-frequency transducer is often necessary. For adults, mean frequencies of 3.5 and 5 MHz are most commonly used. Occasionally, very large patients may require a lower-frequency transducer such as 2 MHz for analysis.

When Doppler studies are performed, the Doppler frequency may differ from the imaging frequency. Diagnostic information should be optimized while keeping total ultrasound exposure as low as reasonably achievable.

▶ **Quality Control and Improvement, Safety, Infection Control, and Patient Education Concerns**

Policies and procedures related to image quality, equipment performance monitoring, infection control, and patient safety as well as patient education with regard to the FAST examination should be developed and implemented in accordance with either the *AIUM Standards and Guidelines for the Accreditation of Ultrasound Practices* or the *ACEP Emergency Ultrasound Guidelines* and the *ACEP Ultrasound Imaging Criteria–Trauma*.

AUTHORS

David Bahner, MD

Michael Blaivas, MD

Harris L. Cohen, MD

J. Christian Fox, MD

Stephen Hoffenberg, MD

John Kendall, MD

Jill Langer, MD

John P. McGahan, MD

Paul Sierzenski, MD

Vivek S. Tayal, MD

Effective October 1, 2007—AIUM PRACTICE GUIDELINES—Focused Assessment With Sonography for Trauma 3.

4 Effective October 1, 2007—AIUM PRACTICE GUIDELINES—Focused Assessment With Sonography for Trauma.

SUGGESTED READINGS

Blaivis M, Debehenke D, Phelan B. Potential errors in the diagnosis of pericardial effusion on trauma ultrasound for penetrating injuries. *Acad Emerg Med.* 2000;7:1261–1266.

Dolich M, McKenney M, Varela J, Compton RP, McKenney KL, Cohn SM. 2,576 ultrasounds for blunt abdominal trauma. *J Trauma.* 2001;50:108–112.

Hahn D, Offerman S, Homes J. Clinical importance of intraperitoneal fluid in patients with blunt intra-abdominal injury. *Am J Emerg Med.* 2002;20:595–600.

Jehle D, Guarino J, Karamanoukian H. Emergency department ultrasound in the evaluation of blunt abdominal trauma. *Am J Emerg Med.* 1993;11:342–346.

Kimura A, Otsuka T. Emergency center ultrasonography in the evaluation of hemoperitoneum: a prospective study. *J Trauma.* 1991;31:20–23.

McGahan J, Richards J, Fogata M. Emergency ultrasound in trauma patients. *Radiol Clin North Am.* 2004;42:417–425.

McGahan JP, Rose J, Coates TL, Wisner DH, Newberry P. Use of ultrasonography in the patient with acute abdominal trauma. *J Ultrasound Med.* 1997;16:653–662.

Melniker LA, Leibner E, McKenney MG, Lopez P, Briggs WM, Mancuso CA. Randomized controlled clinical trial of point of-care, limited ultrasonography for trauma in the emergency department: the First Sonography Outcomes Assessment Program Trial. *Ann Emerg Med.* 2006;48:227–235.

Plummer D, Brunnette D, Asinger R, Ruiz E. Emergency department echocardiography improves outcome in penetrating cardiac injury. *Ann Emerg Med.* 1992;21:709–712.

Scalea TM, Rodriguez A, Chiu WC, et al. Focused assessment with sonography for trauma (FAST): results from an international consensus conference. *J Trauma.* 1999;46:466–472.

Soudack M, Epelman M, Maor R, et al. Experience with focused abdominal sonography for trauma (FAST) in 313 pediatric patients. *J Clin Ultrasound.* 2004;32:53–61.

Tayal VS, Beatty MA, Marx JA, Tomaszewski CA, Thomason MH. FAST (focused assessment with sonography in trauma) accurate for cardiac and intraperitoneal injury in penetrating chest trauma. *J Ultrasound Med.* 2004;23:467–472.

Note: Page numbers followed by *f* indicate figures; and page numbers followed by *t* indicate tables.